ISF
(Tho)

Standards
and
Learning Disability

Standards
and
Learning Disability
SECOND EDITION

Tony Thompson
MA, BEd(Hons), RMN, RNMH, DipN(Lond), Cert Ed, RNT
*Director of Practice Development, Institute of Forensic Care,
Ashworth Hospital Authority, Liverpool*

and

Peter Mathias
PhD, MSc, MA, BSc
Director of Joint Awarding Bodies, London
London Philadelphia Toronto Sydney Tokyo

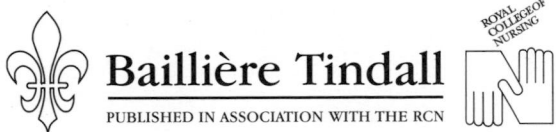

Baillière Tindall
PUBLISHED IN ASSOCIATION WITH THE RCN

Baillière Tindall   24–28 Oval Road
London NW1 7DX, UK

The Curtis Center
Independence Square West
Philadelphia, PA 19106-3399, USA

Harcourt Brace & Company
55 Horner Avenue
Toronto, Ontario, M8Z 4X6, Canada

Harcourt Brace & Company, Australia
30–52 Smidmore Street
Marrickville
NSW 2204, Australia

Harcourt Brace & Company, Japan
Ichibancho Central Building
22–1 Ichibancho
Chiyoda-ku, Tokyo 102, Japan

First published 1992 as *Standards and Mental Handicap*
Second edition 1998

A catalogue record for this book is available from the British Library

ISBN 0–7020–2203–9

Typeset by J&L Composition Ltd, Filey, North Yorkshire
Printed and bound in Great Britain by The Bath Press, Bath, Avon

Contents

Contributors

Owen Barr BSc(Hons) RGN, RNMH, CNMH, PG DipCoun, Ad DipEd, Lecturer in Nursing – Learning Disabilities, School of Health, University of Ulster, Coleraine, Northern Ireland.

Carol Baxter PhD, MSc, RGN, SCM, DN, FETC, HV, Senior Lecturer, Department of Health Studies, University of Central Lancashire, Preston.

Simon Biggs BSc, PhD, CPsychol, CQSW, Reader, Department of Applied Social Studies, Keele University, Keele.

Giles O.M. Blower BA(Hons), Specialist Welfare Rights Officer for People with Learning Disabilities, Nottingham Welfare Rights Service, Nottingham.

James Churchill BA, MA, PGCE, Chief Executive, Association for Residential Care, Chesterfield.

Stephen J.G. Clarke BA, BA(Hons), CASS, CQSW, Lecturer, Department of Social Policy and Applied Social Studies, University of Wales, Swansea.

Haydn Davies Jones BA, LLB, LLM, Formerly Director of Further Professional Studies and Dean of Education, School of Education, University of Newcastle Upon Tyne.

Jan Gilbert RMN, DMS, MBA, Executive Director, ONIS, London.

Leslie Hall BA, MEd, Former Headteacher of SLD School, Suffolk.

Mick Lloyd MSc, CQSW, Senior Training Officer, Lincolnshire Social Services, Lincoln.

Karen Lowater BA(Hons), Welfare Rights Officer, Nottinghamshire Welfare Rights Service, Radford, Nottingham.

Peter Mathias PhD, MSc, MA, BSc, Director, Joint Awarding Bodies (CCETSW and City & Guilds), London.

Mike Musker RMN, DPSN, BA(Hons), MSc, Clinical Team Leader, Ashworth Hospital, Maghull, Merseyside.

Ruth Prime RGN, CQSW, BA, 15 The Grove, London N13 5LQ.

Karen Rea MA, BA(Hons), RNMH, DPSN, Cert Ed, RNT, Lecturer/Practitioner, Ashworth Centre and Senior Lecturer, Liverpool John Moores University, Liverpool.

Peter Rippon Welfare Rights Officer, Bassetlaw CST, Worksop, Nottinghamshire.

Steven Rose MSc, RNMA, RMN, Chief Executive, Southwark Consortium, London.

Marc Saunders RNMH, DPSN, BSc(Hons), MA, General Manager, LEA Castle Centre, North Warwickshire NHS Trust, Kidderminster.

David Sines PhD, BSc(Hons), RMN, RNMH, RNT, PGCTHE, FRCN, Head of School of Health Sciences/Professor of Community Health Nursing, University of Ulster, County Antrim, Northern Ireland.

Paul Stafford BA(Hons), Nottinghamshire Welfare Rights Service, Warsop Town Hall, Warsop, Mansfield, Nottinghamshire.

Andrew R.A. Stevens MA, CQSW, Divisional Head – Learning Disability, School of Community Health and Social Studies, Anglia Polytechnic University, Chelmsford, Essex.

Gwen Swire (deceased) Formerly Assistant General Secretary, British Association of Social Workers, Birmingham.

Carl Thompson BA(Hons), RGN, Research Fellow, Centre for Evidence-Based Nursing, University of York.

Tony Thompson MA, BEd(Hons), RMN, RNMH, DipN(Lond), Cert Ed, RNT, Director of Practice Development, Institute of Forensic Care, Ashworth Hospital Authority, Maghull, Liverpool.

Joan Vagg, Parent, 14 Domonic Drive, New Eltham, London.

Jenny Weinstein, DPhil Social Work, MSc, Head of London and South East Regional Office, CCETSW, London.

Acknowledgements

Since the first edition of *Standards and Learning Disability* (which had the title *Standards and Mental Handicap*) those who are concerned with the development of services and the preparation of competent practitioners continue to be subject to a variety of pressures. For this reason we are privileged to be invited by Baillière Tindall to explore the pressures and to examine theoretical insights and developments which have grown from and contribute to practice.

Our debts as editors of the second edition are numerous. We would like to acknowledge the wide variety of help we have received – it is always the busiest people who find yet another demand difficult to refuse and so our sincere thanks go to the expert contributors who have put so much effort into bringing the book to completion.

We thank Jacqueline Curthoys of Baillière Tindall for her wise guidance and her colleague Karen Gilmour for responding so quickly to so many requests for help. Alison Smith and Hilary Jamieson have provided impressive backup throughout.

Sadly the field of learning disability has lost good friends since the first edition including Gwen Swire, Stephen Brown, Ann Craft and Albert Kushlick.

This edition is dedicated to their memory.

Tony Thompson and *Peter Mathias*

Chapter 1

Trends in Education and Training for Health and Social Care

Peter Mathias and Tony Thompson

Key Issues

- Interprofessional shift
- Standards
- Competence
- Trends
- Content of the book

Interprofessional Shift

Since the publication of the first edition of this book in 1992 reforms in health and social care and in education and training have continued, driven by government policy and shaped by service managers, practitioners and educationalists. The purchaser–provider separation, the push towards primary care, the increasing use of occupational standards, the introduction of local management of schools, the rise of vocationalism in education and training and the language of lifetime learning have created new conditions and shifted the interprofessional debate in learning disabilities so that it is now much broader than the nursing and social work exchange which was the dominant feature of the first edition.

This increase of interest and scope, the emergence of a plurality of provision and the involvement of a wider circle of professions and occupational groups make agreement and publication of standards as an expression and communication of expectation and possibility, ever more important. Of especial use would be standards which capture the aspirations of people with learning disability and their carers, which offer specialist perspectives to those involved in both general and specialist provision and which can be used for a variety of purposes including specification of competence, the design of education and training and the creation of personal portfolios of expertise and experience.

We argue, therefore, that key groupings in the field of learning disability should work together to map out, agree and publish the standards which should apply to practice and publish them so that those involved in workforce planning, in commissioning, providing and designing services or education and training can use them in their plans and practice. The argument is drawn from and supported by many of the chapters in this book.

A learning disability interest group itself drawn from the key groupings already in existence could sponsor the standards and the values associated with them and monitor their use in the services and by the various professional and occupational groups working in the field.

The main purpose would be to preserve and develop the specialist expertise and practice developed by practitioners, managers and researchers of the variety of disciplines and professions thus far involved in learning disability, some of which seems to be in danger of being lost in the rearrangement of services and education and training. The standards developed could inform groups such as nursing, social work, the remedial and therapeutic professions and those interested in both academic and vocational education.

They might also be the basis for a new sort of practitioner able to move more freely within the broad field of health and social care and education, housing and community development.

Standards

In 1993, 34 organizations, including statutory, regulatory bodies, professional associations, trades unions and employers, met in conference to discuss the relationship between professional and occupational standards in health and social care (Joint Awarding Bodies, 1993). Since then it has become clear that standards, however expressed, are set to become the vehicle through which purchasers, providers, employers, educationalists, and the professions express aspirations and requirements of the services and of learning, training and

qualification. The use of occupational standards will be promoted by (for example) the National Health Service Executive, the Local Authority Associations and the new National Training Organizations which will emerge from 1998 onwards. National Training Organizations will include representatives of the private and voluntary sector alongside those from the statutory sector in designing qualifications sensitive to the purpose and workforce requirements of an occupational sector.

In health and social care standards are variously applied to

- professional conduct and codes of behaviour and practice, and
- work, job performance and competence.

Whilst most organizations and practitioners have an interest in both applications of standards there may be division of interest, responsibility and authority between employers, professional associations, trades unions, educational authorities and representatives of service users or consumers.

For example, employers in health and social care may be particularly interested in standards as applied to work functions and as a basis for work organization and job definition and description. Professional associations and regulatory bodies find an application of standards to codes of practice useful alongside competence as a basis for registration and discipline. Trades unions and educationalists may be variously interested in standards as a basis for learning, qualification, certification and the negotiation of rewards and contracts. Standards as a basis for various charters or for judging adequacy of service have been developed by user groups to frame negotiation with service providers.

Standards take different forms according to purpose. The Department for Education and Employment (DfEE) has been promoting the use of standards of occupational competence, usually referred to as occupational standards, for some years. The argu-

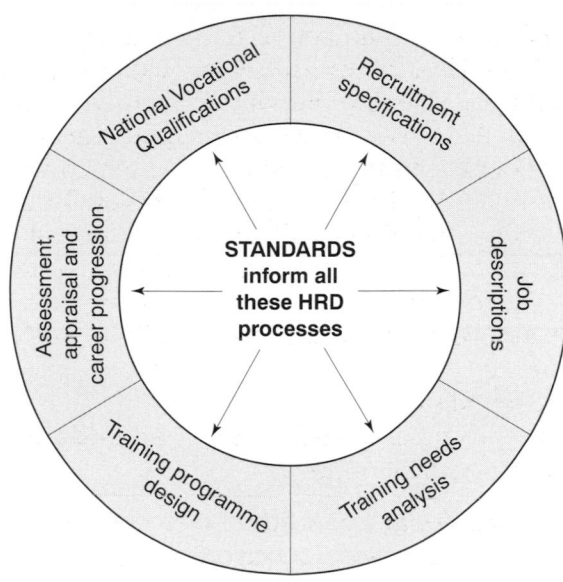

Figure 1.1 Standards. HRD, Human resources development. From Bulletin 1 (1996), with kind permission of the Care Sector Consortium, London.

ment is that occupational standards can inform academic and vocational qualifications particularly National Vocational Qualifications (NVQs), and can be used for a variety of other organizational purposes such as recruitment, job definition, work organization, tendering, contracting and quality assurance (see Figure 1.1).

Occupational standards developed within the DfEE framework have, to date, usually been expressed in terms of units and elements of competence, each of which is accompanied by performance criteria and related knowlege (Box 1). However, more recently, occupational standards are emerging which do not follow this one structural model and it is anticipated that future occupational standards will be written in a form which best fits the sector.

There are other ways to express standards of practice and make statements about competence, capability, ethics or values. For example, the United Kingdom Central Council for Nursing, Midwifery & Health Visiting (UKCC), in its code of conduct, published 16 target behaviours as the standards required for practitioners to justify public trust and confidence and safeguard the interests of patients and clients (Box 2).

Competence and NVQs

Closely related to the idea of occupational standards in current DfEE thinking is the idea of competence.

In terms of NVQs a competent person is someone who has the ability to perform to a standard required in employment. NVQs themselves attest to competence because they are made up of occupational standards. In a slightly more expanded version competence is defined by the National Council for Vocational Qualifications (NCVQ)* as the application of knowledge, skills, values and understanding to work as defined in the occupational standards. An NVQ is made up of a number of units of competence and the national framework allows for five levels of qualification (1–5) (Box 3).

The Care Sector Consortium has used the NCVQ framework to produce a range of awards at levels 2, 3 and 4 in health and social care. The draft units for the proposed NVQ in Social Care at level 4 are shown in Box 4. The British Psychological Society is experimenting with the use of standards and has work in hand for the development of qualifications at level 5 based on standards in (i) applied psychological research, (ii) educational psychology, (iii) clinical

---

* The NCVQ has merged with the Schools Curriculum and Assessment Authority to become the Qualifications and Curriculum Authority (QCA). The QCA counterpart in Scotland is the Scottish Qualification Authority. Similar organizations will be established for Wales and Northern Ireland.

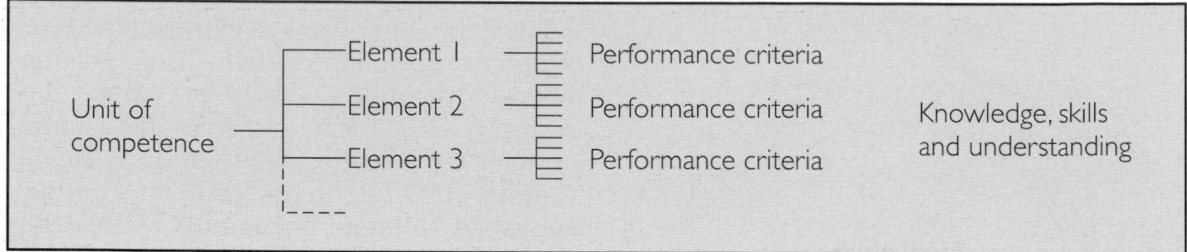

Box 1 The structure of a unit of competence

The registered nurse, midwife or health visitor shall, at all times, act in such manner as to justify public trust and confidence, to uphold and enhance the good standing and reputation of the profession, to serve the public interest and the interests of patients/clients.

In fulfilment of professional responsibility and in the exercise of professional accountability the nurse, midwife or health visitor shall:

1. Comply with the law of any country, state, province or territory in which she works, and have due regard to custom.
2. Be accountable for her/ practice and take every reasonable opportunity to sustain and improve her knowledge and professional competence.
3. Have regard to the customs, values and spiritual beliefs of patients/clients.
4. Hold in confidence any information obtained through professional attendance on a patient/client. Such information must not be divulged unless judged necessary to discharge her professional responsibilities to the patient/client; normally the consent of the patient/client should be obtained. Exceptionally the professional practitioner may be required by legal process to divulge information held: she should seek advice before responding.
5. Avoid any abuse of the privileged relationship with patients/clients or the privileged access to their property, residence or workplace.

6. At all times act in such a way as to promote and safeguard the well being and interests of patients/clients for whose care she is professionally accountable and ensure that by no action or omission on her part their condition or safety is placed at risk.
7. Have regard to the environment of care (physical, psychological and social) and to available resources, and make known to the appropriate authority if these endanger safe standards of practice.
8. Accept a responsibility relevant to her professional experience for assisting her peers and subordinates to develop professional competence.
9. Have due regard to the workload of and the pressures on professional colleagues and subordinates and take appropriate action if these are seen to be such as to endanger safe standards of practice.
10. Make known to the appropriate authority any conscientious objection she holds which may be relevant to her professional practice.
11. Refuse to accept any gift, favour or hospitality which might be interpreted as seeking to exert undue influence to obtain preferential treatment.
12. Avoid advertising or signing an advertisement using her professional qualification(s) to encourage the sale of commercial products, or services. Any nurse, midwife or health visitor who
continued opposite

wishes to use her professional qualifications to advertise her professional services or to take part in any form of commercial advertising should seek advice at the UKCC offices. Notes to be read in association with the preceding Code

1. It is expected that the nurse, midwife or health visitor will perform her professional duties in accordance with any nationally approved guidelines or codes of practice, and (provided they do not conflict) in accordance with approved local policies.
2. Where the guidelines, codes or policies are found to be such as to impede the safe and effective performance of those duties, proposals for change should be initiated through the appropriate professional channels.
3. Where, from a professional stance, a law is considered bad or inappropriate it should be challenged through the due processes of democracy. Where a practice is considered unsound it should be challenged through the appropriate professional channels. Such actions would be accepted as proper expressions of professional concern and responsibility.

Box 2 The UKCC Code of Conduct (1983)

All NVQs must be positioned in one of the following five levels of the framework:

Level 1 – competence which involves the application of knowledge in the performance of a range of varied work activities, most of which may be routine or predictable.

Level 2 – competence which involves the application of knowledge in a significant range of varied work activities, performed in a variety of contexts. Some of the activities are complex or non-routine and there is some individual responsibility and autonomy. Collaboration with others, perhaps through membership of a work group or team, may often be a requirement.

Level 3 – competence which involves the application of knowledge in a broad range of varied work activities performed in a wide variety of contexts, most of which are complex and non-routine. There is considerable responsibility and autonomy and control or guidance of others is often required.

Level 4 – competence which involves the application of knowledge in a broad range of complex technical or professional work activities performed in a wide variety of contexts and with a substantial degree of personal responsibility and autonomy. Responsibility for the work of others and the allocation of resources is often present.

Level 5 – competence which involves the application of a significant range of fundamental principles across a wide and often unpredictable variety of contexts. Very substantial personal autonomy and often significant responsibility for the work of others and for the allocation of substantial resources feature strongly, as do personal accountabilities for analysis and diagnosis, design, planning, execution and evaluation.

Box 3 The five levels of National Vocational Qualifications (NVQs) (NCVQ, 1995)

SOCIAL CARE LEVEL 4

ALL OF THESE 8 UNITS ARE MANDATORY FOR THE ACHIEVEMENT OF THE AWARD

O2   Promote people's equality, diversity and rights

O3   Develop, maintain and evaluate systems and structures to promote the rights, responsibilities and diversity of people

CU7   Develop one's own knowledge and practice

SC14 Establish, sustain and disengage from working relationships with clients

SC15 Develop and sustain arrangements for joint working with other workers and agencies

SC16 Assess clients' needs and circumstances

SC17 Evaluate risk of harm, abuse and failure to protect

SC18 Plan and agree with individuals service responses to meet their identified needs and circumstances

6 of these optional units are required

W5   Support clients with difficult or potentially difficult relationships

SC19 Co-ordinate, monitor and review service responses to meet individuals' identified needs and circumstances

SC20 Contribute to the provision of physical, social and emotional environments for group care

NC2   Enable individuals, their family and friends to explore and manage change

NC11   Contribute to the planning, implementation, and evaluation of programmes to enable individuals to manage their behaviour

CJ4   Represent agency at a formal hearing

CJ5   Contribute to the development of agency policies and practice

CJ14   Assist individuals with negotiations and formal hearings

SNH4U4   Promote the interests of client groups in the community

SNH4U6   Develop control for people who are at risk to themselves and others

D1301   Select, develop and coordinate volunteers

MCI/B3   Manage the use of financial resources

MCI/D4   Provide information to support decision making

AGCP/B5 Structure learning opportunities with individuals

CU8   Contribute to the development of the knowledge and practice of others

MCI/C5   Develop productive working relationships

MCI/C8   Select personnel for activities Develop teams and individuals to enhance performance

MCI/C13 Manage the performance of teams and individuals

Box 4 The unit titles in the draft level 4 National Vocational Qualification in Social Care (Care Sector Consortium, 1997)

neuropsychology, and (iv) health psychology (NCVQ, 1997).

Outcomes in social work and nursing

The regulatory bodies responsible for nursing and social work have not used the DfEE or NCVQ approach to design qualifications and have not developed NVQs for nurses and social workers but do express expectations in terms of outcomes, either as competences (social work) or learning outcomes (the learning disability branch of nursing).

The revised requirements for the Diploma in Social Work identify six competences and a set of values for the beginning social work practitioner, the competences are based on a

---

There are six core competences in social work:

1. *Communicate and engage*
Communicate and engage with organizations and people within communities to promote opportunities for children, adults, families and groups at risk or in need, to function, participate and develop in society.

2. *Promote and enable*
Promote opportunites for people to use their own strengths and expertise to enable them to meet their responsibilities, secure rights and achieve change.

3. *Assess and plan*
Work in partnership to assess and review people's circumstances and plan response to need and risk.

4. *Intervene and provide services*
Intervene and provide services to achieve change through provision or purchase of appropriate levels of support, care, protection and control.

5. *Work in organizations*
Contribute to work of the (employer) organization.

6. *Develop professional competence*
Manage and evaluate own capacity to develop professional competence.

The Values Requirements

In order to achieve the award of Diploma in Social Work, students must demonstrate in meeting the core competences that they:

- Identify and question their own values and prejudices, and their implications for practice.
- Respect and value uniqueness and diversity, and recognize and build on strengths.
- Promote people's rights to choice, privacy, confidentiality and protection, while recognizing and addressing the complexities of competing rights and demands.
- Assist people to increase control of and improve the quality of their lives, while recognizing that control of behaviour will be required at times in order to protect children and adults from harm.
- Identify, analyse and take action to counter discrimination, racism, disadvantage, inequality and injustice, using strategies appropriate to role and context.
- Practise in a manner that does not stigmatize or disadvantage either individuals, groups or communities.

Box 5 Social work: expectations of the beginning practitioner (CCETSW, 1995)

1. Identify factors that may lead to disability and associated mental handicap in the context of the life continuum of the individual paying regard to his/her family unit, friends, community and society.

2. Examine and evaluate the factors which contribute to adverse physical, social and mental experiences. Initiate and co-ordinate actions to create positive growth-enhancing experiences for people. To play an active part in the development of a facilitative environment.

3. Use existing knowledge base to inform nursing practice.

4. Evaluate the influence of social and cultural factors in relation to the personal service system. Be proactive in the process of change to benefit the individual.

5. Understand the requirements of legislation relevant to practice.

6. The therapeutic use of self in the network of care systems.

7. Acquire and utilize skills and knowledge to maximize own health and that of others.

8. Identify and utilize principles that guide nursing practices in services for people with a mental handicap.

9. Understand and interpret contemporary philosophies of care by demonstrating professional and interpersonal skills within the context of multi-agency provision and life-planning.

10. Develop a partnership with people to enhance each other's quality of life via approaches that are planned, rational and lead to shared interventions that pay positive regard to individuality and differences.

11. Function effectively in a team and participate in multiprofessional approach. Use the full resources available within an individual's local community to most effectively meet that person's needs.

12. Develop and utilize the skills and knowledge required to supervise, teach and monitor others.

Box 6 Nursing: outcomes of the learning disability branch programme (ENB, 1989)

set of occupational standards which were used to develop the requirements but which have not yet been published (Box 5). The English National Board's learning disability branch in nursing continues to express its expectation in terms of learning outcomes which indicate something of the competence expected of the beginning nurse practitioner, these statements were drawn up just as interest in competence was emerging (see Box 6).

Competence in dispute

In moving from a description of the DfEE/NCVQ approach to a description of the work of nursing and social work we begin to move away from standard and com-

monly agreed definitions of terms and enter into the disputed and contested world of vocational education with commentators and protagonists arguing about the concept of competence and the case for and against the use of occupational standards as the basis for vocational education.

For example, Eraut (1996), in a paper offering a conceptualization of the link between theory and practice in nurse training, discusses various models for characterizing expertise including that proposed by Dreyfus and Dreyfus (1986) which has its own five levels with competence at level 3.

Hyland (1994) gives a dissenting view about the value of competence and NVQs as

Level 1   Novice
Rigid adherence to taught rules or plans
Little situational perception
No discretionary judgement

Level 2   Advanced beginner
Guidelines for action based on attributes or aspects (aspects are global characteristics of situations recognizable only after some prior experience)
Situational perception still limited
All attributes and aspects are treated separately and given equal importance

Level 3   Competence
Coping with crowdedness
Now sees actions at least partially in terms of longer-term goals
Conscious deliberate planning
Standardized and routinized procedures

Level 4   Proficient
See situations holistically rather than in terms of aspects
See what is most important in a situation
Perceives deviations from the normal pattern
Decision-making less laboured
Uses maxims for guidance, whose meaning varies according to the situation

Level 5   Expert
No longer relies on rules, guidelines or maxims
Intuitive grasp of situations based on deep tacit understanding
Analytic approaches used only in novel situation or when problems occur
Vision of what is possible

Box 7 Summary of Dreyfus model of skills acquisition

the proper basis for vocational education arguing that the DfEE/NCVQ approach is lowering national standards rather than lifting them. Mansfield and Mitchell (1996) argue for the competence approach tracing its history and describing methods of functional analysis, standards development and qualification design setting out a model for job competence which suggests there are four important aspects to all work roles. These are:

- the technical expectations
- the ability to cope with uncertainty when things go wrong

- the ability to manage the different and sometimes conflicting demand of the work role
- the ability to manage and work within environmental constraints such as the culture of the organization and physical environment.

However, despite the arguments, the language of occupational standards, of competence and of learning outcomes runs through health and social care and as we noted earlier both the National Health Service Executive and Local Authority

Associations are likely to advocate the use of occupational standards to help state expectations, measure performance and support the management of human resources.

But just exactly what is the occupation(s) of health and social care to which standards might apply?

The Occupational Sector

Health and social care is carried out by some 2.8 million paid workers and millions more carers, partners, children, brothers, sisters and friends at a cost running into billions (40+ in 1997). It is subject to political, legal, economic, social, philosophical, ethical and moral concerns and extends, includes and is informed by the social sciences and the sciences of physiology and biochemistry extending through medical, remedial and social care professions to the worlds of community work, criminal justice and special needs housing. The world of health and social care has its own internal interprofessional and interdisciplinary challenges and problems but also intersects with other sectors such as housing, education and the law. People with learning disabilities will, of course, make use of a variety of general and specialist services within this overall provision.

Those involved in education for health and social care must wrestle with this complexity as must students and practitioners preparing for work in what may be private, public or voluntary sectors.

Purpose in Health and Social Care

The Care Sector Consortium, the Occupational Standards Council for Health and Social Care explored role and function

V Promote and implement values of good practice
A Enable individuals, families, groups and communities to take greater control over their own health and social well-being
B Enable individuals, families, groups and communities to optimize their health and social well-being according to their needs or stage of development
C Develop and improve the ability of people and organizations to optimize the health and social well-being, of individuals, families, groups and communities
D Commission, co-ordinate and facilitate the provision of care services and facilities
E In partnership with a population, assess health and social well-being to develop strategies and structures for its improvement

Box 8 The main functions of health and social care from the Functional Map of Health and Social Care: Working Document (Care Sector Consortium, 1994)

within its very diverse sector and produced a functional map with six domains (Box 8). Coats and Mitchell (1997) provide a fuller description of the functional map.

Trends

Underpinning the statement of function from the Care Sector Consortium are trends and influences such as moves from a focus on illness to one on health and the emergence of primary care and community programmes to offset or prevent social problems.

Other trends obvious at the time of writing can be shown in two triangles of influence, the first based on shorter term

Education

The Education Reform Act (1997)

The National Committee of Inquiry into Higher Education (1997)

The Professions
The Review of the Professions Supplementary to Medicine Act and the creation of a Council of Health Professions

The creation of a General Social Services Council/Voluntary Code of Conduct Group

The Health and Social Care Provision

The NHS & Primary Care Act (1997)

The White Paper on Local Authority Social Services (1997)

Box 9 Some of the short-term legislation and policy trends affecting education, health and social care provision and the professions (see other chapters for fuller descriptions)

Technological
Communication technology
The Internet
Telemedicine
Tele-learning and assessment

Political/economic
Structure of the public sector and the future of NHS and local government
European and world health initiatives in health, social care and learning

Human
People and their changing relationship with
■ work and careers
■ health and social care

Box 10 Longer term trends: technological, human and political/economic

legislative and policy trends, the second in longer term trends (Box 9 and 10).

At least three imperatives seem to emerge from these trends for policy makers, managers and professionals involved in education for health and social care.

■ Recognize that the future demands negotiation and discussion between all those involved in education, the provision of services and the professional bodies

about standards, competence, curricula, numbers, value for money, fitness for purpose, workforce planning and perhaps establishment of a common core curriculum for health and social care.

■ Establish a set of qualifications or certificates within a comprehensive national framework using vocational, academic and occupational opportunities to allow a variety of routes and opportunities for practitioners and potential practitioners to acquire and demonstrate competence but also recognize that much learning is likely to remain uncertificated; and to be expressed in personal portfolios.

■ Work with public health interests in the population including community groups, patients/clients, carers and advocates to agree standards and the action necessary to develop and maintain them.

In addition, beginning practitioners could usefully consider continuing the portfolio of their interests, expertise and achievements developed in initial training throughout their early career and beyond.

This book intends to provide material to support students, candidates, practitioners and educationalists respond to the challenges set out previously. Since the first edition the requirements of the beginning social work practitioner have been rewritten and the numbers in training have remained constant. For learning disability nursing, however, the numbers have declined. This is in common with training of nurses generally. This reduction in training generally is leading to a shortage of trained nurses in the health service.

There may be particular reasons for the reduction in learning disability nurses separate from the general trend, reasons associated with the radical reforms in health and social care and the constant tussle to decide which side of the health and social care line nursing falls.

However, it has always been important in our minds that the skills and understanding developed through learning disability nursing and the specialist branches of other professions is maintained and developed further as understanding grows and services change. Unfortunately, this is not always the case and some changes have removed skills and removed essential services.

As we argued in the opening paragraphs, we think it is particularly important that we seize the opportunity to use ideas of standards and competence within health and social care to mark out the specialist, confirm the general and specify the components of effective practice. We argue that a body of practice is emerging from interprofessional working in the field of learning disability which will be of interest to practitioners from different professions and services as a reference point for personal development.

We think that this body of practice and the standards which apply to it could influence and be influenced by the various strands of the national framework of qualifications which will emerge after the Education Reform Act 1997, and the outcomes of the National Committee of Inquiry into Higher Education (1997). Practitioners, employers, user groups and the various professional associations and interest groups could build a new shared professionalism around this area of pratice sharing ideas for learning, development, ethics and research and setting standards for services.

A body of practice and standards promoted through a reformed educational system, practised in whole or part by various occupational and professional groups and sustained by new methods of communication is possible and is arguably the most effective way to maintain special interests and expertise in today's world. This body of practice will be distinctive because it draws insights from education, community work and housing as well as health and social care.

New Statements about Practice

But what emerges from the field of learning disability – what new skills, competence and understanding flow from the intense interprofessional explorations of recent years?

Many reports show that it has proved useful to share ideas and practice and to become acquainted with various perspectives and approaches in order to be more effective in teams, in liaison or in joint projects or to learn how to transfer or apply skills in new settings.

But we think something more has emerged or is emerging – a body of practice which is by turn habilitative, therapeutic and educational, enabling and supporting people as they overcome difficulties in development, learning, thinking, perception and emotion.

This emergent practice is continuous with the social pedagogy movement in Europe and the outcomes of the conference 'Opportunities for Change: A New Direction for Nursing for People with Learning Disabilities' organized by the Department of Health in 1993. Five options for change were put to this conference:

- continuation of the learning disabilities branch within the family of nursing;
- assimilation of pre-qualifying nurse training programme for learning disability within the child, adult and mental health branches of Project 2000 and within a revised post-qualifying framework;
- the emergence of a new profession with contributions from social work, nursing and from informal carers specific to the care of people with learning disabilities;
- the concept of a new rehabilitation spe-

cialist with a focus on disability across a range of client groups;
- the assimilation of the Registered Nurse for Mental Handicap (RNMH) programme within the pre-qualifying social work curriculum.

During the consultation exercise which followed the conference a clear preference was expressed for exploration of the possibilities of an NVQ-oriented approach and for training and learning shared across professions and occupational groups (Brown, 1993). The Department of Health noted this finding advising chief nursing officers in the UK to be aware of the possibilities whilst maintaining the learning disability branch of nursing.

After the Department of Health Conference the then MHNA (Mental Handicap Nurses Association: now the Association of Practitioners of Learning Disability (APLD)) published a set of 'Refined Competences' (Thompson, 1994) relating specifically to the field of learning disability (Figure 1.2). We think this work is the starting point from which to draw together new standards for practice.

The final standards could inform the development of qualifications at all levels within the academic and vocational framework influence general specialist programmes, and qualifications for school leavers as well as those involved in continuing professional development.

An outline of the MHNA competence indicating its broad coverage follows. These statements could be added to those from the specialist branches of the various professions and occupational groups to provide a more extensive list. Standards from special needs housing, community, child care and education, management, advice guidance and counselling and health and social care generally could be scanned for relevance. Standards promoted by user groups

Core competence

- promote human development (language cognition, motor, . . .)
- promote learning and skill development
- promote effective communication
- support acquisition of personal relationships and friendships
- promote physical and mental health

through assessment and intervention which recognizes the implications of factors which cause learning disability and which applies key values

Community focus

Promote integration through:

- care management
- provision of home-based activity
- provision of residential support
- supported involvement in general and special educational, health and social services
- facilitation of employment and leisure opportunities
- support of relocation

Specialist focus

Assess intervene and organize care management for:

- people with challenging behaviour
- people with multiple disabilities
- people with mental health problems

Figure 1.2 The Refined Competences. Adapted from Thompson (1994)

and advocates could be included and the whole set then subjected to debate and amendment in the course of producing a map of the standards of practice emerging from and relevant to learning disability.

Education and Training

Previously (Mathias and Thompson, 1997) we argued that opportunities to explore various disciplines and professions and experience interdisciplinary and interprofessional activity could and should be built into the 'educational opportunities available to practitioners as they move along various pathways from school to work, to further and higher education and to professional training, practice and continuing professional development' (p. 103).

These opportunities might have:

- the modest ambition to introduce and describe various perspectives and approaches in health and social care in order to enhance general education and preparation for practice;
- an intent to equip the practitioners with an understanding of the practices, values, underpinnings and frameworks of various professions and agencies in order to equip the practitioners to work with other professions or transfer competence to new contexts and situations;
- the purpose of solving complex problems, setting new ones or to restructive or reframe established wisdom and practice creating new understanding or interventions.

We assumed that in setting the interprofessional purpose and so preventing the fragmentation and separation which can so easily damage those who participate in the services, professions would still rightly strive for differentiation, specialization and development of profession specific as well as common knowledge and skill.

Some commentators extend the interprofessional argument and call for a common, holistic approach to education and training for health and social care and advocate the creation of a common core curriculum as a foundation to help people move into various careers in health and social services.

For example, Lämsä et al. (1994) describe how the reform of the Finnish educational system allowed for just such an approach in Finland. In the UK the report into the future of the healthcare workforce (Conrane Consulting, 1996) argues for the creation of common core training for future healthcare workers whilst a parallel report into social services by the Association of Directors of Social Services and the Local Government Management Board envisages the emergence of a hybrid health/social care worker somewhere in the system of qualification and certification (ADSS/LGMB, 1997).

In the field of learning disability these ideas have been turned into reality by some universities who in association with service providers provide degrees in health or social studies combined with preparation and assessment for either or both nursing and social work.

The reform of the British framework of qualifications, and the debates about life-long learning, career flexibility and continuing professional development lend themselves to continued experiment and innovation in education and at work.

The practitioner of the future will make new pathways through the services and through the various educational opportunities available to create unique configurations of competence and experience on top of basic professional training and registration.

Someone who enters the field through the learning disability nurse branch might find themselves working through various practitioner and management jobs in the health and social services, in one phase working residentially, in another in day provision and in yet another concerned with purchasing services and monitoring or inspecting provision. A social worker or an occupational therapist might follow a similar post-professional pathway and people of all professions become involved in research, general management and education and training. People who enter directly into practice should have work-based opportunities for learning and qualifications as well as those provided through colleges or universities.

Practitioners must have an eye to their future by thinking about the balance of academic and vocational experience best suited to them and their ambitions taking responsibility for their own learning and investing in themselves and their development.

We hope that the opportunities available will address standards of practice in learning disability and interprofessional competence as well as any profession or group specific requirements.

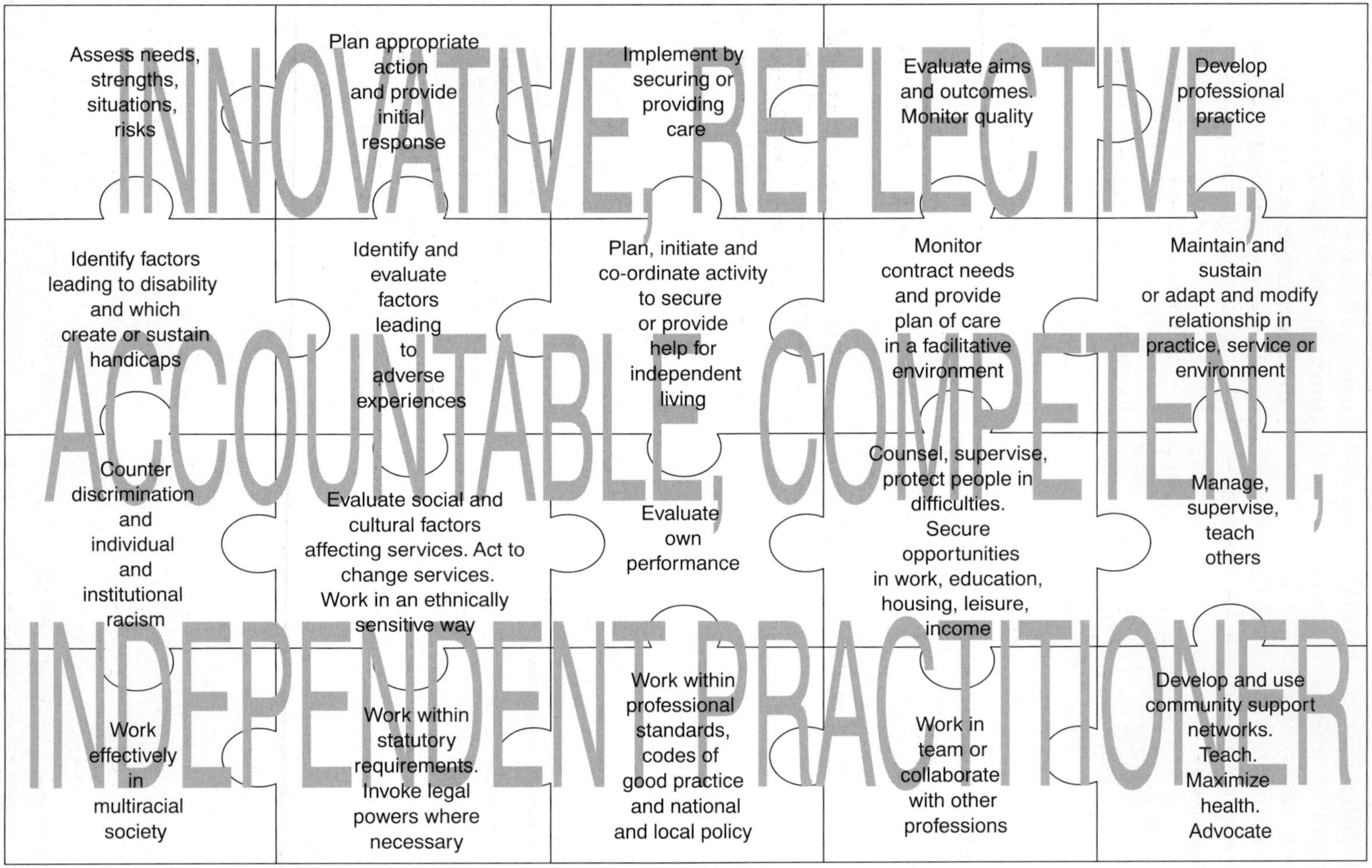

INNOVATIVE REFLECTIVE

ACCOUNTABLE COMPETENT

INDEPENDENT PRACTITIONER

Assess needs, strengths, situations, risks

Plan appropriate action and provide initial response

Implement by securing or providing care

Evaluate aims and outcomes. Monitor quality

Develop professional practice

Identify factors leading to disability and which create or sustain handicaps

Identify and evaluate factors leading to adverse experiences

Plan, initiate and co-ordinate activity to secure or provide help for independent living

Monitor contract needs and provide plan of care in a facilitative environment

Maintain and sustain or adapt and modify relationship in practice, service or environment

Counter discrimination and individual and institutional racism

Evaluate social and cultural factors affecting services. Act to change services. Work in an ethically sensitive way

Evaluate own performance

Counsel, supervise, protect people in difficulties. Secure opportunities in work, education, housing, leisure, income

Manage, supervise, teach others

Work effectively in multiracial society

Work within statutory requirements. Invoke legal powers where necessary

Work within professional standards, codes of good practice and national and local policy

Work in team or collaborate with other professions

Develop and use community support networks. Teach. Maximize health. Advocate

Chart I.

Community focus

Promote integration through:

- care management
- provision of home-based activity
- provision of residential support
- supported involvement in general and special educational, health and social services
- facilitation of employment and leisure opportunities
- support of relocation

Core competence

(i)   Promote human development
(ii) Promote learning and skill development
(iii) Promote effective communication
(iv) Support acquisition of personal relationships and friendships
(v)   Promote physical and mental health

through *assessment and intervention* which recognizes the implications of factors which cause learning disability and which applies key values

Specialist focus

Assess intervene and organize care management for:

- people with challenging behaviour
- people with multiple disabilities
- people with mental health problems

Chart 2.

Discussion Questions

- Chart 1 is an amalgam of statements of competence or the skills and knowledge described in Chapter 1.
- Identify the area(s) most important to you. Are there any missed out? If so add them.
- Assess or rate youself against them:
  1 = totally proficient/competent
  5 = have not yet started
- Make a plan to develop skills and knowledge – are there links/overlaps between the different boxes?
- Consider making a portfolio which contains your plans and evidence of learning or skill or competence.

or
Chart 2 shows the refined competencies proposed by the MHNA.
- Identify the ones most important to you and any that have been missed out.
- Make a Plan to develop your skills and knowledge – consider making a portfolio?
or
- Look at charts 1 and 2 and make up a similar chart for your area of practice or work, then work out how you would like to develop or demonstrate your competence and abilities; again consider a portfolio.

References

Association of Directors of Social Services (ADSS) and the Local Government Management Board (LGMB) (1997). *From Personnel Administration to Human Resource Management*. LGMB, London.

Brown, J. (1993). *Protocol for Progress*. Dept of Social Policy and Social Work, University of York.

Bulletin 1. (1996). *Development of National Occupational Standards for Professions Allied to Medicine*. Care Sector Consortium, London.

Care Sector Consortium (1994). *The Functional Map of Health and Social Care: Working Document*. Care Sector Consortium, London.

Care Sector Consortium (1997). *Draft for the Revised Level 4*. Care Sector Consortium, London.

Central Council for Education and Training in Social Work (1995). *Assuring Quality in the Diploma in Social Work – Rules and Requirements for the DipSW*. CCETSW, London.

Coats, M. and Mitchell, L. (1997). The Functional Map of Health and Social Care. In *Inter-professional Working for Health and Social Care* (eds J. Ovretveit, P. Mathias and T. Thompson), pp. 157–185. Macmillan, London.

Conrane Consulting (1996). *The Future Healthcare Workforce*. University of Manchester.

Dreyfus H.L. and Dreyfus S.E. (1986). *Mind Over Machine: The Power of Human Intuition and Expertise in the Era of Competence*. Oxford, Basil Blackwell.

English National Board for Nursing, Midwifery and Health Visiting (1989). *The Learning Disability Branch of Nursing*. ENB, London.

Eraut, M. (1996). *Mediating Scientific Knowledge into Health Care Practice: Evidence from Pre-Registration Programmes in Nursing and Midwifery Education, and Recommendations for Future Curriculum Design*. Research report available from the English National Board for Nursing, Midwifery and Health Visiting, London.

Hyland, T. (1994). *Competence, Education and Dissenting NVQs Perspectives*. Cassell, London.

Joint Awarding Bodies (JAB) (1993). *Professional and Occupational Standards in the Care Sector. Report of the Awarding Bodies and the Care Sector Consortium Conference*. Available from JAB, Derbyshire House, St Chad's Street, London WC1.

Lamsa, A. Hietanen, I. and Lämsä, J. (1994). Education for holistic care: a pilot programme in Finland. *Journal of Inter-professional Care (International Issue)* **8** (1), Spring.

Mansfield, B. and Mitchell, L. (1996). *Towards a Competent Workforce*. Gower, Hampshire.

Mansfield, B. and Matthews, D. (1985). *The Components of Job Competence*. Bristol, Further Education Staff College.

Mathias, P. and Thompson, T. (1997). Preparation for inter-professional work: trends in education, training and the structure of qualifications in the United Kingdom. In *Inter-professional Working for Health and Social Care* (eds J. Øvretveit, P. Mathias and T. Thompson), pp. 103–115. Macmillan, London.

National Committee of Inquiry into Higher Education (1997). *Higher Education in the Learning Society: Report of the National Committee*. HMSO, London.

National Council for Vocational Qualifications (NCVQ) (1995). *NVQ Criteria and Guidance*. NCVQ, London.

National Council for Vocational Qualifications (NCVQ) (1997). *Case Studies of Higher Level Vocational Qualifications*. NCVQ, London.

Thompson, T. (1994). *Refined Competences*. MHNA, Kidderminster.

United Kingdom Central Council for Nursing, Midwifery and Health Visiting (1982). *Code of Professional Conduct for Nurses, Midwives and Health Visitors (based on ethical concepts)*, 1st edn. UKCC, London.

Part One

The Services

Chapter 2

The National Health Service

Carl Thompson

Key Issues

- The continuing place of the NHS in the lives of people with a learning disability
- Structural change in the NHS
- The components of the NHS
- How the NHS works
- Purchasers – an introduction
- Providers – an introduction
- Contracts and contracting
- *The Health of the Nation* and people with a learning disability
- User consultation in services and purchasing

Introduction

The National Health Service (NHS) was for many years the primary form of statutory social protection and support for people with a learning disability. Large-scale institutional provision and unsophisticated needs analysis of local and national popula-

tions prevailed. It would be easy to assume, since the re-emergence of 'community care' on to the policy and service agendas, that the NHS's importance to the lives of people with a learning disability has been negated somewhat. The evidence, however, suggests that whilst some forms of NHS provision (such as in-patient beds) have declined, others (such as out-patient facilities) have increased (Table 2.1). Moreover, the resources that are given over to learning disability are being used more efficiently. In short, NHS provision is changing.

Given this continuing significance to the lives of people with learning disabilities the aims of this chapter are four-fold:

- To enable the reader to appreciate the historical legacies which have led to the current NHS.
- To gain an understanding of the structure, roles and responsibilities of the NHS in relation to people with a learning disability.
- To enable the reader to make the link between the role of the NHS and ideas of 'health' in the learning disability population.
- To show the routes through which people and money move within the NHS and to

Table 2.1 The numbers of learning disability beds[1] within the NHS and selected activity statistics

(a) No. of learning disability beds

	1993/94	1994/95	1995/96
Number of beds available	16 269	13 211	12 676

(b) In-patient activity[2] – mental handicap (sic) excluding community units

	1981/82	1986/87	1991/92	1993/94
Finished consultant episodes	34 000	58 000	62 000	61 000
In-patient episodes per bed	0.6	1.2	2.6	2.8
Mean stay (days)			553.5	317.1

(c) Out-patient activity[2]

	1981/82	1986/87	1991/92	1993/94
New attendances	3000	4000	4000	6000
Average attendance per new patient	6.6	4.6	11.5	10.8
Day care attendances	1000	4000	1000	2000

[1] The Department of Health Statistics Division.
[2] *Social Trends 1996* HMSO, tables 8.12 and 8.13.

tentatively outline ways in which they might usefully contribute to services.

This chapter addresses these aims by examining the structural changes over time which have led to the current NHS, by looking at how the NHS operates, and the basic separation of purchasing from the provision of services. Moreover, it also introduces the mechanisms by which strategic intent becomes service reality; namely, the processes of contracting and contracts. The role of the NHS in promoting a new, broader conceptualization of 'health' is outlined, as is the promotion and incorporation of users' and carers' views in the service delivery agenda.

What is the NHS?

In order to understand the composition and operations of today's NHS it is essential to understand its heritage. The NHS has enjoyed an almost 'organic' development during its history with a bitter-sweet legacy of large-scale structural change, heart-felt political debate, and subtle (as well as not so subtle) policy shifts.

The NHS came into the world on 5 July 1948 following the passing of the National Health Service Act (1946) in November 1946. This innovative piece of legislation compelled the Minister of Health:

To promote the establishment of a comprehensive health service designed to secure improvement in the physical and mental health of the people and the prevention, diagnosis and treatment of illness, and for that purpose to provide or secure the effective provision of resources.

(National Health Service Act (1946) Chapter 81: Part I, Section I: I)

What this meant for the British populace was a declared policy intention to move away from the old system of limited coverage for all but the most needy. A shift away from an inequitable system made up of prestigious teaching hospitals, and unevenly distributed voluntary and municipal hospitals, the latter having their roots in the workhouse system of the Poor Law. The shift was toward a system of free health care for all, regardless of whether they had contributed moneys to the national purse in the form of National Insurance or not. The NHS would be planned, rational, comprehensive and, above all, based on clinical need as opposed to ability to pay.

The Structure of the NHS

The beginning

The new NHS was to comprise several linked organizations all acting within the statutory framework of the 1946 Act. This new NHS would be comprehensive but right from its conception would be split into three separate arenas:

- Hospital services – which pulled in the old voluntary, municipal and teaching hospitals, although teaching hospitals retained separate management arrangements largely due to the influential composition of their Boards of Governors.
- Community services – these were the preserve of the Local Health Authorities (county councils and municipal borough councils). These included services such as immunization, environmental health, health visiting and, perhaps most importantly for this discussion, the majority of care and after-care of people with a learning disability.
- Family practitioner services – these were general practitioners (GPs) supported by administrative Executive Councils.

This initial NHS structure is outlined in Figure 2.1.

The creation of the NHS and the development of the hospital services sector gave medical consultant leaders the opportunity to further their stake in the provision of health services for the population. From 1946 onwards the number of hospital

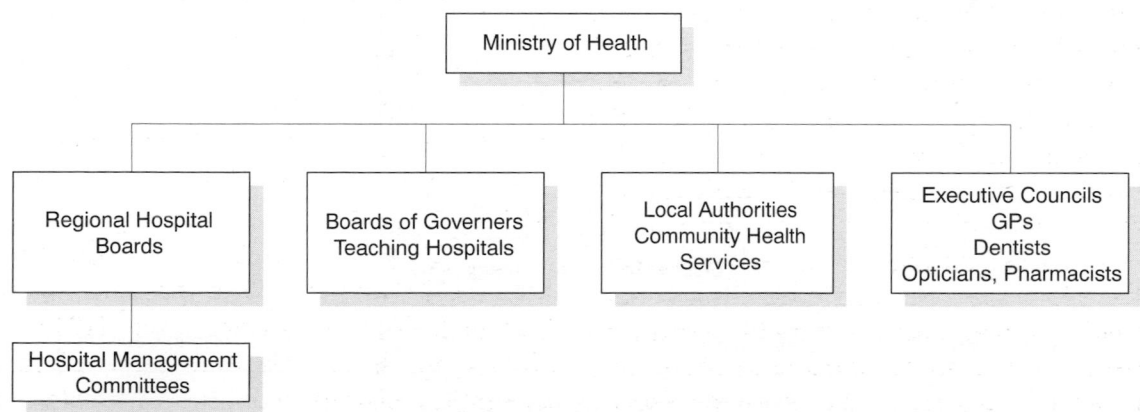

Figure 2.1 Structure of the NHS 1948–1974.

clinicians gained ground steadily so that by 1968 there were more hospital-based medical staff than GPs, a trend which has continued up to the present day.

GPs were often located in poor quality accommodation. They also worked within a payment mechanism which offered little incentive to deliver care of anything other than basic adequacy. Acknowledging the family practitioner service's lack of ability to match the developments in the hospital sector a GP's charter was introduced in 1966. This opened the way to an incentive-based payment system and loans and helped reinforce the more holistic approach to health which the Royal College of General Practitioners had been encouraging since 1952.

The common bond between GP services and the hospital sector was the Health Centre, which was administered under the aegis of the Local Authorities. Health Centres aimed to bring together the work of family doctors, health visitors and district nurses. They proved a vital link between hospital and primary care sectors.

The 1974 reorganization

This picture continued, apart from the development of the District General Hospital concept in the 1960s, through to the early 1970s. The increasing split between hospital and primary care sectors, as well as the separate status attached to the teaching hospitals, meant the two sectors were becoming increasingly disparate.

In 1974, Area Health Authorities with District Management Teams (DMTs) were created to plan broader services around the District General Hospitals. Teaching hospitals also lost their separate status. Clinical hospital staff were also given the power of veto over DMT decisions. This effectively meant that the predominant mode of change in the NHS was on a consensus basis; that is, all the stakeholders had to agree before services could change. This would prove significant later with the introduction of General Management in 1983. This new structure is represented in Figure 2.2.

GPs, dentists, opticians and pharmacists kept their separate administrative structure at District level but a degree of co-ordina-

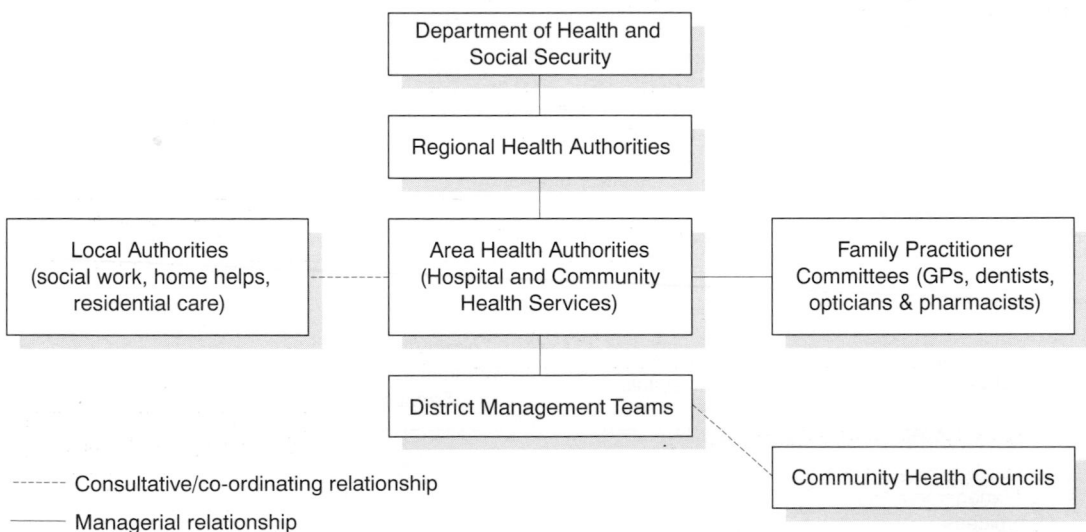

Figure 2.2 The structure of the NHS 1974–1982

tion was assumed by making the Family Practitioner Committees accountable to the new Area Health Authorities.

Crucially for people with a learning disability, the 1974 reorganization led to the establishment of Community Health Councils (CHCs). These were tasked with giving patients and potential patients an independent voice which would be listened to, and as a structurally located form of advocacy for 'vulnerable' groups who's share of NHS resources had been neglected thus far.

The 1974 reorganization was not as strong a force for unification as had been hoped for, despite the introduction of a planning system which compelled Health Authorities to act according to national guidelines. The oil crisis of the 1970s, recession and prolonged inflationary pressure meant that the Treasury had, for the first time, to introduce cash-limits in public expenditure (only the GPs escaped unscathed). Plans to redistribute resources to those under-funded groups, such as those with a learning disability, were either 'diluted' or shelved.

The financial reality of service provision, however, was not the only constraint on developments seeking to move away from the *status quo*. The power of veto afforded to clinical staff meant that consensus management at DMT level was hugely inefficient. This attracted criticism, not least from the opposition Conservative party. A new Government, with a new ideology, and a leader prepared to implement it, was imminent.

The Thatcher years

The 90 Area Health Authorities were replaced in 1982 with 200 District Health Authorities (DHAs) in the hope that decisions taken closer to the front-line in services would be more sensitive and encourage greater accountability (Figure 2.3). Accountability, however, was a two-edged sword, as the Department of Health and Social Security (DHSS) introduced performance reviews which made administrators accountable for pre-established targets. Outputs from services had entered the policy-funding arena and began to shift away from crude indicators, such as waiting lists, towards more detailed specifications, such as number of surgical operations completed.

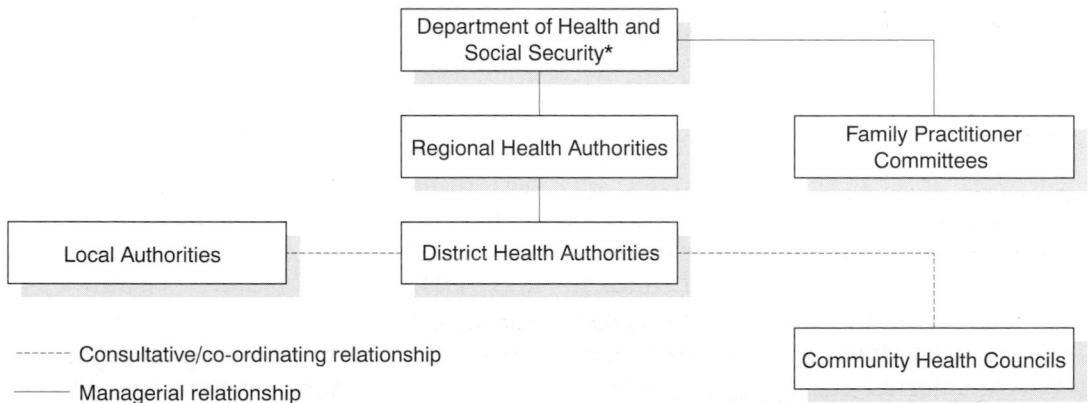

Figure 2.3 The structure of the NHS 1982–1990. *The Department of Health split from the Department of Social Security in 1988

Alongside the setting of targets came the rise of the hospital *manager* as opposed to the simple *administrator*. The Griffiths Report of 1983 ensured that a new breed of manager was in place at every level in the NHS, from the Regional Health Authority (RHA) downwards. This new breed would depend on continuing performance for employment and would become widely perceived as the instrument of the 1980s reforms. Clinical staff lost their power of veto and non-clinical services such as laundry were put out to competitive tender. Consensus management was now over and the language of the commercial world made its first tentative forays into the health care arena.

The shift towards general management was not, in itself, sufficient to secure the revenue savings which the Conservative Government desired. Managers still had no say on spending at the micro level by individual clinicians. And at local level decisions could be held up by the local CHC who were to be consulted before change could be put in place.

The huge growth in the cost of the NHS, although still efficient (as a proportion of gross domestic product) was beginning to take centre stage on the governmental policy agenda. Pay awards were no longer fully funded by the centre and Health Authorities were required to make up the difference from funds that would have been spent on direct patient care. By 1987 the situation was critical and culminated in severe unrest within the NHS. The campaign centred on ward closures, cancelled elective operations and widespread concern from the Health Authorities that the NHS funding shortfall had gone beyond the point where internal savings and redistribution could mask the impact on patient services. Box 1 highlights four of the major flaws that contributed to what was perceived as a failing NHS by many commentators.

The situation inspired a Prime Ministerial review of the NHS and the development of the most far-reaching and radical reforms the NHS had yet experienced. The review took evidence from a variety of sources but was most heavily influenced by the ideas expressed by the American economist Alan Einthoven (1985). He proposed that by separating the purchasing of health care from its provision and management and by making providers compete for limited contracts then incentives would be in place for cost-cutting, quality improvement and consumer responsiveness. Einthoven's views formed the basis of the White Paper *Working for Patients* (DOH, 1989) and the development of an 'internal', or quasi, market. More significantly for people with a learning disability, Einthoven's ideas also found favour with Sir Roy Griffiths and his proposals for community care (Griffiths, 1988).

The 'new' NHS

The NHS and Community Care Act (1990) made a number of radical changes to the ways in which health services in England, Scotland and Wales were organized. These are summarized in Box 2.

Following the royal ascent of the NHS and Community Care Act (1990) the NHS had in place purchasers, providers, a policy board and a management executive (the NHSME). The RHAs were still in existence and DHAs and Family Health Service Authorities (FHSAs) remained separate. In 1993 the Government proposed to rationalize this structure further by abolishing RHAs, and merging DHAs with their local FHSAs. The current NHS structure is shown in Figure 2.4.

Poor matching of funding to workload

- Funding to DHAs via RHAs was needs-based and was termed the RAWP (Resource Allocation Working Party Formula). This was adjusted for factors such as teaching, research, regional specialties and flows of patients between RHAs (cross-boundary flows). There were serious problems attached to this mechanism:
  (i)   there was a 2-year adjustment to a DHA's RAWP figure instead of cash compensation for cross-boundary flows
  (ii) day- and out-patients were not included in the RAWP calculations and often these were very cost effective (and their numbers were increasing)
  (iii) calculation was on average specialty cost and did not take into account the varied and complex nature of referrals especially to teaching hospitals.
- all of this meant RAWP-based financial headaches for DHAs

Disincentives for managers and clinicians

- The efficiency trap – cash-limited budgets meant efficient DHAs (those that treated most patients) increased costs and not revenue. At the end of each financial year surgeons and beds unused.
- The quality trap – shorter waiting times and clinical excellence equals more referrals but not more money. Conversely, those that lost referrals through poor quality had less work and therefore more money.
- Clinicians who kept lengthy waiting lists increased demand for their private services. Those that reduced their lists just got more work.

Lack of consumer responsiveness

- A cross-discourse consensus (right wing, feminist and Marxist amongst others) emerged regarding the oppressive and paternalistic nature of the route that health services were taking
- On a less academic level, the introduction of General Management meant that the language of providers and consumers began to take hold.

Few incentives to innovate

- The bureaucratic controls in place to protect public moneys led to unnecessary caution in services – management strengthening still meant those who spent the money were not the same people who were having to account for it.
- Clinicians were left untouched and managers of hospitals could do little – their contracts were held at DHAs.

Box 1 The flaws of the NHS leading to the NHS review 1988 (Ranade, 1994)

Management arrangements

- Streamlined RHAs and DHAs were created
- FHSAs were directly managed by RHAs
- Non-executive members of Health Authorities and Family Health Service Authorities (FHSAs) could now be paid (not just chairpersons)

Funding and audit arrangements

- RHAs get funds from the DOH and then through them to DHAs and FHSAs
- Health Authorities and FHSAs have accounts audited by the Audit Commission

NHS contracts

- Health Authorities and FHSAs could provide goods and services via NHS contracts, i.e. one NHS body (the commissioner) purchases goods and services from another NHS body (the provider)
- These arrangements did not, however, confer contractual rights and liabilities on the bodies concerned
- The Secretary of State has the power to resolve disputes within the system

NHS Trusts

- The label Self Governing Trusts covered a range of services including hospitals, ambulance services, community services and services for people with a learning disability
- Chairman and non-executive directors of Trust Boards were paid
- Each Trust sets out its duties in its initial approved order from the Secretary of State but this can be amended by him/her if necessary
- Trusts carry out work under contract but are reimbursed by relevant DHAs for treatment given to people not covered by contracts
- Trusts can also treat patients privately
- Trusts could dispose of assets such as land and employ staff on such terms as they saw fit
- Trusts can retain surpluses and borrow funds from the Secretary of State and other sources

Fundholding practices

- GPs could apply to the relevant RHA to be recognized as fundholding practices, as long as they met certain conditions (such as minimum numbers of patients on their list)
- RHAs pay GPFHs allotted sums for them to purchase specific goods and services
- Amounts available for individual patients were fixed and any extra funds from the patients DHA

Community care

- Local Authorities (LAs) were required to publish community care plans for services in their area
- LAs had a duty to assess people in need and decide if they required services
- LAs were given the power to employ voluntary organizations for the provision of welfare services to disabled or elderly people

continued opposite

- The Secretary of State could make grants available (via RHAs) to meet the social services costs for caring for the mentally ill

Others

- The establishment of a Clinical Standards Advisory Group
- Crown immunity was removed from NHS purchasers and providers
- NHS income was exempted from income tax

Box 2 The National Health Service and Community Care Act, 1990

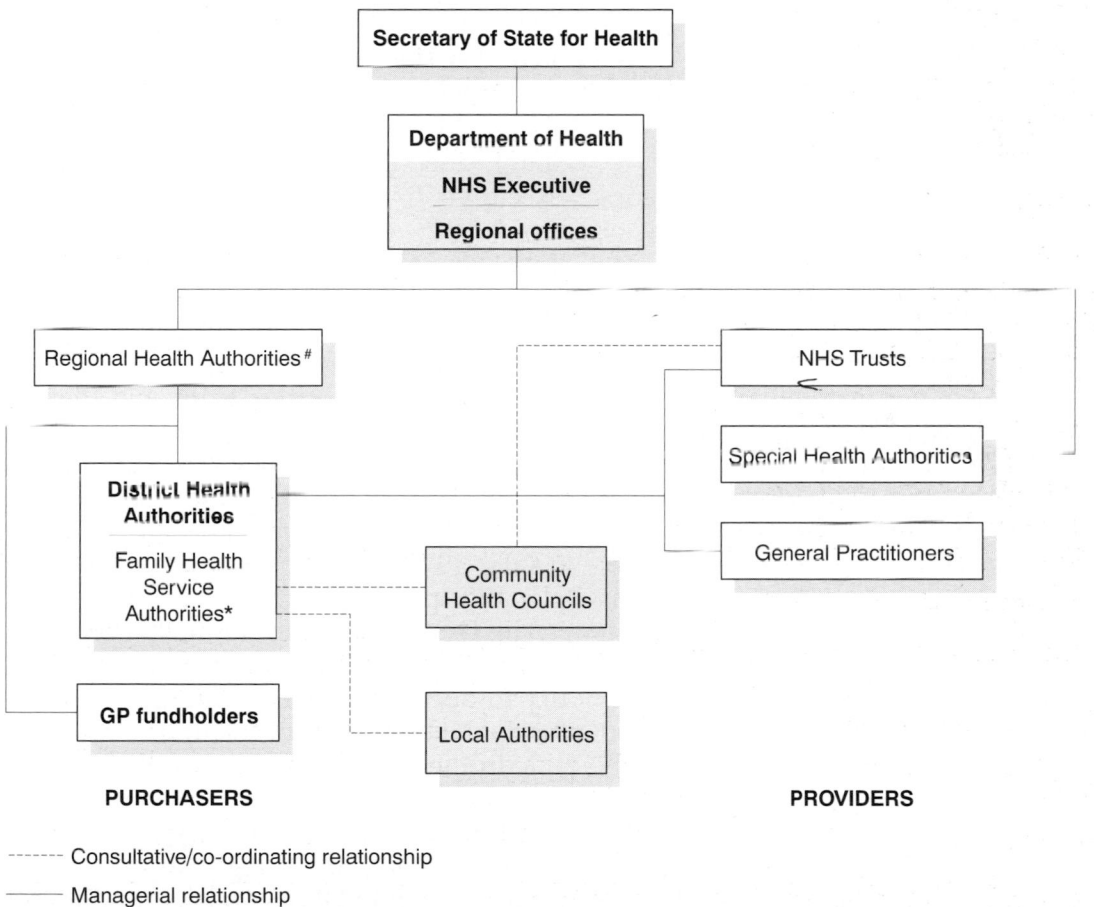

Figure 2.4 The structure of the NHS 1990–present. [#]Regional Health Authorities were abolished in 1995. Their functions were taken over by the NHSE regional offices. *District Health Authorities were also merged with local Family Health Service Authorities in the same year

The Sum of Its Parts: The Functional Components of the NHS

The NHS's components have several roles and statutory duties which they are expected to fulfil in order to successfully deliver the service. These are outlined in this section.

The influence of Parliament

Parliament oversees the work of the Secretary of State for Health and ensures that he/she is accountable to the state via a number of mechanisms. These include:

- *Parliamentary questions*, correspondence and debate. MPs can ask questions or raise points with the Secretary of State and he/she is expected to respond. This might include requests for information the Department of Health (DOH) might otherwise have not made available.
- *Parliamentary Select Committee*. The two main ones influencing the NHS are:
  (i) *the Public Accounts Select Committee* which examines the allocation to and spending of finances by the NHS;
  (ii) *the Health Select Commiteee*. This examines the work of the DOH and inputs into major policy issues.
- *The Health Service Commissioner* (Ombudsman). This post is charged with the task of investigating complaints of failure to deliver services or maladministration on the part of NHS Health Authorities and Trusts. The Commissioner publishes an annual report detailing complaints and whether or not they were upheld. By and large the Commissioner is excluded from examining complaints involving clinical judgement. He/she has 13 clinicians available to draw on to help decide whether a complaint has a clinical judgement element attached.
- *The Audit Commission* is a body established by Parliament (but is separate from it) to examine Local Authority accounts in England and Wales. Throughout the 1980s and 1990s it has seen its role extended and broadened to include the NHS. Its recommendations often go far beyond simple auditing and their reports have acted as significant change-agents in areas such as community care and hospital management.

The DOH and the NHSE

The DOH has two main elements: the NHS Policy Board (chaired by the Secretary of State) and the National Health Service Executive (NHSE). The Policy Board sets broad NHS strategy and the NHSE operationalizes this strategy in the form of Executive Letters (ELs) and Health Service priorities and planning guidance (HSGs). These are documents sent out to Trusts and Health Authorities to enable them to plan services in line with national policy. Major changes in policy are outlined via White Papers; for example, *The National Health Service: A Service With Ambitions* (DOH, 1996), which sets out Government plans for primary care.

The DOH negotiates annually (known as the public spending round) with the Treasury to decide the level of funding available for the NHS. Details of the figures are available in the Public Expenditure White Paper published annually. Most of the DOH's allocated funds from the Treasury are devolved down to the NHSE's regional offices, and through them to DHAs and GP fundholders (GPFHs). The Special Health Authorities get their funds direct from the DOH.

During the 1990s the DOH has come to play an increasingly important role in the research and development (R&D) field of the NHS. Following the appointment of Professor Michael Peckham as Director of R&D in 1991 and the Culyer review of 1994 (DOH, 1994) large-scale R&D funded by the DOH has come under the aegis of the Central R&D Committee based at the NHSE's central office. Their function is to co-ordinate research in the NHS around key policy areas such as *The Health of the Nation* (DOH, 1992) targets. Each regional NHSE office has a Director of R&D and an R&D Manager. These support specific research-based working groups and projects drawing on central R&D funds.

The DOH plays a key quality assurance role in the NHS via the NHSE's setting of corporate contracts with DHAs and the annual review process within which DHAs are expected to account for their performance towards national policy. The NHSE's regional offices also monitor Trust performance in meeting statutory financial requirements (such as making a 6% return on the value of their capital assets, such as buildings, annually) and towards policy criteria such as *The Patients' Charter* (DOH, 1991) targets.

The regional offices of the NHSE

These have replaced RHAs and absorbed some of their functions. The eight NHSE regional offices act as one of the primary vehicles for translating central health policy into forms that address regional contexts. The main functions of the NHSE's regional offices include:

- resource allocation to DHAs;
- overseeing the appointment of non-executive members of DHAs and two of the non-executive members of NHS Trusts in their region;
- resourcing and planning non-medical education and training;
- managing the NHSE's R&D programme;

- monitoring the performance of purchasers and providers in the region through *Patients' Charter* returns.

The Purchasers – An Introduction

DHAs and GP fundholders

There are 103 DHAs in England and Wales and these act as the purchasers for hospital and community health services for local populations. Since April 1996 they have also been responsible for primary health care in the shape of non-fundholding GPs, as DHAs and FHSAs formally merged. DHAs (and GP fundholders) are the cornerstones of the new NHS and the Conservative Government's vision of a responsive, effective, internal market. The Government in a response to the Health Select Committee's first report on *Priority Setting in the NHS: Purchasing* suggested:

Health Authorities [and GP Fundholders] assess the needs of people they serve and decide what treatments and services are required to meet those needs. This process should be informed by proper consultation with the public.

(DOH, 1995a)

DHAs move towards assessing these needs by compiling health profiles of their local populations. These profiles are the result of analysis of data sets such as the census or the public health data set and discussions with local GPs, Local Authorities, voluntary agencies and community groups. An effective purchaser in the eyes of policy makers is seen as one which:

- takes strategic as opposed to short-term views;
- develops and places robust contracts;
- is responsive to the needs of local people;
- has mature relations with local providers

(moving towards partnership and long-term agreement but with a healthy level of creative tension);

- nurtures local alliances around health-care;
- possesses organizational fitness (effective and efficient internally) (Mahwinney and Nichol, 1993, p. 21).

Because of the merger with FHSAs the DHA also has responsibility for the following:

- managing the contracts of general practitioners (non-fundholding);
- remunerating the same practitioners in line with their contracts;
- information provision to the general public on health services in their area;
- dealing with complaints about GPs, hospital or community services;
- the allocation for funds for certain capital-based developments in GP and hospital services.

The tools by which DHAs purchase services are contracts and more is said of these later in the chapter as they are crucial to understanding the process of service provision in the NHS.

GP fundholders (GPFHs)

GPs (or groups of GPs) who have more than 3000 patients registered with them, and who meet certain other criteria, can apply to adopt fundholding status. There are three separate levels of fundholding services:

- community fundholders; this enables GPs to pay for staff, drugs and community health services in practices with a list of more than 3000 people;
- mainstream fundholding; this enables GPs with more than 5000 patients to purchase a more comprehensive range of services;
- total purchasing; this is at the pilot stage

at present and involves GPFHs purchasing almost all services for their list, including accident and emergency care.

Fundholding status means GPs can purchase a range of services and enjoy greater degrees of managerial autonomy and flexibility than their non-fundholding counterparts. The range of services GPFHs can purchase is predefined and established centrally at the DOH. These limitations on purchasing are set out in Health Service Guidelines (HSGs). Conventional services which GPFHs may purchase at present include:

- out-patient services
- X-rays and laboratory services
- some in-patient and day-case treatments
- medicines and drugs
- certain community health services.

DHAs make up the 'gaps' in services by purchasing services for GPFH patients where necessary. There are many variables which can impact on a purchasing decision and these are summarized in Figure 2.5.

The Providers – An Introduction

NHS Trusts

Almost all NHS services are provided by NHS Trusts. Trusts came into being in 1991 following the accension of the NHS and Community Care Act (1990). They are officially classed as self-governing and have relative freedom to organize their own structures and processes in order to adjust to local service contexts such as staffing availability or the demands of different purchasers.

The constraints on Trust activity come in the form of legal duties and contractual frameworks with purchasers. The NHSE's

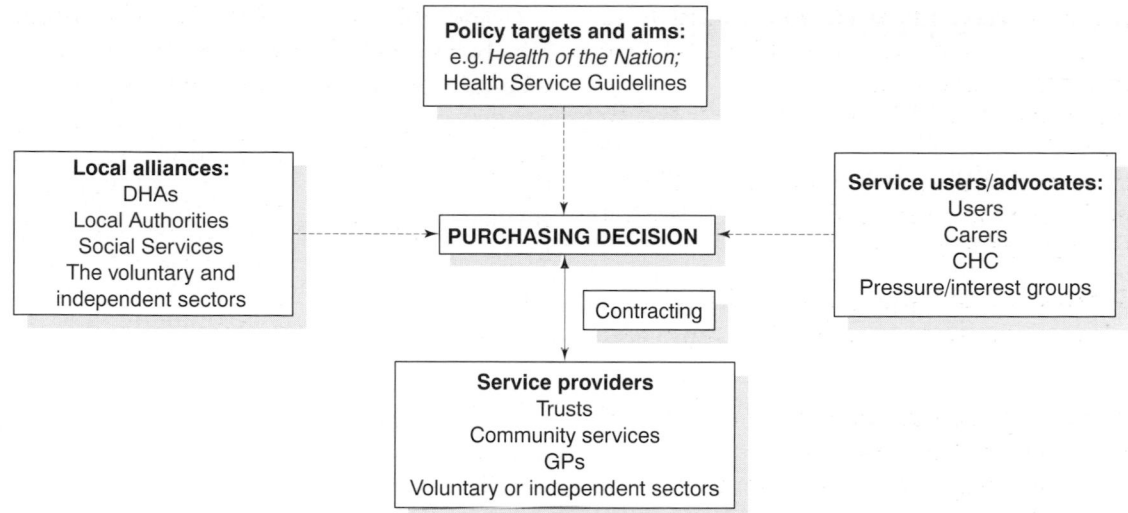

Figure 2.5 The major factors and influences on purchasing decisions. DHAs, District Health Authorities; CHC, Community Health Council

regional offices also monitor the performance of Trusts through the use of performance indicator league table data and *The Patients' Charter.* As well as these quality measures the NHSE also ensures the financial probity of the Trust by compelling Trusts to prepare:

- proposals for developing services
- proposals for capital investment
- a business plan.

Trusts have a number of financial duties:

- to break even
- to earn at least a 6% return on the value of their capital
- to operate within the external financing limit (EFL) set by the DOH.

The EFL represents the amount that each Trust can borrow in order to finance its capital developments. These limits are derived from the DOH's assessment of a Trust's business plan (its income flow, capital plans and so on). The EFL can be positive, negative or zero loaded.

If the EFL is positive it means the trust can borrow money up to the value of the EFL. If the EFL is negative then the Trust must pay back any surplus to the revenue or invest in future schemes. A zero EFL entails the Trust financing schemes directly from internally generated revenue.

Most revenue for Trusts derives from selling their services to purchasers via contracts with GPFHs or DHAs. Smaller amounts come from extra contractual referrals (ECRs – treating patients from other areas without a contract); the private sector (e.g. insurance firms), the DOH, and other Trusts.

The NHS still has a number of short- and long-stay beds as well as treatment centres dedicated for people with a learning disability. Many of these come under the aegis of NHS Trusts. Whilst the average number of available beds is declining there is still significant NHS activity in relation to learning disability, as was seen from Table 2.1.

Community Health Councils (CHCs)

Purchasers, providers and the DOH are not the only organizations involved in services provided by the NHS. CHCs have been in existence since 1974 and their role is to represent the public's interest in the system. There is usually one CHC for every DHA. They have little statutory power to draw on in order to effect change. They can, however, influence the policy process through advising DHAs on the views of the public. They gain funding from the local NHSE office.

In order that CHCs can usefully input into the policy process they have had several rights conferred on them. These include the right to:

- relevant information from the NHS (DHAs, Trusts, GPs);
- access certain NHS premises (e.g. NHS Trusts);
- be consulted on substantial developments or variations in services;
- observer status at DHA meetings.

CHCs are expected to produce an annual report which acts as the basis for discussions with local purchasers.

The Tools for the Job: Contracting

Contracting for what?

The contract is the mechanism through which purchasing strategy is operationalized. Contracts represent the 'business' of the NHS at the micro level of individual services. As such, the nature, tone and values enshrined within, and reinforced by, contracts strongly influence the character of local services for people with a learning disability.

Contracts, in the NHS sense, are not legally binding; they represent a form of service agreement between commissioner and service provider. The contract specifies the service required. It does this by outlining the levels of quality, cost and volume in services purchased. The contracting process in the NHS is still relatively naive when compared to contracts placed in commercial and private sector environments and thus far the primary challenges facing managers have been largely of a reactive nature (i.e. muddling through the process of contract negotiations without worrying about the details of proactive health gain achievements).

Costs in NHS contracts are based around the twin maxims that price (what it costs the purchaser) must equal cost (what it costs the service provider) and services must not subsidize other services through contracts, a process known as cross-subsidization.

The volume of services is commonly defined in terms of service activity. Indicators of volume in contracts include 'the number of finished consultant episodes'; 'the numbers attending out-patient departments' or 'community learning disability team contacts'. It is these twin tenets of volume and quality, and the relationship between them, which assist commissioners in determining value for money.

The quality dimension

The concept of quality is notoriously difficult to represent in contracts. A number of commentators (Pfeffer and Coote, 1991; Ovretveit, 1992; Harrison and Pollitt, 1994) have highlighted the complex and contested nature of this concept and this complexity has manifested itself in NHS contracting. Each of the aforementioned commentators have recognized that quality is, to some extent, determined by the standpoint of the person in relation to NHS services. A person's judgement of quality in a service, and the emphasis they might wish to operationalize through contracts may be very different according to whether they are professionals delivering technical care within the service; managers attempting to balance technical excellence with finite resources and meet policy aims and objectives; or consumers/carers at the receiving end of service delivery or purchasing decisions.

Service contracting thus far appears to have taken the lowest common denominator route to developing quality. Quality in most contracts is restricted to the monitoring of *Patients' Charter*-related issues of waiting times; privacy; dignity and, lately, the issue of mixed-sex units. Where quality specifications are not detailed in relation to *Patients' Charter*-related standards then the other primary means of promoting quality in service through contracts is through the use of proxies. The presence of quality initiatives and quality mechanisms in place within provider settings is often used as indicators of quality as opposed to the effects of these approaches on individuals or client groups. Initiatives or frameworks such as patient fora or councils, clinical audit and total quality management all act as proxy indicators of quality in services for the purposes of contracting.

Over the past 2 years the debate has become more sophisticated with service and clinical outcomes beginning to enter the contracting-quality equation. This is particularly crucial to the area of learning disability provision, where the boundary between treatment and care is often hard to discern. Outcomes in other NHS areas, such as acute surgical care, are relatively easy to develop. Treatments such as hip replacements or coronary bypass operations can be measured in terms of survival or failure rates and whole packages of indicators for acute hospitals as a whole have been piloted on a large scale (such as the

Maryland Outcomes Indicators in Northern Region). Such 'measures' of success or failure are not as easy to develop in the field of learning disability. There is, however, a growing recognition that the monitoring of clinical and service outcomes is an important part of contracting in learning disability services. At an academic level money has been made available from the DOH R&D 'pot' to enable managers and academics to come together to discuss the usefulness of outcome information in routine practice (Quereshi, 1996). The outcome of such a shift has been the funding of ongoing research into the area of outcomes in community care, including learning disability. Some outcomes are already being piloted for learning disability services by purchasers. These include:

- reduction of admissions to hospitals for behavioural reasons;
- reduction of placement breakdown for behavioural reasons;
- reduction in the use of psychotropic drugs to control behaviour;
- reduction in intensity, frequency and duration of challenging behaviour;
- improved quality of life;
- improved ability to self-manage;
- improved ability of carers to manage behaviour;
- increased engagement in meaningful activities.

(Pilot outcomes derived from informal contact with one DHA in the Midlands.)

Types of contracts

Getting the balance between cost–volume and quality right requires different frameworks according to the nature of the client groups and the shape of existing services. These frameworks come in the form of contract types. There are three primary types of contract in use in the NHS at present and each lends itself to different types of service and client. These contract types are termed:

- block
- cost per case
- cost–volume.

It is only really necessary to discuss two of these (block and cost per case) as cost–volume contracts are essentially an amalgamation of the other two.

Block contracts

In the block contract the purchaser agrees to pay the provider for services which are only broadly defined and in which the price is fixed. The contract lays down simple performance targets which often are based around process indicators of activity rather than desired outcomes, although this is changing, as was seen in the last section.

Block contracts can promote 'information asymmetry' (Glynn and Perkins, 1995). Simply put, this means providers know more about their activity than purchasers and block contracting mechanisms do not always develop monitoring systems which are sensitive enough to overcome this flaw. Consequently, there is a reliance on trust between purchaser and provider. When this trust is abused or absent then the provider can engage in opportunistic behaviour if it wishes and seek to further its own interests as opposed to the interests of the purchaser. This is significant for people with a learning disability as the *raison d'être* for the NHS reforms was the development of the purchasing function as the means of better representing the consumer interest in the process of delivering health services. This opportunism can manifest itself in various ways but the most common is either over- or under-performance, where Trusts alter their activity rates as a response to pressure (or lack of it) on budgets.

This is a real problem within block contracts as most of the risk in the purchaser–

provider relationship is located at the provider's end. Whilst providers have the ability to establish contacts based on pre-set volumes, circumstances can change for providers. Policy changes, service-structural alteration and staffing or recruitment crises can all serve to alter the volume–cost equation. Block contracting has evolved in order to account for this background operating context. Volume and quality 'triggers' are being placed within contracts where more money is paid if activity or standards increase. Block contracts in learning disability appear to be the preserve of Trust contractual relations with corporate and large-scale purchasers such as DHAs.

Cost per case contracting

In cost per case contracts an agreed price is paid for each procedure, therefore the more procedures a Trust carries out within these types of contracts the more money a Trust receives. A procedure might constitute a Community Learning Disability Team contact, or an out-patient clinic episode with a consultant in psychiatry. Prices in cost per case contracts are set in order to enable Trusts to reach their statutory 6% return on assets each year.

The lack of information relating to the actual cost of treatments within learning disability can be a real problem within services. Although as providers 'learn from experience' and for groups of clients with similar needs then this should improve. The tying in of initiatives such as clinical guidelines, protocols and more reliable outcomes-based knowledge into contracts should also play a part in reducing some of the margin of error for Trust cost setting.

Cost per case contracts are expensive to draw up and implement because both parties require detailed information on cost and activity and enforcing them can be problematic due to the extensive marketing required (Glynn and Perkins, 1995). There are few economies of scale in these contracts and consequently their use tends to be in the realm of small-scale purchaser–provider relations; for example, in the case of GPFHs and NHS Trusts.

Cost–volume contracts

Cost–volume contracts involve the partitioning off of some of the moneys paid by the purchaser. These are then released according to the levels of activity reached. This is essentially a combination of block and cost per case contracting. To some extent the increasing sophistication of block contracting mechanisms is reducing the advantages of such contracts.

Contracts then represent the means by which NHS services are purchased for people with learning disabilities. But what services for people with a learning disability come under the aegis of the NHS?

A Comprehensive Health Service?

People with a learning disability have the same rights to access NHS services as any citizen of the UK. There are occasions though when health services not specifically catering for the needs of people with learning disabilities can act to deny those people the access they are entitled to. The NHSE is quite clear on the responsibilities of the NHS in relation to meeting the special requirements of people with a learning disability:

Purchasing authorities should include in their contracts specific provision to enable people with learning disabilities to obtain NHS health care services and to ensure that, where necessary, that special provision is made where the health care needs of people with learning disabilities cannot be met through the ordinary range of services.

(NHSME, 1992)

Box 3 details the responsibilities of the NHS in relation to the special requirements of the population with learning disabilities.

In addition to its responsibility to people with a learning disability, the NHS also has a series of obligations to Local Authorities (Box 4).

Both of these sets of responsibilities take on board the recognition that health services cannot purely concentrate on treatment alone and that the distinction between health and social care in learning disability is a tenuous one. If the health profile of the population with a learning disability is to be raised in any meaningful way then it is essential that health services work with other agencies in an attempt to produce health gains. This, in part, is the rationale behind that part of the NHS contracting process called 'Joint commissioning'.

Joint Commissioning

Joint commissioning, at its simplest, is the purchasing of services by more than one agency, although most commonly this has been interpreted in learning disability to mean DHAs and Local Authorities. Wertheimer and Greig (1993) identify a number of features of joint commissioning (Box 5).

Joint commissioning can occur at macro and micro levels of purchasing. Macro-level joint commissioning is seen in centralized budgets, large-scale population needs assessment and block contracting. At its most visible, macro-level joint commissioning is observable in the production of Community Care Plans which detail the services and plans of local agencies in relation to community care.

Micro-level purchasing takes place at the level of individual needs assessments and commonly entails the tailoring of Local Authority care plans and resources to local

---

Purchasers should:

- Ensure that service specifications for health care include appropriate provision for meeting the needs and promoting the health and well-being of people with learning disabilities.
- Use contracts with provider units to ensure that wherever possible people with learning disabilities are enabled to use ordinary health services.
- Consider contracting for additional services for people with learning disabilities, including:
  (i)   *alternatives to the ordinary services*. For example, where local NHS dental practitioners are unable to treat patients with severe learning disabilities, DHAs should arrange alternative services.
  (ii) *specialist assessment and treatment services*. For example, some people with learning disabilities need treatment for psychiatric illness or severe behaviour disturbance. If it is not possible adequately to meet these patients' needs within the general psychiatric services, specialist assessment and treatment services will be needed in hospital or community settings.
- Wherever possible contract to provide continuity of care and contact; taking into consideration the preference of the patient and carers.

Additionally, DHAs should:

- Consider contracting for residential and respite care. This is seen primarily as being for those 'small number of people with severe or profound learning disabilities and physical, sensory or psychiatric conditions . . .'. Such admissions should be the result of multiprofessional assessments and consultation with parents or carers. Where such care is normally provided by families there may be a need for short-term respite care arrangements to be provided by the NHS.
- Contracts for service provision should include a requirement on providers to inform GPs and other members of the primary health care team what services are available in their locality.
- Ensure that during the transition to community-based services, the improvement in the quality of care in specialist mental handicap hospitals at least matches general improvements in health provision.

Box 3 NHS responsibilities for people with learning disabilities (NHSME, 1992)

circumstances and the special requirements of separate clients. Initiatives such as the pooling of funds between care managers and fundholding GPs (Glynn and Perkins, 1995) may act to increase the sensitivity of such micro-level co-operation. If increases in health gain are to be realized then the ideas behind, and processes of, joint commissioning will have to be broadened to encompass a much broader conceptualiza-

tion of health in relation to people with learning disabilities.

A Healthier Learning Disability Population?

This broader conceptualization of health and the actions needed to promote it lie behind the Government policy enshrined in *The Health of the Nation* (DOH, 1992).

- Local Authorities will look to Health Authorities to secure through their contracts the services of professional staff, including psychiatrists, mental handicap nurses, psychologists and therapists, to help assess the needs of individuals with learning disabilities and to provide the health services for them. Health services professional staff will also need to be made available to provide training, advice and support to Local Authority staff.
- Health Authorities will also need to contribute to the preparation of Community Care Plans and consider with local authorities how resources can jointly best be used to provide care. FHSAs will also need to ensure that the views of all GPs and other members of the primary health care team are properly reflected in these considerations. Additionally, GPFHs will need to be aware of the overall approach to and of the principles underlying Community Care Plans in order that they can take these into account when contracting for health care.
- Full use should be made of the arrangements for joint finance.

Box 4 NHS responsibilities to Local Authorities (NHSME, 1992)

- Agencies make joint decisions about how money is spent.
- Money spent comes from the same 'pot', although financial systems may not necessarily be shared or formally merged.
- Joint commissioning is primarily the means to the end of improving outcomes for users and carers and as an expression of commitment to improved quality in services.
- Agencies share a set of values and operate in a context of mutual trust.
- Greater coherence at all levels of commissioning.
- Both sides recognize that joint commissioning may involve concession, gains and losses, as well as potential reductions in authority and autonomy in decision-making.
- Joint commissioning means retention of accountability for individual agencies whilst carrying out their individual statutory responsibilities.

Box 5 Features of joint commissioning (Wertheimer and Greig, 1993; Glynn and Perkins 1995)

The main document issued in 1992 made little mention of the special needs of people with a learning disability, a situation that was rectified in 1995 with the publication of *The Health of the Nation: A Strategy for People with Learning Disabilities* (DOH, 1995b). This document was intended to:

. . . help commissioners of health and social service to implement the strategy for health by addressing the particular needs of people with learning disabilities within five key areas – coronary heart disease and

stroke; cancer; HIV, AIDS and sexual health; accidents; and mental illness . . . [the document] looks at ways of ensuring that people with learning disabilities are included in action taken for the whole population.

(DOH, 1995b)

The main points of the strategy are outlined in Box 6.

The Health of The Nation: A Strategy for People with Learning Disabilities set few objectives or targets for people with learning disabilities. This was surprising given that its parent document (DOH, 1992) was accompanied by key performance targets in areas such as teenage pregnancy and suicide.

The document recognizes that some health problems are more common in people with learning disabilities, such as:

- communication problems
- hearing problems
- eyesight problems
- obesity and poor levels of cardiovascular fitness
- behaviour problems
- epilepsy
- psychiatric illness
- respiratory problems
- orthopaedic and mobility problems.

It suggests that joint working and collaboration should be based around the idea of 'health alliances':

Every agency responsible for an aspect of services should seek to improve joint working, with involvement of users and carers, to plan, develop and review services. This should be part of the process of commissioning services. (p. 10)

Alliances might comprise two or more of the following:

- Local Authority Social Services Departments
- Housing Departments and Housing Associations
- Education Authorities and schools
- Health Services:
  Primary care
  Hospitals
  Community Services – including specialist learning disability services
- Voluntary and private services
- Family and friends.

The three main conclusions are that service commissioners 'might consider' specifying in their contracts:

- Health surveillance and health promotion programmes which ensure that people with learning disabilities are included in programmes for the rest of the population, and health surveillance and health promotion programmes specifically for people with learning disabilities.
- Health services which enable people with learning disabilities to use health services available to everyone else; and specialist health services where necessary.
- Learning disability support services which use their expertise to help their clients to use resources that everyone else uses, and which meet needs of people with learning disabilities which would not otherwise be met.

At the practical level this should mean commissioners of health and social care having a portfolio of contracts including:

continued opposite

Community support

- housing
- education
- vocational training
- employment
- leisure activity
- social activity
- programmes for personal and social development
- Health Services.

Specific programmes for additional needs arising from:

- sensory impairments
- motor impairments
- communication problems
- behavioural problems.

Specialist health care by

- promoting access to general health services
- ensuring that needs are met through alternative services when it is difficult to meet them through general health services.

Forensic services for offenders with learning disabilities (p. 11).

One objective it did set was that commissioners should:

Choose services with high quality individual assessment of needs and care delivery, which facilitate the inclusion of people with learning disabilities.

(DOH, 1995b, p. 13)

The challenge of including people in a meaningful way in services is currently one of the major issues facing commissioners and providers alike within the NHS.

Involving Users and Their Carers

In latter years one of the most fundamental shifts to occur within the NHS has been the recognition that successful services are the ones that best meet the requirements and needs of the people whom they serve. Learning disability services have been at the forefront of this new feature of the service commissioning and delivery processes. Initiatives such as citizen advocacy, user forums, patient councils and carer representation in services have been around for a long time in the most innovative services for people with learning disabilities. In the 1990s, however, these arrangements for getting service users' voices on to the macro- and micro-policy agendas have become more formalized and the claims regarding the desirability of such initiatives given added impetus by the role of policy, and guidance from the centre.

The incorporation of user's perspectives

on services are already a feature of many services with patients councils in settings as diverse as the secure environment of NHS Special Hospitals such as Ashworth, and in NHS Trusts with resident populations primarily catering for clients with profound and challenging disabilities.

The DOH has in recent years invested much in the way of resources in implementing and researching the incorporation of user's and carer's views into local services. The reasoning behind this intervention from the centre can be seen, in part, as a recognition that locally led initiatives, whilst well meaning, have sometimes failed to grasp the essential values behind consultation – namely, that effective consultation depends on an 'equal partnership' between agency and carers/users. The DOH sees effective consultation as being based on the following values:

- dialogue
- liaison
- communication
- participation
- respect
- listening
- appreciation
- understanding (DOH, 1996, p. 8).

It is clear from the earlier discussions of contracting, joint commissioning and promoting health in relation to people with a learning disability that the idea of consultation and partnership with local populations of people with a learning disability and their carers is one of the fundamental challenges and shifts in practice facing all the components involved in the commissioning and delivery of services to people with a learning disability in the short–medium term.

Moving Through the System

Ideally, within the NHS–Local Authority interface the money is supposed to follow the patient as they progress from care manager or GPFH to provided care or treatment. However, in reality the lack of sophistication in the early days of contracting and service planning has led to criticism that patients tend to follow money. Figure 2.6 illustrates funding flows through the NHS. In general these follow the patterns of service provision for people with learning disabilities.

Perhaps the biggest problem in moving through this complex system of gateways as a means of having your needs met is that some of the gatekeepers (care managers, DHA purchasers and GPFHs) and almost all service provider professionals adhere to a traditional, and professionally ingrained, approach to needs analysis. When a care manager or a GPFH assesses a client's needs they are asked to draw on a 'holistic' conception of what it means to be healthy or to lead a 'normal' life. Similarly, within care planning carried out by Community Learning Disability Nurses the overwhelming discourse is one of comprehensive and holistic health assessment. Flynn *et al.* (1995) suggest that this breadth and holism in assessment is the antithesis of the contracting for health approach:

. . . the activities of community health services workers are by definition undertaken within the homes and social contexts of local people for whom health needs are defined holistically in a way which is difficult to specify in contractual terms. The paradox is that the mechanism of the NHS quasi-market at one level compels commissioners (purchasers) to stimulate competition and adversarial contracting, which may be incompatible with these characteristics and may even undermine objectives and injunctions at other levels of the NHS to pursue healthy alliances, seamless care, and interagency collaboration.

(Flynn *et al.*, 1995, pp. 548–9)

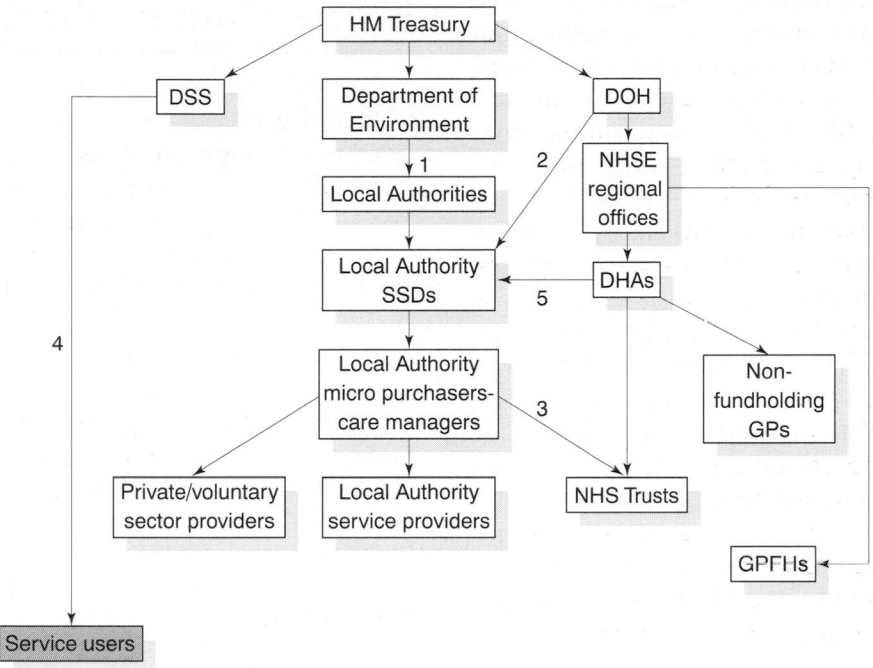

Figure 2.6 Funding at the NHS–Local Authority interface. 1, Revenue support grant; 2, special transitional grant and specific grants (e.g. mental illness); 3, where Trusts provide social care; 4, social security funding via individual claimants; 5, joint finance/section 28a money. DSS, Department of Social Security; SSDs, Social Services Departments.

It remains to be seen whether contracting and the mechanism of the quasi-market will ever catch up and encompass the sensitivity of individual needs assessment that only prolonged and informed contact with individuals and their families provides.

Conclusion

Clearly, the picture of social support and protection for people with a learning disability is one that suggests a shift away from the medical model of disability which traditional NHS services have promoted. However, the NHS is still a significant component in the lives of many people with a learning disability, not least as the NHS has gradually recognized that accessibility to general medical services rather than the automatic creation of segregated 'disability' services is an aim worth striving for.

The new emphasis within the NHS on joint working and collaboration, coupled with the broader conceptualization of health as promoted by *The Health of the Nation* holds much promise for people with a learning disability. Perhaps for the first time the NHS is beginning to recognize that barriers to health in people with a learning disability are rooted in societal prejudice as opposed to rational difference. The fact that these barriers are being challenged suggests that the social model of disability is finally being recognized within policy-making for people with a learning disability, and that the NHS is beginning to address some of its former criticisms. Initiatives such as formalized user consultation, innovation in contracting, and the recognition that contracts represent more than just pieces of paper – they are an expression of values – all suggest a shift towards the positive valuation of the lives of disabled people.

Practitioners can play a part in this shift by recognizing the importance of NHS services, assisting clients or service users to take full advantage of their rights to access and redress within the NHS and to ensure that conventional services adapt themselves to the needs of disabled people rather than disabled people having to adapt to outmoded services. The healthiest alliance of all is between the NHS and the people who use its services and who can judge its ability to promote health from the most meaningful perspective of all – their own.

Discussion Questions

- How can health care professionals promote more user-focused NHS services?
- How can the views of stakeholders from outside your service (such as a local advocacy group) be incorporated into better planning or service delivery?
- How does your relationship with your service's purchasers measure up to the ideals of the NHS reforms?
- Is there potential for increased collaboration between agencies in your service area? If so, what can you do to encourage it?
- How would you advise your local CHC or client representative group to best maximize their chances of impacting on your service (off the record of course!)?

- How well does contracting for your service mirror your values as a professional? and as a service generally?
- If there's a gap in response to the last question what can you do to close it?

References

DOH (1989). *Working for Patients*, Cmnd 555. HMSO, London.

DOH (1991). *The Patients' Charter*. HMSO, London.

DOH (1992). *The Health of the Nation: A Strategy for Health in England*. HMSO, London.

DOH (1994). *Research and Development Task Force: Supporting Research and Development in the NHS* (Culyer Report). HMSO, London.

DOH (1995a). *Government Response to the First Report from the Health Committee: Priority Setting in the NHS: Purchasing: Session 1994–95*, Cmnd 2826. HMSO, London.

DOH (1995b). *The Health of the Nation: A Strategy for People With Learning Disabilities*. HMSO, London.

DOH (1996). *Consultation Counts: Guideline for Service Purchasers and Users and Carers Based on the Experiences of the National User and Carer Group*. HMSO, London.

Einthoven, A. (1985). *Reflections on the Management of the National Health Service*. Nuffield Provincial Hospitals Trust, London.

Glynn, J. and Perkins, D.A. (1995). *Managing Health Care: Challenges for the 1990s*. Saunders, London.

Griffiths, R. (1983). *The NHS Management Inquiry, DHSS*. HMSO, London.

Griffiths, R. (1988). *Care in the Community: An Agenda for Action*. HMSO, London.

Harrison, S. and Pollitt, C. (1994). *Controlling Health Professionals: The Future or Work and Organisation in the NHS*. OUP. Buckingham.

Mahwinney, B. and Nichol, D. (1993). *Purchasing for Health: A Framework for Action*. NHS Management Executive, Leeds.

National Health Service Act (1946). HMSO, London.

National Health Service Management Executive (NHSME) (1992). *HSG(92) 42*.

Ovretveit, J. (1992). *Health Service Quality: An Intro-*

duction to *Quality Methods for Health Services.* Blackwell Scientific Publications, Oxford.

Pfeffer, N. and Coote, A. (1991). *Is Quality Good for You?*, IPPR, London.

Quereshi, H. (1996). Outcomes in service for people with learning disabilities – the heart of the matter. *Tizard: Learning Disability Review,* **1** (3), 36–43.

Ranade, W. (1994). *A Future for the NHS: Health Care in the 1990s.* Longman, London.

Wertheimer, A. and Greig, R. (1993). *Report on Joint Commissioning for Community Care.* National Development Plan, Manchester.

Further Reading

Klein, R. (1996). *The Politics of the NHS*, 3rd edn. Longman, London.

Levitt, R. and Wall, A. (1994). *The Reorganized National Health Service.* Chapman & Hall, London.

NAHAT NHS Handbook (published annually). JMH Publishing, Tunbridge Wells.

Ovretveit, J. (1995). *Purchasing for Health.* OUP, Buckingham.

Robinson, R. and Le Grand, J. (1994). *Evaluating the NHS Reforms.* Kings Fund, London.

NHS changes are best observed by reading journals regularly. In relation to the NHS and the NHS–LA interface the best journals are:

- *The Health Service Journal*
- *NHS Manpower Review*
- *British Medical Journal*
- *British Journal of General Practice*
- *Primary Care Management*
- *Journal of Social Policy*
- *Sociology of Health and Illness*
- *Social Science of Medicine*
- *Journal of Quality in Health Care*
- *Policy and Politics*

Chapter 3

The Independent Sector

James Churchill

Key issues

- Composition of the independent sector
- Organizational structures
- External controls
- Motivation
- Philosophy of care
- Financing of residential homes
- Future of voluntary sector

Introduction

A new phrase has come into use in the late 1980s and early 1990s which refers to the 'independent sector' of the residential care industry. This is an umbrella term meaning any provision which is not provided by statutory agencies such as Health Authorities or Local Authorities.

Like many umbrella terms it is a little confusing. Broadly speaking, there are two parts to the independent sector – the private sector and the voluntary sector. Some have argued that residential provision based on projects run by Housing Associations or by newly created charities, often called simply Trusts, which have been formed out of Local Authority or Health Authority provision constitutes a third element situated somewhere between the voluntary and statutory sectors.

This confused status for Housing Associations is probably a reflection of the high level of financial and administrative control demanded by Central Government in the form of the Housing Corporation administration. So, whilst most Housing Associations are charities or Friendly Societies, and could reasonably claim to be voluntary sector bodies, the level of Central Government influence on their services is so high as to place them in the no-man's land of not being a truly independent voluntary sector body yet obviously not a commercial concern. In theory the new ex-Local Authority Trusts and the NHS Trusts created by the sweeping changes to the NHS are more autonomous than the Housing Associations. In practice, this may not be so because many representatives of their parent agencies still hold positions of power in them and the culture of 'independence' has yet to flower within many such agencies. One of the potential levers of change in the future is the extent to which these new groupings adapt to and exploit the freedoms the independent sector offers. They are a useful potential seedbed for new ways of interprofessional working, but most have, as yet, to develop their new role. However, for the purposes of this chapter we will assume that the 'voluntary sector' includes Housing Associations, charities, voluntary agencies, Trusts, and not-for-profit agencies.

Any consideration of the independent sector must include a clear understanding of the various legal and organizational frameworks with which people try to provide services. We will be considering mostly the provision of residential and day services to this client group because they make up the preponderance of activity in this area, though there are some vigorous campaigning charities in this area.

Organizational Structures

There are a wide variety of 'legal vehicles' which carry the burden of providing services for this client group. For example, an independent sector residential home could be run by any one (or more) of the following:

- public limited company
- private limited company
- registered charity
- Housing Association
- Friendly Society
- Industrial and Provident Society
- sole trader
- partnership
- consortium (which would also have to have some other legal form such as a charitable status and/or a voluntary association)
- voluntary association

- company limited by guarantee
- trade union
- professional association.

Many of these categories are not mutually exclusive. For example, a trade union or professional association may run a home for its members using a company limited by guarantee which is also a registered charity. At some stage this home might also become part of a local consortium and the property sold to a Housing Association to help with maintenance and gain access to Special Needs Management Allowance whilst the charity retains management control of care. It is important to note that 'ownership' of a home does not necessarily imply management.[1] This is often delegated to any one of the above categories by any other of them, or handed to a specialist managing agency on a profit or not-for-profit basis. The managing agency can then obtain access to Central Government funds for its residents and the Authority can specify a contract, retaining its statutory obligation to inspect and maintain good standards of care.

So, in dealing with registered homes, it is important to understand who the owner is and who is in day-to-day control of the home. For example, whilst some homes might be run for the benefit of clients in a particular area, they may also be part of a national organization (e.g. Elizabeth Fitzroy Homes, Walsingham Community Homes, Mencap Homes Foundation) and be responsible to a central management.

Equally, a home may, as a matter of policy or of economic necessity, have accepted residents from all over the country but be responsible to a local volunteer board of management (e.g. Leonard Cheshire Foundation, Ark Housing Association Homes). The care industry, and in particular the voluntary sector, contains a wide diversity of organizational structures. Some national organizations are highly centralized, others have decentralized to the point where most decisions affecting individual homes are dealt with locally or regionally. Individual voluntary sector homes may have their own management committee drawn from the locality or provided from a regional office, or even a central office or have some mixture of local management under the overall guidance of central policy directives. 'Management' itself as well as care staff may be professional and salaried, or unpaid and voluntary, or a mixture of the two.

In dealing with such a diversity of structures, professionals should have a clear understanding of how an organization works – at least with regard to the management of its services. For example, it does no good complaining about the poor state of a building to a volunteer or worker or even a local member of the management committee who has no ability to effect the desired change. The message needs to go where it can be most effectively dealt with – perhaps a regional manager, or the chair of the local Social Services Committee, or a director at the head office of the charity. In the voluntary sector the 'normal' lines of management accountability which usually exist in statutory sector agencies cannot be assumed. The professional must 'know their agency' in order to be effective.

In addition to varying organizational structures, each voluntary organization develops its own 'culture'. This may reflect the ideals and attitudes and practical capabilities (or lack of them) of the organization's 'founding-fathers'. It may be strongly hierarchical with complex consultative committee structures or almost a co-operative enterprise where all staff are regarded as having equal status and all shades in between. A particular characteristic of smaller voluntary agencies is their volatility. They may be overly dependent upon the vision and energy of one or two key indivi-duals and go into decline when these people leave. Alternatively, they may grow rapidly with the arrival of new staff and/or volunteers.

Equally some of the larger voluntary sector agencies (e.g. Mencap and Barnardos) have a degree of 'permanence' and independence which many professionals in the statutory agencies would envy, with all the advantages of comparability of conditions of service plus the freedom to innovate without the burden of statutory responsibilities to weigh them down.

External controls

'Freedom' is a relative term and it would be wrong to assume that independent sector agencies are totally free to pursue whatever objectives they choose without any control (apart from the obvious constraint of inadequate finance). Many of them are regulated by a number of external bodies as well as internal controls or oversight exercised by their boards of trustees or directors.

Registered charities

Registered charities are under the control of the Charity Commission[2] and must make an annual return to the Commissioners. Their reports and accounts are publicly available and their activities must reflect their stated aims and objectives. All charities are controlled by a board of trustees who are technically responsible for the activities of the charity. In day-to-day terms, this will probably be delegated to various directors, officers or employees. Names of the trustees should be available from the Charity Commissioners. The disposal of assets (particularly property) by a charity is subject to strict controls and any activity outside its stated field may bring a rebuke from the Commissioners and even, ultimately, the loss of charitable status. After considerable consultation new controls on the ways charities record and present their finances were introduced in 1996. The Statement of Recommended Practice (often known by the acronymn SORP), adopted by the Charity Commission, lays down specific reporting and recording requirements which vary according to the size of a charity, bringing a new level of clarity to the often hitherto obscure world of charity accounting.

Limited liability companies (public or private)

Limited liability companies are subject to scrutiny by the Registrar of Companies at Companies House to whom annual returns are made.[3] The records at Companies House should show who owns the company and who the directors of the company are. It should also list the auditors, and a copy of audited accounts should be available so they are also subject to Company Law. It should be noted that, whilst the vehicle of a limited liability company may provide protection for the directors of the company against unlimited personal financial liability in the event of a failure, the directors of that company are severally and individually liable for the safe conduct of that company's business (see the prosecution of directors arising from the *Herald of Free Enterprise* ferry disaster). This can be significant when dealing with matters of safety with regard to residents in homes which are known to be in some way defective by managers.

Friendly Societies and Industrial and Provident Societies

Friendly Societies and Industrial and Provident Societies are not-for-profit organizations set up with a specific objective – usually for the benefit of a particular group within society or their dependants – and they are controlled by and report to the Registrar of Friendly Societies and the Registrar of Industrial and Provident Societies.[4]

Housing Associations

In addition to their varying accountability as charities, Friendly Societies or Industrial and Provident Societies, Housing Associations are directly accountable to the Housing Corporation for the management of projects on which Housing Corporation funds have been expended.[5] Housing Associations often have local committees of volunteers who manage the work of the Association within an overall framework provided by the Housing Corporation and in line with the specific objectives for which that Housing Association was set up (e.g. housing for young single people and sheltered housing for the elderly). Some Housing Associations are very large with many thousands of housing units under their direct management, whilst others are tiny and operate only in one area with a few houses. It is important to recognize the strengths and weaknesses of the particular Housing Association you are working with, especially their capacity to cope with complex administrative matters relating to 'special needs' housing projects which may be outside their previous experience.

All the above is in strong contrast to the owner/occupier who will, typically, be a married couple or a single person. They may have the financial protection of a limited liability company or they may be a 'sole trader' or a partnership. They have total freedom to operate as they see fit within the constraints of the law and the 'marketplace' of care. This is often not the case for charities who are prevented from providing services to certain groups by the limits placed on them in their founding charter or Memorandum and Articles of Association (a term which refers to the legal document describing the range of activities to be undertaken by a particular limited liability company). For example, some major national charities were set up specifically for the benefit of children and they find themselves unable to continue to provide services when children grow up and become adults. Co-operation with another charity or setting up a sister charity is often the only way round such constraints.

Big is beautiful?

Looking at the residential care market as a whole, the pattern of development for the largest client group of residential homes (for the elderly) clearly shows the proliferation of a large number of owner/occupiers. Over the years, a number of public limited companies have moved into this market[6] and the more successful private operators have developed chains of homes (usually at the top end of the market with rates well above the national minimum).

It is possible that this pattern of development will occur within the sphere of learning disability and there are already some signs that, where costs are high and alternatives to residential care non-existent, private operators feel that there is a place for them. This is particularly so in the case of 'difficult to place' clients who display anti-social and/or aggressive tendencies and who would previously have been placed in hospitals.

Whilst there are undeniable advantages in an organization and economics in such developments, care must be taken to ensure that these are not offset by tendencies towards inflexibility and the depersonalization of large-scale enterprise (e.g. bulk purchasing of supplies). Large voluntary agencies have also had to guard against the sort of institutional hardening of the arteries which size often brings with it. The organization's operational structure as well as its collective 'culture' can play an important part in this.

Consortia – here today and gone tomorrow?

A final organizational structure is that of a consortium. In response to a complex pattern of financial and other pressures, many statutory and voluntary agencies are coming together in various parts of the country to set up a local consortium to manage the provision of residential and day services. Typically, this will involve the creation of a shell legal vehicle (sometimes a charity, or an Industrial and Provident Society) through which residential and day-care services are channelled. Participating members of the consortium (which acts as the controlling body for the shell) are usually the Local Authority, Social Services Department, the Health Authority, one or two local Housing Associations and some local voluntary associations.

By passing the provision of services through a voluntary agency shell, Central Government resources were maximized (before April 1993) in terms of income support levels for residents. Many agencies therefore worked to transfer all their residential provision to such shells as a method of increasing the amount of revenue funding available to them post April 1993.

Another virtue of a consortium is that it encourages agencies to work co-operatively rather than competitively in the provision of a range of services and increases the chance of attracting funding from other agencies (e.g. the Housing Corporation). In some areas, housing departments have joined the consortium and District Councils can contribute significantly to the housing needs of this client group.

Consortia can only work when all the participants co-operate fully with each other. For example, where a new development depends on a financial contribution from five players (a District Council, a County Council, the Housing Corporation, a voluntary organization, a District and/or Regional Health Authority) it only requires one of these to back out or simply fail to meet a deadline for the whole project to fail. Even when projects are up and running, the potential for confusion over responsibilities is much greater than normal unless very great care has been taken with operational planning.

In short, consortia can be compared to 'self-build' cars – difficult to construct and get going, as strong as their weakest component and not renowned for their comfort or ease of maintenance, often requiring constant attention to keep in the best of trim. They are not, perhaps, the best vehicle for delivering services to people with disabilities. Their track record has, to date, been uneven with the lack of success being mostly due to stresses within the consortia as member agencies are variously affected by events largely affecting only one or two members (e.g. the reduction in funds available to the Housing Corporation, changes in local authority financing, National Health Service (NHS) reorganization, etc.). In short, consortia are vulnerable to the fact that their member organizations have their attention focused elsewhere and learning disability services are not top of everyone's agenda. As in the commercial world, there is often value in an agency being dedicated to one activity or industry. It helps to get things done!

Motivation

Social workers and nurses must recognize that independent sector organizations make provision for this client group for a variety of motives. Motives may well be mixed and their relative order of importance may change from time to time as organizations change.

It is up to individual professionals to make their own assessment of the effect of motivation upon the nature of care provision. The acid test of a service is how it is perceived by the user. Care professionals must be on their guard against moralizing over the various motivations they perceive amongst care providers. 'Bad care' is unacceptable even if it is provided with the best of all possible motives with no thought of personal or financial gain. Let us examine some current motivations: for profit, not for profit, charities or voluntary organizations, religious orders and parents.

For profit

Profit is a deceptively simple motivation. A private home owner may provide care 'for profit' as a way of earning a living and/or providing a home for a disabled relative. Public limited companies are obviously in business to make profits for their shareholders (as are some private companies), but to suggest that private/for profit agencies are in some way 'inferior' to other agencies like charities or Housing Associations is an over-simplification.

For example, a single unit owner/occupier investing life savings in providing care for a disabled daughter and others (perhaps as a reaction against the poor quality of services available elsewhere) may be grateful to clear £15000 'profit' at the end of a year. When this figure (with all its attendant risks, worries and anxieties) is compared with the pay and conditions of service of officers in charge in statutory agency homes (and some of the larger voluntary organizations), the so-called 'profit' of £15000 before income tax, National Insurance, pensions, etc., begins to look positively altruistic.

Of course, there will be situations where a straight choice has to be made between the quality of the service provided and the level of the 'profit margin' obtained at the end of the year. The application of open market disciplines post April 1993 has acted as a restraining effect on those who would seek to increase margins at the expense of quality. Indeed, quality control provides a useful mechanism for assessing value for money in all forms of care (not just private). Another influence to restrain the excesses of the profit motive and promote good care is the operation of the Inspection Units run by Local Authority Social Service Departments. Interestingly enough, it is often these same Inspection Units which try to force up standards by demanding service improvements by providers. These in turn then demand extra money from the same Local Authority and the true 'independence' of the Inspection Unit is then revealed. As many authorities have found their community care budgets woefully inadequate, the struggle between financial prudence in the Treasurer's department and the Inspection Unit's desire to improve standards is short and unequal, resulting in a stark choice for all providers – become more efficient and improve services with nil or minimum cost increase or go out of business. For commercial providers profitability is essential and hard bargaining is to be expected, for some charities this financial rigour comes as something of a shock.

There is an important message here for all providers (not just for profit ones) about their organizational competence. With money very tight and standards under scrutiny the margin between success and failure has narrowed; those agencies who survive will do so by maximizing the utilization of staff and their skills. Under such circumstances the role of the learning disability professional (either as provider or as a purchaser of specialist services) is the key to identifying the essential elements in a service for an individual and purchasing or providing them in a cost-effective way. Of course, some agencies may be able to get by for a while using reserves, donations (see below) or deliberately achieving market share by adopting a 'loss leader' approach, but ultimately this cannot be sustained in a market where price and value for money (VFM) rather than sentiment or perceived motivation increasingly dictate purchasing decisions.

Not for profit

A recent development has been legal vehicles (typically limited companies with carefully controlled shareholdings) whose motivation is said to be 'not for profit'. This is often a device to avoid the difficulties and delays of obtaining charitable status as a means of progressing quickly to the provision of services. 'Not for profit' agencies are a confusing new creation. They are not, strictly speaking, voluntary bodies but they aim to operate in a way reminiscent of the voluntary or charitable ethos. Any surpluses are ploughed back into the company and not taken as dividends by the shareholders. Such agencies are a useful addition to the range of vehicles but there is scope for concern over the control of management, consultancy or directorial fees which may be levied to reduce or eliminate any profits. This is a type of organization which lacks many of the controls charities are subject to.

Charities or voluntary organizations

It is a well-known adage in the voluntary sector that 'you don't make a profit but an operating surplus'. These agencies often do make quite legitimate surpluses arising out of fund-raising efforts, donations, appeals, etc. They are precluded by their charitable status from paying dividends and usually use their donated funds to expand the scope of their operations by the purchase of new properties, etc. Some of the very large voluntary organizations are able to make significant contributions from their donated funds to subsidize the care costs of individuals. Whilst this is, no doubt, a welcome contribution to the provision of care, it should not be seen as a requirement by care professionals and purchasing authorities. Many small or medium-size agencies do not have such financial resources available and are totally dependent upon fee income to cover the running costs of their home. It should not be necessary to use donated income to balance revenue accounts (and to do so discourages donors) nor is it an appropriate and reliable way of providing secure services for clients.

Religious orders

Given the history of care of people with learning disabilities in England, it is hardly surprising that there is a significant number of religious orders providing a range of residential services for this client group. Religious motivation is often a strong factor in the founding of new agencies and provides a continuing source of support as they develop. Just as many parents seek to have their children educated in denominational schools, so many feel it equally appropriate that their disabled children should be cared for within the same tradition. It would be a mistake, however, to assume that merely because a home is run by a religious order or a religiously motivated voluntary agency, that their objective is to turn everyone into a practising member of that religion. Before making such judgements care professionals should get to know the agency concerned and evaluate its services on a home-by-home basis, since many such homes vary widely in practice.

Parents

Many parents of disabled children become heavily involved in voluntary agencies. This may take the form of starting a new charity to meet local needs (including that of their own child) or contributing in some way to existing agencies. Many management committees of voluntary agencies are domi-nated by parents of children with learning disabilities.

Whilst this motivation can be clearly understood and the debt to the contributions of such parents is enormous, it must be said that sometimes parental concerns can cloud judgements. Voluntary agencies can find themselves the battlefields for conflicting views on the way forward where an individual's perception of need is based on their own experience as a parent rather than as an objective observer. As a professional providing, advising on, or perhaps even controlling, access to services for people with learning disabilities, it is a salutary and necessary thought for nurses and social workers alike to realize that so many parents have so often been so dissatisfied with what 'the State' has seen fit to provide for their child that they have attempted to do it better for themselves.

Self-help

Given the paucity of resources (and the often poor quality of resulting services) it is hardly surprising that there is a strong tradition of self-help within the field of learning disabilities (see for example the work of the charity Contact a Family).[7] This is something which all professionals would do well to encourage and be aware of because, without countless contributions from self-help groups of varying sorts, existing services would be totally overwhelmed by demand.

The challenge for professionals is how best to encourage and promote good practice amongst such groups of highly motivated people who may not share your views on many issues affecting their child. This is particularly difficult when parental concerns lead to over-protection and it may actually inhibit the full development of an individual. Professionals need to be able to work in and through independent sector agencies as a means of moving their services in the right direction. Obtaining agreement with parents as to what the 'right' direction is provides social workers and nurses with a sometimes difficult task and a challenge to their powers of communicative skills. After all, not everyone starts off from the same point of view and some individuals have given much thought to how best to provide for people with learning disabilities in modern-day society and can produce arguments that are difficult, if not impossible to refute.

Philosophy of Care

The wide variety of styles of care provision are not just an accident of history. They grew up because of a particular way of looking at 'mental handicap'. Just as the arrival of new ideas can transform the political or economic scene, so the same is true in the field of learning disability. There are several ideas around today (normalization, service brokerage), which have a strong impact on the direction of future services. They may also have an equally strong impact on the way existing services are viewed. This section attempts to review the way in which the voluntary sector has coped with these changes.

Many independent sector agencies have no distinctive philosophy of care of their own. They may sometimes reflect some residual aspects of their founding fathers (which is often a Christian or other denominational viewpoint) but the effect this has on the actual delivery of services is often negligible. Irrespective of the degree of such religious influence, these agencies still need to have some guiding principles. These are often taken from current thinking about what constitutes 'good care' and the reasoning behind it. In doing so they are often in an identical position to the statu-

tory authorities for whom mainstream positions are easier to defend against their critics than the adoption of a very distinctive (and debatable) philosophy.

The dominant philosophy of the 1980s has been that of 'normalization' (or 'social role valorization').[8] It would be inappropriate here to attempt any in-depth consideration of this way of thinking, but it is important to note two things. First, 'normalization' has often been misunderstood and misapplied. Second, normalization is not an immutable credo fixed in stone. Wolf Wolfensberger[9] and many of his followers have refined the original idea (hence the later jargon term 'social role valorization'). Professionals should be aware of the dangers inherent in an uncritical and incomplete appreciation of this extremely useful approach to care services. They might best regard it as a useful tool or measuring stick, rather than the answer to all their problems.

In essence, normalization proposes that people with learning disabilities will only cease to be devalued and put down when they are seen to be living their lives in ways perceived by the rest of society not merely as 'normal' but also as positively socially valued. So it is seen as important for people with learning disabilities to exercise choice as far as possible over how and where and with whom they live, to control their daily routine, and to have meaningful employment and/or recreation. This requires professionals to ask themselves questions about what are 'valued ends' and 'valued means' and disciplines like PASS and PASSING workshops[9] enable carers to see their services through the eyes of the user. The results can be quite a challenge to service providers. As a result of ideas like normalization, liberal considerations are filtering through to those who inspect and regulate services.

Normalization was only part of a strong movement towards making the individual the centre of the service rather than merely its recipient. Other associated notions (notably those of 'empowerment' and self advocacy)[10] have chimed in with 'normalization' to strike a strong note for valuing and encouraging the individual and placing him/her above and before whatever handicap they may have. Slogans such as 'people first' and advertising campaigns across a range of disability groupings have reinforced this message – 'look at the individual not the disability'.

Service brokerage/individual funding packages

A more recent manifestation of this trend has been the Canadian concept of 'service brokerage' in which a 'broker' acts as the agent for those unable to speak for themselves and 'buys in' the various services needed for the care requirements of an individual. The point here is that the purchasing power lies with the individual (or his/her agent/broker) to buy rather than ask the statutory agency to provide on a 'take it or leave it' basis a spread of services which they think are appropriate.[11]

These ideas were reflected in the White Paper *Caring for People* which spoke vaguely of individualized packages of care. However, the idea of having an individual assessment, followed by the offer of a range of services designed to meet that individual's need leads inexorably to the *real* service user (i.e. the client, not the Local Authority) demanding the power to choose and use a service of his/her own. Here is one movement in service development which the Government has found impossible to halt or refute, since it so closely reflects the 'consumer-is-the-customer' approach it has endorsed in so many other areas of life (e.g. schools, Health Services, etc). Recent legislation has opened the way

for direct purchasing of services to become a reality for many in 1997 but the detailed regulations on implementation show that it will not be easy for many people with a learning disability to access this scheme.

At the time of writing it is difficult to estimate the impact that large-scale adoption of individualized funding could have on services. If direct payments are widely taken up it may diminish the power of social workers to 'direct' people to services their authority already has contracts with. Whilst (at present at least) direct payments are not permissible for long-term residential care services, if they are successfully adopted, there will inevitably be pressure for the scheme to be extended to embrace other care services. That will indicate a real revolution in customer power. One thing which is clear is that the professional(s) making the assessment of need and subsequently putting a financial 'value' on that assessment must be capable of defending such decisions against the demands of clients, their families and/or advocates. There would be no shortage of demand for learning disability specialists with such skills – on either side of the fence.

Some individuals have in the past obtained 'individual funding packages' with which they can hire (and fire) staff to meet their needs, but there were difficulties to be overcome. For example, to avoid problems with income tax liabilities and questions over the appropriate use of public funds, such individual funding packages had to be channelled through a voluntary agency or a specially created trust fund – with all the legal, procedural and technical complications that can be involved. Some of the campaigning voluntary organizations saw this as the way forward. At first sight it appeared to be in harmony with the 'individualized packages of care' described in *Caring for People* – and has found logical expression in the Direct Payments legislation. It is the conclusion to the process of individual assessment and is a major step towards the creation of a true 'market' for care services. Problems of application and administration lie ahead.

A new role for the hospitals?

'Normalization' has been a very strong influence in care philosophy during the 1980s and no voluntary agency has been immune to it. Even so, there are those who regard notions of normalization and the like as doing damage not only to the English language but also to the prospects of the clients they seek to serve. Some see the policy of closing the hospitals as a big mistake and would prefer to see the hospital sites redeveloped as 'village communities' along the lines of some examples on the Continent (notably Holland). Care in the community is 'not suitable for everyone' according to organizations like Rescare.[12] Some handicapped people would be better served by retaining long-stay hospitals and developing services on those sites.

Campaigning voluntary agencies such as Via (Values into Action, formerly the Campaign for Mentally Handicapped People) and many direct care providers and their umbrella organization ARC (the Association for Residential Care) would strongly resist such a reversal of policy and prefer to direct efforts and resources to making community care work.

However, it does remain legitimate to ask 'how wide is the spread of the spectrum of services for people with learning difficulties?' This must also prompt further questions such as 'are there any patterns of services which would be "off the end" of the spectrum – that is, totally unacceptable? If so, what is it about these services which make them so fundamentally "unacceptable"?'

Social workers and nurses may find themselves in some difficulty with each other on this issue. Protagonists of hospitals and of the perpetuation of the medical model of care are mostly (but not exclusively) drawn from the nursing profession and they can point to the fact that there will always be a small number of patients who will require the 'sort of treatment offered by the hospitals'. From this it is a small step to move the argument over into how large this group should be rather than to question whether anyone who is not sick should be in hospital care.

Social workers, trained perhaps in a different tradition, may reject the current role of the hospitals and yet be compelled to see them as a 'place of last resort' for clients for whom they cannot find suitable placements in the community. In this role they may find themselves at odds with their own professional beliefs, being driven to use a service which they feel is fundamentally inappropriate. This is an area where independent sector agencies can play a useful role by providing specialist services – given support from the statutory agencies. It does not absolve professionals from the need to sort out their thinking on the nature of the important 'residual' role left to Health Authorities and to question whether existing long-stay hospitals are the best way of fulfilling that role.

Care in the community

The phrase 'care in the community' or 'community care' as it applies to learning disabilities has always meant care in 'non-institutional small homes in the community' as opposed to putting people away in large mental hospitals.

Elsewhere, especially with regard to the care of the elderly, care in the community means something slightly different. It is usually taken to mean 'care in the home of the individual client' as opposed to 'residential care for that person in a registered residential home'. This differing usage can lead to confusion and it is important to understand which interpretation is being referred to when the phrase 'community care' is used.

Distinctive philosophies of care

In addition to mainstream ideas like 'normalization' there are other carefully thought out philosophies care, which may to a greater or lesser extent have absorbed ideas like advocacy and normalization but still retain a significant and separate identity. Such ideas are usually to be found in the voluntary sector, although some small private sector homes may also reflect elements of these ideas too.

L'Arche communities

The Christian religion has always provided a strong moral challenge to those to put their beliefs into practice for the benefit of people with learning disabilities. The results are not always 'comfortable' for the secular minded and can challenge the often lazy assumptions of others. One such example is the steady development of the L'Arche communities all over the world.[13] Their founder, Jean Vanier, has inspired many people to copy his vision of 'handicapped' and 'non-handicapped' living and working together in a community. In such communities all are regarded as having equal worth and it is recognized that all have strengths and weaknesses, capabilities and handicaps. They use local housing and promote strong ties with the local communities. They provide a home for as long as someone needs it and positively encourage disabled members of the community to 'move on' to other accommodation with the help of the community when they are ready.

Camphill communities

Another distinctive philosophy of care is that espoused by the Camphill movement.[14] It came to Britain just before World War II when a group of children with disabilities moved with Rudolf Steiner to Scotland from Germany. The philosophy of 'anthroposophism' which underpins all the Steiner schools and communities deserves careful study in its own right.[15] It has been extremely influential and inspired others to establish numerous care homes with strong links with the Camphill Village movement. Steiner's educational ideas have also been very influential at primary school level and there are many nursery and primary schools which follow his educational theories.[16]

In the field of learning disabilities Camphill communities provide a natural extension to Steiner's philosophy. Described as 'therapeutic communities living and working with children, young people and adults in need of special care and understanding' they offer a distinctive type of care where disabled and non-disabled live together in mutual respect. It is a fundamental principle of all Camphill communities that no one receives remuneration in the usual sense of the word but that needs are met on an individual basis.

CARE (Cottage and Rural Enterprise) and Home Farm Trust

Both these organizations have come to prominence in the field of residential and day-care services by having a clear philosophy of care. Whilst there are considerable operational differences between them, they both aim to provide a stable caring environment in communities of around 30–50 which are in turn broken down into small domestic-sized units.[17]

It is interesting to note that both organizations were started by parents who wished to provide a safe, secure and lasting care environment for their children. There was a strong tradition of rural settings and the development of horticultural and agricultural skills in both organizations and considerable importance on the contribution which people with learning disabilities could make to the life of their community and the dignity which fruitful employment can give to each individual. Even so, the original ideas of both organizations have been modified in the light of recent thinking and both are now pursuing smaller developments and the use of 'satellite' houses in the local communities.

There are many other smaller organizations which have distinctive philosophies of care, and space does not permit us here to investigate them but their existence reminds professionals that they should always be ready to consider new ideas and not dismiss a small home with its own ideas as 'cranky'. Equally, they must be prepared to make and defend a professional judgement on the merits of a particular style of care in any home (irrespective of who is running it) – especially if they consider that it is harming the residents it purports to care for.

Legal constraints versus a 'real' life?

These examples do provide alternatives to the monolith of mainstream thinking. They also present a challenge to the regulation of residential care. By starting from differing standpoints and having different objectives from the majority, the sort of services they provide frequently fall foul of registration and inspection routines which are often designed and implemented in an unthinking way and are based on the care needs of the elderly.

Under such circumstances it is hardly surprising that many independent sector agencies have had to argue their case strongly over the nature of their services against those who would wish to force them into the straitjacket of regulation. There is some evidence that the force of their arguments has been largely accepted and that, in future, Registration Officers will be urged to consider all aspects of care in a home (its 'climate') rather than concentrating on measurable items such as room sizes and menus.[18]

There is a paradox about much of the law relating to residential care as it applies to learning disabilities. On the one hand, the law and its attendant regulations and enforcement agencies seek to establish a minimum norm of care support which is based on a perception of client dependence (e.g. so many staff on duty, certain types of safety precautions). Yet the thrust of much modern care is totally at variance with such concerns. The ideas of risk-taking, normalization, self-determination and normal housing, generate friction with those who wish to control things carefully. How can someone 'in care' be allowed to go unsupervised for a period of time? Can you really take 'controlled risks' with someone else's safety while at the same time providing care for them?

Such friction is not the preserve of the independent sector though much of it is generated there. Even statutory agencies can outrun the capacity of the regulations to keep up with them in thinking how to monitor and control care services. For example, the All Wales Mental Handicap Strategy (originating from the Welsh Office) required statutory agencies to provide residential care in homes no larger than four or five residents on the grounds that small family settings provided an individual with a greater degree of choice and control over their lives than larger homes. In some areas of Wales the very idea of residential care in a 'home' has been superseded by placing people in families and providing a network of paid carers to support people in their own homes and communities. Ideas like this have challenged accepted mainstream thinking and regulatory practices and provided hope that one day services may be 'user led' rather than 'provider led'. It is a sign of the times that the All Wales Mental Handicap Strategy is now ending amidst general recriminations and uncertainty, with many current purchasers unwilling or unable to buy expensive services in such small-scale provision. The potential impact of individualized funding being used in any possible future extension of the direct payments system on such a situation may provide an illuminating scenario on what users really want and who really makes such decisions.

Innovative patterns of care services often fall foul of the constraints imposed on existing services. The most obvious of all these is the question about what sort of person/ qualification is suitable to run a registered home. For example, is a qualified nurse or social worker necessarily automatically equipped by virtue of their qualification to run a residential home? Many independent sector agencies would argue that such qualifications are at best marginal and at worst often inimical to the successful delivery of innovative services – and yet in many areas such qualifications are mandatory for those in charge of a 'home'. Care professionals need to be aware of these issues and to have worked out what their own contribution can be to the debate.

The financing of residential homes

The development of care in small community homes has been greatly assisted by the financial arrangements available to independent sector agencies to fund this. Although the costs of care are now often

well above Income Support limits (in the region of £250 per week) there was a period of time in the middle to late 1980s when state funding via the Supplementary Benefit System was available for good-quality care. Under such circumstances small charities such as Elizabeth FitzRoy Homes, Walsingham Community Homes, United Response, and Christian Cause for Concern, were able to flourish. Royal Mencap was also able to launch its well-known Homes Foundation scheme.[19]

Under the Homes Foundation scheme, parents were encouraged to donate their home to Mencap who would in turn provide lifelong care for their child (but not necessarily in the parental home). The scheme was very successful, and Homes Foundation homes are now to be found all over the country. Such rapid growth did not come without drawbacks and Mencap does now have the large problem of administering and supporting these homes, but they are undeniably a very significant contribution to the spread of care options open to professionals. It shows clearly that, given the right conditions, parents can make a significant contribution to care provision through voluntary agencies – something which professionals will in future overlook to their cost.

For a number of reasons there has been a consistent rise in the number of independent sector homes for people with learning disabilities since the 1980s (from 15 776 homes in 1989/90 to 38 083 in 1995 according to the latest Department of Health statistics). In spite of all the recent cutbacks in finances, numbers continue to rise and there seems little sign of the sector shrinking as statutory agencies continue to close down hospitals and/or Local Authority homes. The Local Authorities, which were given 'lead responsibility' for learning disability in the community care reforms, are increasingly being seen as purchasing and commissioning agencies of all community care services rather than continuing to act as providers. In learning disabilities services this trend is quite marked in residential services, although statutory provision still forms the vast majority of day services.

April 1993 saw the end of 'open cheque' for residential services from Income Support. Those within the system at that time now have 'Preserved Rights' to higher rates of Income Support and constitute a significant element of continuing funding in all community care services, but particularly so within learning disability services because of the relatively slow rate of turnover compared with other client groups. This does mean that, at some future stage, as those with Preserved Rights lose them, local authorities will need to find new community care funds merely to maintain the level of services with new clients using them who do not have Preserved Rights.

Other parts of the benefits system, notably Housing Benefit, have been exploited to the full since April 1993 as agencies have struggled to find ways of providing the 'housing + care' packages so many need. Many independent sector providers have made use of the 'lighter regulatory touch' offered by the 1991 Registered Homes (Amendment) Act which imposed some regulation on homes for three or fewer people. All these services are very sensitive to the way the benefits system works because they are operating at the edges both of benefit and viability. Consequently, the changes proposed to Housing Benefits aimed at single people under 29 (or, more recently, 49) may have a very damaging effect upon many services. Equally, local authorities are very aware of how Social Security benefit changes (many of which are funded from Central, not Local, Government) may adversely affect their own finances. Consequently, over a period of time services may be asked to register or deregister as a Regis-

tered Home in order to maximize central funding. Whereas in the 1980s and early 1990s the motivation for this came from owners, it now comes from funding agencies.

In 1996 the National Health Service Executive (NHSE) moved to begin to claw back from District Health Authorities (DHAs) in England the total of £614 million which had been included in the DHA's annual allocation for what was termed 'old long stay hospital residents'. In effect, the funds that had been allocated to DHAs for the care of people with mental illness or learning disabilities who had been in hospital since the early 1970s are going to be progressively withdrawn as patients die or move into other forms of care. At present the money clawed back will be put back into the general allocations with no ring-fencing of these funds for either client group. The result will, over time, be a loss in revenue terms of over £600 million to the care of these two client groups, with, in the case of learning disability, no compensating payments being made to social services who will in future be required to fund such services. This is part of an unspoken but clear pattern within the NHS to pass this client group on to local authorities, but to retain as much capital and revenue funding as possible within the NHS. There are some honourable exceptions to this trend but in general the long-term consequences can only complicate the funding of care.

So, the question is not always 'how much does this cost?' but rather, 'how much does this cost *my agency* and what can we fund from other sources?'. No learning disability professional can afford to be ignorant of the complex web of funding sources which may influence both service design and deliverability and how these may be subject to change (or, at least, non-renewal!). For those operating in the independent sector accessing other sources of finance can make all the difference between a Local Authority signing the contract or not.

Lifelong care or long-term care?

An enduring thread in the care of people with learning disabilities down the ages has been that of concern for their safety and (moral) welfare. Indeed the original meaning of the word 'asylum' was a place of safety into which people could retreat (as in political asylum). The major parental concern has always been 'who will look after our disabled child when we are both dead?'

Organizations offering 'lifelong' care seemed to provide the answer but experience has showed such agencies how difficult it can be to achieve. Many independent sector agencies are now wary of making commitments because they may not be able to fulfil them in any individual case where personality changes and/or physical care needs alter to the point where a home or organization can no longer cope. The absence of such a commitment should imply no criticism of the philosophy of care of any particular agency – it may simply reflect the care facts of life. There are voluntary agencies and schemes specifically set up to help parents round the problem of providing lifelong care.[20] It is a complicated problem often involving trusts, wills and taxation considerations. It should not be undertaken without specialist advice.

Access to services

Parents have not always liked what services have been on offer for their child in their locality and have frequently looked for alternatives. The traditional pattern was to find a service which suited the needs of your child and to persuade 'the State' (in the form of the Local Authority and Central Government) to pay for it.

Usually, this meant money for residential or day services in a private or voluntary agency which was often outside the geographical area of the parents' Local Authority. Having obtained the offer of a place the parents often then had to persuade the Local Authority to 'top up' their child's entitlement to State Benefit to cover the full cost of care. In effect this amounted to a very large degree of Local Authority control over the access to care simply by controlling the purse strings. Another obstacle to 'open access' was that some voluntary agencies have entrance criteria (e.g. a local catchment area) and/or long waiting lists.

The residential home boom of the mid-1980s, for a brief period, handed considerable purchasing power to clients by giving them access to State funding as of right by virtue of their disability. As a result in the latter half of the 1980s the size and vigour of the private sector increased dramatically whilst voluntary sector provision increased slowly and statutory sector provision actually contracted. All this was possible because of the huge influx of funds to residential care provided as of right by the Supplementary Benefit System.

Before controls were imposed in 1986 and tightened further a year later, there was virtually unlimited access to residential care. The support of Social Services Department was not necessary to obtain a place in a home – indeed it was often necessary to obtain written proof of refusal to pay for an individual's residential care before Supplementary Benefit was payable. Whilst access to residential services became notably easier, access to other services (notably day and respite care) was still difficult and these services came under increasing pressure as people moved out of long-stay mental handicap hospitals with insufficient commensurate increase in services to meet their needs. Since Supplementary Benefit could not pay directly for such services it is hardly surprising that there was a short-fall compared with the rapid growth else-where.

As Central Government began to curb the cost and kept increases lower than inflation it once again became uneconomic to run small homes on Income Support limits and Local Authority 'top-up' again became necessary. This became more and more difficult to obtain in new cases and the White Paper *Caring for People* in 1990, released by the Government as a belated response to Sir Roy Griffiths' proposals about community care, foreshadowed the end of unlimited central funding for residential care.

The question of the control of access to services remains crucial. Access to any services is now via an assessment of individual need of a client by the local Social Services Department. The 'perverse incentives' to move into residential care which Sir Roy Griffiths had pointed out have now been removed by a funding system which gives Local Authorities total control over their community care budget. Money is now being spent on 'individual packages of care' from a cash-limited budget to meet local needs and provide choice for the client, and there is no longer any financial incentive to put someone in residential care.

There still remains the vexed question of who chooses the service? In theory the Government's Choice Directive, issued in a guidance letter to Local Authorities, requires a Local Authority to offer someone who has been assessed as needing a service a range of service provision from which to choose. In practice, many independent sector providers doubt that this actually happens and that users and their families are 'guided' into accepting services which may well have been prepaid for by the Local Authority under a block-purchasing arrangement with the provider. Whilst this may represent good value for money and ensure the viability of the provider, it does significantly reduce client choice. This practice may be more prevalent in services for the elderly, but it does reflect the basic flaw in a service designed on the principles of the market-place but which denies those same principles by withholding the power of purchase from the service user.

In future this may change (see page 55 on individualized funding) and the changes may even reach learning disability residential services, eventually. However, as many have already learned, access to services means meeting (what seems to be ever higher) 'eligibility criteria'. These are the means by which Local Authorities control access to services and the threshold is raised or lowered according to resources available and funds are channelled into what are perceived as the local priorities in community care.

The Role of the Professional

What roles will be open to nurses and social workers in the brave new world of assessments, contracts and cuts?

Access to services will arise from the results of an individual assessment of need. Those professionals with a specialist knowledge of learning disability are best placed to fulfil the role of assessor who must define an individual's need and others who must respond to it 'within the resources available' by making appropriate purchasing decisions. In the field of learning disability this could best be done by someone who not only knows 'the market place' for services for this client but who also can make an informed judgement on their appropriateness for an individual's case.

A market-orientated approach has been equally applied by the Government to the NHS and to Local Government and Social Service Departments. A whole new world of contracting and tendering has developed. It is equally appropriate for an assessor or budget holder to be either a social worker or nurse since both should be equally familiar with these new concepts.

However, there remains an area of ambiguity about the role of the professional here in relation to their client – are they acting as the advocate for the client or are they protecting the interests of their Department and looking after their own budget? In a time of scarce resources, there will always be situations where the professional has conflicting loyalties which can undermine the effectiveness of their performance. For example, how would a professional feel undertaking an assessment on a client in January knowing that the Department's budget was already overspent and that money for a move into residential care was out of the question?

In becoming the gatekeeper to services there is the danger that professionals will be seen as an obstacle rather than a guide to services by those seeking help. Their performance will also be keenly observed by service providers (e.g. residential home owners and those who run day services).

An important question must be 'how impartial is the advice given?'. Some doctors are already under criticism for being less than candid about their own financial interests in the nursing home they are recommending to their patients. Care professionals could easily be faced with the same dilemma in recommending residential care to a client.

Also, should the professional carer encourage and enable client choice? An assessment of client need could result in an agreement to pay for a place in a residential home or a day centre. Exactly which services, homes, etc. are recommended (if at all) will be a matter of professional judgement – but the client or family may have other ideas. Their choice might be for some-

where regarded as 'unsound' or 'unfashionable' with ideas or philosophies outside the mainstream of care. Such places are most likely to be found in the independent sector and it will be a matter of considerable professional skill to negotiate such a situation to an appropriate conclusion.

The rhetoric of current Government policy does place a premium upon widening client choice and the power of consumer pressure in the so-called 'market place' for services. It is debatable how (if at all) the providers need to bend to accommodate themselves to the current fashions and how far professional advisors can go in 'persuading' their client to choose 'appropriately'. Client choice must mean the freedom to choose something which goes against a Local Social Services Department's preferences for patterns of service provision. The professional must be wary of being driven to say (on behalf of the so-called enabling authority) to clients 'You can have any home you like as long as it's on this list'. They must also be able to demonstrate that the client made (as far as was possible) an informed choice and was not pushed into a particular decision by a dominant individual. Making a reality of client choice and client access will present a challenge to all future professionals – providers and advisers alike.

The Future of the Independent Sector

As regards learning disability services some broad themes can be drawn out from the situation in the late 1990s.

The policy of care in the community will continue and there will be no return to the establishment of large hospitals as a means of providing care. The closure of hospitals will also continue but greater attention will be paid to ensuring that what is on offer outside the hospital is better than what was available to the clients inside. In practice this may contribute to slowing down the closure programme (along with other factors such as shortage of finance within the NHS and lack of funding within Local Authorities for care in the community projects).

The role of the independent sector will increase whilst that of the Local Authority will shrink to a largely monitoring, purchasing function with some residual ability to staff and run residential services. The range of services provided by the independent sector will widen as Local Authorities encourage them to take on additional functions – more day services, domiciliary care, information services, etc. The traditional role of the voluntary sector as in some way 'representing the true interests' of the client (or at least being closer to the client than statutory sector providers) will be under threat as funding for such potentially 'awkward' activities as advocacy and campaigning is cut in favour of retaining or developing adequate baseline services of other kinds. If this does happen it will be all the more vital for the professionals in the independent sector to be aware of this change and to make allowances for it.

The pattern of service provision in the independent sector will change. Providers will have to become more flexible to meet the very specific service needs that clients have had identified for them (or more cynically, those which Local Authorities are able to fund). This means that homes might have to develop as a matter of routine the capacity to support people with learning disabilities living in their own homes nearby for 'x' hours per week. Day services may well move away from a 'bricks and mortar' approach where clients are 'contained/entertained/put to work' in a special building. New services will develop which may

be smaller and more localized in their scope, perhaps more informal and with clearer aims and objectives than at present.

In such new services there will be a clear role for the care professional (nurse or social worker) to provide a lead in defining objectives and planning and delivering new types of service. The independent sector with its usual flair for innovation and urgency will be ideally placed to provide the diversification that is needed. The problem for users may well be the lack of appropriate day services to meet the needs of care in the community. If the professionals fail to win that debate and those needs remain unmet, then the future for care in the community seems bleak. Perhaps the resulting crop of bad publicity over some 'community care horror stories' will be the only way of obtaining necessary resources. It will be up to future professionals to be able to demonstrate the need for such resources and to find new ways of providing good day-care services.

The pressure to use small units of accommodation often will continue – even though financial considerations may mean that such units are grouped together to make them viable as 'care homes'. Whilst some in the independent sector may claim to have led the way in care innovation, there is a danger that in future the severe limitations of care in the community funding will tend towards the standardization of residential care patterns within a known safe and costed spectrum of provision.

Perhaps the most significant change for the future of the independent sector is the effects of the 'contract culture'. There are many different types of contract which independent agencies may enter into but in the field of learning disability they are typically concerned with the provision of day services and residential care (together or separately).

One advantage of the new contract culture is that it gives independent organizations an opportunity to provide the client with a contract which reflects the financial and physical reality of residential (or day) care. Such a contract is essentially three-way, involving the client at the centre but also including the care provider and the monitoring sponsoring agency.

The nature of inspection and regulation is again under review. Following a consultation paper, *Moving Forward*, the Government commissioned a wide ranging report[21] on the scope and nature of inspection and regulation, at the very same time as it was also pursuing a parallel agenda of deregulation across every aspect of industry and commerce. The consensus in the industry which the report has generated will make it difficult to reduce regulation and monitoring in community care services. On the contrary, it is likely that inspection and regulation will increase in scope to cover day and domiciliary services. Additionally, consistent pressure from the independent sector for a truly independent inspectorate is likely to bear fruit, although the ideal of a separate national inspectorate operating locally to national standards seems some way off yet.

Even so, with all the changes being mooted there is an opportunity for learning disability services to secure an improved recognition of the special needs of this group. The proposals in the Burgner Report[21] for National Benchmark Standards for services for different client groups provide an ideal opening for the development of a new nationally recognized description of services. With these in place it would be difficult for Local Authorities to deny to independent sector providers the right to operate services which meet these National Benchmark Standards.

It will still be very important for the independent sector to secure a voice on the Advisory Committee of each Local Authority. Such committees have the chance to influence the work of the Inspection Units and to broaden the understanding of the scope of the independent sector. In future the independent sector must therefore be much more adept at a local level in promoting the whole spectrum of its services (and the various rationales behind them) to the statutory sector agencies responsible for inspecting, specifying and purchasing those services. They will also need to reach the real customer, the client and/or his/her advocate/family to make them aware of what they have to offer. Those who have their light under a bushel may find that the force of circumstances will extinguish it completely.

The final area of change for the independent sector concerns staff training. Vocational qualifications in the form of N/SVQs[22] and the Diploma in Social Work from Central Council for the Education and Training Social Work (CCETSW) have become well established, but they are generalist qualifications and may contain little or no knowledge of or contact with people with a learning disability. The NHS is now the major provider of specialist qualifications for staff working with this client group and the future continuance of NHS-based specialist training is essential to maintaining a viable specialist workforce. The challenge for the learning disability specialist is to seize the opportunity provided by the open nature of vocational qualifications and to ensure through effective assessment of staff competence in the workplace that a new group of staff emerges from the N/SVQ process skilled at working with people with learning disabilities. The take-up of N/SVQs has been slow, though the independent sector has a better record than the Local Authority sector, probably because of the length and complexity of the whole assessment process required to achieve a full qualification.

Funding for such qualifications is also extremely difficult to achieve on any consistent basis, with a variety of sources (Training and Enterprise Councils (TECs), Local Enterprise Companies (LECs), Further Education Funding Council (FEFC) funding, etc.) offering partial opportunities to selected groups. This is the long-term Achilles heel of the independent sector, where the short-sighted purchasing policies of many authorities purchasing on price alone will undermine those agencies that do invest in staff development.

The learning disability professional will be a valuable (and increasingly scarce) resource for independent sector agencies, wherever they are located. At first sight this might appear reassuring to the professional trainee who can be confident that their rare skills will always be sought after. It does, however, place the burden of the future upon the collective shoulders of those specialists who will probably increasingly be working in the independent sector as statutory sector provision contracts in size. It is a moot point as to whether or not the current professional qualification structure can survive in its current form of either social work or health care training. Already there are some moves to join together the 'two tribes' in learning disability training with joint social work and nurse training courses. The future needs of the independent sector market place might well increase pressure to produce a new breed of learning disability specialist, capable of straddling the health/social care divide in the interests of meeting the real needs of clients. The future policies of the local educational training consortia within the NHS and the influence of the independent sector upon their purchasing strategies for NHS-funded training may yet prove to be highly influential in the future of the learning disability specialist practitioner.

Discussion Questions

- There are many different kinds of agencies in the independent sector, what differences might you expect to find in workplace attitudes and practice in the different agencies? To what extent do you think they might impinge on your professional practice? What would you do if they did?

- How can you most effectively regulate services and support staff in an increasingly diverse market? What are the arguments for and against separating those who inspect and regulate services from those who provide them?

- Service provision is always changing and adapting to professional, political, organizational and financial pressures. What is the role of the learning disability professional in all this?

- What right does a service user have to choose a service which is seen by many as outdated, unfashionable or a little paternalistic? If you conclude that this choice really does reflect a (reasonably) well-informed decision by the client (irrespective of any pressures from family/friends or the provider) what should your attitude be to this?

- Care for people with a learning disability has a long (even lifelong) time scale. What are the implications of this to the various professionals (health, social work, education, etc.)

> ■ who come into contact with a client (typically) for a few months or years at the most?

Notes and References

1. See Part I Section 3 of the 1984 Registered Homes Act which takes care to identify the 'person in control' as needing to be registered as well as any absentee owner/manager/corporate body.
2. For more details of controls over charities contact the Charity Commission, St Albans House, 57/60 Haymarket, London SW1Y 4QX, Tel. 0171 210 3000.
3. There is a series of offices covering the country providing a service for the Registrar. They are all under the control of the Department of Trade and Industry from whom further details can be obtained.
4. More information on the work of these two types of organization can be obtained from the Registrar of Friendly Societies. Their activities are subject to the Friendly and Industrial and Provident Societies Act 1968 and the Friendly Societies Act 1974.
5. The Housing Corporation, 149 Tottenham Court Road, London W1P 0BN, Tel. 0171 387 9466. Housing Associations have their own federation at NHF, 175 Gray's Inn Road, London WC1X 8UP, Tel. 0171 278 6571.
6. For example, Care First plc, Cresta Care, Westminster Health Care.
7. Contact a Family, 16 Strutton Ground, London SW1P 2HP, Tel. 0171 222 2695.
8. There have been many books and articles written about normalization and it is often difficult to put into practice. See: Williams, P. and Race, D. (1988). *Normalisation and the Children's Society.* CMHERA London. Also Wolfensberger, W. (1980). The defi-nition of normalisation. In *Normalisation, Social Integration and Community Service* (eds R.J. Flynn and K.E. Nitsch). Baltimore University Park Press, Baltimore.
9. Wolfensberger, G.W., Glen, L. *PASS 3. Programme Analysis of Service Systems: a method for the quantitative evaluation of human service.* Toronto National Institute for Mental Retardation; 1975.
10. See the LASA pack *Learning about Self Advocacy* (Via publications, 5 Kentings, Comberton, Cambs CB3 7DT).
11. See articles on service brokerage in *Community Living* **2** (4), April 1989 (Good Impressions publishing, Hexagon House, Surbiton Hill Rd, Surbiton KT6 4TZ).
12. Rescare, Rayner House, 23 Higher Hillgate, Stockport, Cheshire SK1 3ER.
13. L'Arche Secretariat, 10 Briggate, Silsden, Keighley, West Yorkshire BD20 9JT.
14. Camphill Village Trust, Delrow House, Hillfield Lane, Aldenham, Watford, Herts WD2 8DJ, Tel. 01923 856006.
15. Anthroposophical Society, Rudolf Steiner House, 35 Park Road, London NW1 6XT.
16. Committee for Steiner Special Schools, Philpots Manor, West Hoathly, Sussex RH19 4PR.
17. CARE, 9a Weir Road, Kibworth, Leicester LE8 9LQ; Home Farm Trust, Merchants House North, Wapping Road, Bristol BS1 4RH.
18. See the recently issued Distance Learning Pack for training Registration Officers issued by CESSA/ Department of Health.
19. Mencap Homes Foundation, Royal Mencap, 117–119 Golden Lane, London EC1 0RT.
20. The Lifecare Charitable Trust c/o Stewarts, 63 Lincoln's Inn Fields, London WC2A 3LW. Mencap also have a Trustee Scheme and a Visitors Scheme.
21. *The Future of Regulation and Inspection*, compiled by Mr Tom Burgner, known as the 'Burgner Report'.
22. i.e. National/Scottish Vocational Qualifications.

Chapter 4

Local Authorities

Mick Lloyd

Key Issues

- Structure of Local Authorities
- Funding Social Services
- The reforms of the 1990s
- Responsibilities, power and duties
- Targets and priorities
- Philosophy of care and provision
- Controls and influences
- Training and qualifications
- Referrals and transitions
- The future

Introduction

Primarily through their Social Services and Social Work Departments, Local Authorities maintain a significant and lifelong involvement for some of their learning disabled population, while for others the involvement is peripheral. This chapter focuses upon some of the key issues of the duties, tasks and challenges faced by Local Authorities. A brief description of their functions and structure is provided along with comment on how the philosophy of care and controls and influences serve to shape the Local Authority contribution to the lives of people with learning disabilities and their carers with particular consideration given to the reforms of the 1990s.

The Structure of Local Authorities

The brief history of Local Authority Social Services Departments (SSDs) and Social Work Departments in Scotland, is one that is associated with significant change. Since their formation in 1971 they have had to respond to continual changes driven both nationally (through legislation, policy and boundary changes) and locally (by prioritizing, reorganization and partnership arrangements with other agencies). These changes are reflected in the nature of services for people with learning disabilities who, as a significant group of service users, can be seen as benefiting or otherwise from such developments at different times.

As a result of the Local Authority Services Act of 1970, Social Services Departments took over the existing work of Local Autho-

1948   National Assistance Act.
Empowered Local Authorities to promote the welfare of people with a range of disabilities and needs, including the capacity to delegate certain responsibilities to the voluntary sector.

1962   National Assistance (Amendment) Act
Permitted Local Authorities to provide services such as meals within their own homes.

1968   Health Services and Public Services Act.
Increased powers to promote welfare of older people and people with mental health problems.

1970   Local Authority Social Services Act.
Made Local Authorities set up a single department with a director and committee to replace 'related but separately administered services'.

1970   Chronically Sick and Disabled Persons Act.
Provided additional duties and powers relating to information and services.

1977   National Health Service Act.
Related to the care of people defined as being 'mentally disordered'.

1983   Mental Health Act.
Consolidated the 1959 Act and 1982 amendment Act, affecting the 'reception, care and treatment of mentally disordered patients'.

1984   Registered Homes Act.
Drew together Local Authorities' duties relating to the registration, running and inspection of residential homes.

1989   Children Act.
Brought together public and private law relating to children, including specific, new provision for children with disabilities.

1990   NHS and Community Care Act.
Emphasized keeping people in their own homes as long as possible, separated functions of purchaser and provider imposing duty to develop mixed economy of care.

1995   Carers (Recognition and Service) Act.
Concerned with carers who provide 'substantial amount of care on a regular basis', and entitles them to an assessment which should be taken into account when decisions are made about the service user.

rities such as social work within Children Departments and Welfare Departments as well as the transfer of hospital social workers, or almoners. The aims of this legislation were to clarify responsibility and to distinguish Social from Health Services. Needless to say, such aims were ambitious and it could be argued that these issues continue to bedevil services some decades later.

Local Authorities are geographically defined, each has a council of elected councillors and paid staff. Council members appoint a chairperson and carry out their functions via various committees and subcommittees. By law where they have responsibility for the services, they must have dedicated committees for Social Services, and may then appoint as many other committees and subcommittees as they see fit. For its Social Services function, for example, there may be subcommittees for both Adult and Childrens' services.

Of the paid staff, the most senior officer will be the chief executive who is appointed by council members. Each main function of an authority, such as Social Services, has a director who traditionally heads a hierarchical pyramid of various senior and middle managers through to the junior staff.

Within a Local Authority, Social Services continue to represent one arm of a much larger provision of locally governed services as diverse as education, fire brigades, housing and libraries. Some authorities are responsible for a wide range of services – while others operate at county and district level.

At first glance, the national structure of local authorities can appear fragmented and confusing; the Audit Commission in England and Wales describes the map of local authorities as a 'patchwork quilt' of councils of varying size and functions (Audit Commission, 1996) as listed in Box 2. It should

County Councils
Unitary Metropolitan Authorities
London Boroughs
District Councils
English Unitary Councils
Scottish Unitary Councils
Welsh Unitary Councils
Parish and Community Councils

Box 2 Local government in England, Scotland and Wales

be noted that Northern Ireland operates a joint agency approach through Health and Social Services Boards.

Funding

Finance for Local Authorities is raised from three main sources, funding direct from Central Government, contribution from the local population raised from the council tax, and income from charges for services.

In order to assist the implementation of community care, specific additional funds were made available by the Government, including the Special Transitional Grant, transferring funds from social security to be spent specifically on community care. This arrangement was to be set for the 4 years up to April 1997, after which time it is included within the general Revenue Support Grant, meaning that it can be used for other Local Authority provision.

An important difference in the administration of Social Services provision and National Health Service (NHS) provision, is that the former have a discretionary power to charge for services, while it remains a key principle of the latter that it is free at the point of delivery. Policy expectation on Social Services from the Department of Health is that 'Local Authorities will institute arrangements so that users of services of all types pay what they can reasonably towards their costs' (DOH, 1992). The practice of charging has increased and provides practitioners in the field of learning disability with what Bradley and Manthorpe (1997) refer to as 'the conundrum of applying charges to people whose consumer position in a social care market may be weak and inexperienced'. Who is charged for which service and how much, is subject to great variation, and service users may be means tested or charged a flat rate.

Charges to service users; case examples

Mr and Mrs Davis have a daughter, Laura, with a learning disability who lives at home and attends the local social education centre (SEC). From its days as an industrial occupational type Adult Training Centre she receives an 'allowance' of £3.50 each week, which she calls her wages. Although the centre no longer carries out contract work these payments are maintained in all of the authorities SECs at a total cost of over £100 000 per year. The only charge made to Laura is for her lunch. Laura stays at a local hostel for a period of respite care and will be charged for this.

Donna Craig lives with her mother in the same town and as her learning disability is assessed as being more profound than Laura, she attends a day care facility run by the Health Authority. She is also charged for her lunch but does not receive any payment from the centre. When she stays at the Health Authority's respite care facility, no charge is made.

Frank Gillespie lives in a town 15 miles away within the boundary of another Local Authority, attends a Social Services day centre who make no payment to him but charge for his attendance and the transport in addition to the cost of lunch. He also pays for a home care worker who comes to his house once a week to help with housework and washing.

The Reforms of the 1990s

Although the notion of community care is readily associated with reforms of 1990 through the NHS and Community Care Act, the actual practice of caring for people in non-institutional settings can be measured in centuries rather than decades.

The effects of both the Children Act 1989 and the Community Care Act 1990 are described by Langan and Clarke (1994) as 'signalling the break-up of the last of the local state's "bureau-professional" welfare empires and threatened the fragile base of social work itself'. They point not only to Local Authorities changing role from providers to enablers, commissioners and purchasers, but also to the 'transformation' of the very character of the agency itself in which a welfare agency becomes a 'customer centred network of facilities', and professionals become managers. Change in language usage has been very evident in this cultural shift and not only have the mentally handicapped been relabelled as 'people with learning disabilities', but as consumers of Social Services they moved from being clients to customers to service users within a relatively short space of time.

The impact of the reforms is also reflected in the shifts of the role of key personnel. Jones (1991) conceived the new role of social workers as being that of 'inspectors, resource managers and budget holders' and notes the shift from the traditional focus of 'human relation' skills. This had been presaged by the Audit Commission (1989), which stressed the importance of separating the 'distinct roles of care manager and service provider' with the demands of care management requiring 'devolved budgets, improved information systems, safeguards, and new ways of planning'. More specifically, the Audit Commission pointed to the need for care managers 'becoming experts at balancing budgets and finetuning expenditure', which is a far cry from the 'helping' job that people originally came to and were trained for. In the main, Local Authority care managers are drawn from social work although not all social workers are care managers and not all care managers are social workers; for example a number of care managers are occupational therapists by profession.

In response to the legislation and subsequent guidelines, SSDs varied in their approach as to how the challenges were to be met. Some moved with more enthusiasm than others into splitting the functions of purchasing and providing services, some enthusiastically included the independent sector as providers while others actively discouraged them.

In their research into the implications to five Local Authorities in implementing community care, Lewis and Glennerster (1996) observed that 'the pace of change has varied considerably'. Within learning disability services this can partly be explained by the fact that there were very different starting points and the tensions of conflicting priorities. Despite what had appeared to be a rapid pace of change with the closure of long-stay hospitals, the end of the 1980s found '60% of the combined Local/Health Authority budget is still locked up in hospital provision' (Audit Commission, 1989).

The consequences of hospital closure were to affect more than just the former residents, as illustrated in the following practice example.

Practice example

The closure programme of three long-stay hospitals in a rural county was jointly managed by a partnership of Health and Local Authorities and the voluntary sector. The longer term management included a 'no admission' policy. Following detailed individual assessment small groups of residents moved into new group-homes provided by all three agencies in partnership plus private sector homes. Others were to move into existing Local Authority hostels into beds vacated by individuals whose assessments indicated could benefit from the opportunity of smaller community-based group homes. A parallel development was the expansion of existing day services. This included extending the capacity of existing services and the opening of two new centres which involved existing users moving to new centres nearer their homes. Former hospital residents living in their new community based homes were also accommodated in local day centres.

Responsibilities, Power and Duties

As a very 'public' service, there is no shortage of people telling Local Authorities what they should do. From the very highest level of Government to the most vulnerable individual there are demands and opinions.

The responsibilities, power and duties of Local Authorities are outlined by a range of legislation and guidance mainly from the Department of Health. Regulations are constantly updated by Government circulars. Some Local Authorities interpret their powers and obligations broadly and seek to act more proactively than others who, for political or resource reasons, take a more cautious approach.

In their highly informative book *Community Care Practice and the Law*, Mandelstam and Schwehr (1995) explain that authorities have a duty to provide some services and a power to provide others and observe that complications exist because there are different types, for example a duty can be 'towards individual people or it can be towards a local population in general'.

The complexity of need and the nature of services and professions throws up continual tensions. The ever blurring of distinctions betwen 'health' and 'social' care, make it increasingly difficult to accurately define either. Although it may be argued that the question of what is health care and what is social care is ultimately futile and unhelpful for the service user and their carer – for if an individual has an identified need then does it matter who provides it? – it remains of great importance to the agency who becomes responsible for the cost.

Practice example

In planning new service provision to accommodate the closure of two long-stay hospitals, representatives from the Local and Health Authorities worked closely together. Striving to agree criteria of who should provide what and how joint finance should be spent, considerable resources were deployed, compromises made, and decisions agreed. At the same time a placement had broken down for a man with learning disabilities who originated from the area but had been living in a private sector home for some years and now required an alternative, expensive placement. The original placement had been made by the Local Authority but the recommended move was to a specialist health facility. Solicitors were engaged by the two authorities in order to prove that the other was financially liable.

Health and Local Authorities and the non-statutory sector can be found providing similar services for people with similar needs in similar buildings and settings. It has become more difficult to establish which agency exclusively provides any major service, and which professional group exclusively carries out particular tasks.

The map of services within a mixed economy of care finds Local Authorities both in partnership and competition with other agencies in their role as providers, purchasers and regulators. Inevitably, the nature and quality of interagency relationships varies considerably. In their research into social care in a mixed economy, Wistow *et al.* (1994) found that 'Ignorance, misunder-standing, and mistrust between Local Authorities and the private sector were widespread and mutual'. To attribute difficulties in joint-working merely as being problems of communication would be to unhelpfully simplify a more complex analysis. The characteristics of an organization may be a key factor in why individuals decide to work for them or take up a particular profession, but they also contribute to potential barriers of a co-ordinated service.

Hudson (1995) refers to 'cultural fragmentation', in which the interests of individual professions could lead to conflict with and stereotyping of others. It is perhaps revealing that reference to joint agency working frequently includes the term 'collaboration', one definition of which is 'co operate traitorously with the enemy'.

That close joint-working is an unarguable 'good thing' without any drawbacks is not universally accepted. Hudson goes on to suggest that collaboration raises two main difficulties; first, he notes that an agency loses some freedom to act independently, and, second, agencies need to focus scarce resources on the mechanics of the relationships when the benefits are not wholly apparent. Clearly, there will be costs as well as benefits to individual organizations who will need to recognize and monitor the potential dangers of developing an opposition mentality within the relationship as well as a preoccupation with self-interest, for as Booth (1988) suggests 'Collaboration is a self-interested process in which organizations will participate only if it suits them'. Partnership with a true spirit of co-operation placing the needs of service users first and foremost within a prevailing culture of a market economy remains a formidable achievement likely to remain elusive to many.

Targets and Priorities

Within any one Local Authority, people with learning disabilities represent one group of people who are, in effect, competing for resources with other groups and individuals. In the wider definition of social services provided by Local Authorities, that is to say education, housing and personal Social Services, the latter accounts for considerably less of the total expenditure than either of the other two. Within Social Services and Social Work Departments, competition exists with other traditional client groups such as children and older people, a competition that is created by the growth in demand and underfunding. The Chartered Institute of Public Finance and Accountancy (1994) report that services for people with learning disabilities account for 13% of Social Services budgets in England and Wales.

The competition within learning disabilities may occur at different levels. At a macro-level is the competition between types and models of services, while at a micro-level individuals are in competition with each other, either for the more tangible resources such as a bed in a residential facility or a day centre place, or at a more immediate level, for the attention of staff. Where deficiencies exist in provision compared to need, increasing use is made of developing criteria in an attempt to ensure that those with greater need receive priority, but complexities abound as individual need does not remain constant.

A strategic function of Local Authorities is that of planning – deciding how they are to spend their budget. The results of planning decisions in community care are very much in the public domain, for each authority is required to publish their intentions in a Community Care Plan, an annually published document generally produced in partnership with the Health Authority, and in consultation with the local population. Within each plan will be some level of detail regarding targets, strategy, progress and intended action for service activity for people with learning disabilities.

Philosophy of Care and Provision

In common with any other organizations, a Social Services Department will find its philosophy and its ideals tempered by available resources. As a purchaser, enabler and inspector it will seek to identify, pursue and measure high quality service provision. As a provider it will seek to do the same, but will encounter the restrictions of available resources within the context of competing priorities.

How social care should be delivered has gained increased attention, nowhere more so than within the field of learning disability. Challenging discrimination through anti-oppressive practice is central to the training of social workers and other social care workers, with workers having to question their own values and prejudices. Philosophy of care in learning disability has also included influence from the values of normalization and the work of Wolf Wolfensberger and John O'Brien.

The traditional base of SSD services to people with learning disabilities has been in residential and day care provision and field- and hospital-based social work.

Residential care

Throughout the 1970s and into the 1980s the idea of the 20–30 bedded hostels built, managed and funded by SSDs sat quite comfortably in comparison to large long-stay hospitals, but as significant numbers of hospitals closed they exposed hostels, through a comparative view of community care. This was to be more starkly emphasized with the development of smaller homes closer to the principles of 'ordinary lives' developed by the Kings Fund Centre (1980) who set the goal of services for people with learning disabilities in the mainstream life 'living in ordinary houses, in ordinary streets, with the same range of choices as any citizen, and mixing as equals with other and mostly not handicapped members of their own community'.

This change of thinking underlines the speed of change and development, for what appeared as an important forward thinking model of one decade became questioned as a redundant concept in the next.

Within this change was the realization that it is not simply the sheer scale that leads to negative, impersonal institutional practices. The continuing use of larger residential units is largely due to the economy of scale that they seemed to offer, although alternative provision of supported living is now challenging this.

As a compromise, many such establishments adopted the practice of separating the living arrangements into smaller groups. One perceived advantage of larger units for Social Services has lain in flexibility, with many incorporating a respite care function alongside long-term residential care. The hostel model illustrates many of the dilemmas of residential care – is it a home for life, with appropriate support for both the needs and rights of its residents? Is it a flexible resource for the Local Authority to help meet the needs of the wider learning disabled population and their carers? Who or what a residential facility is for is not always easily answered. The resource model approach has developed further in some authorities who use part of a 'home' to offer day care to non-residents or who have designated a building as a suitable

base for work with a wide range of individuals who may have very different disabilities and needs. In adopting a critical view of these developments, we may have some sympathy with attempts to use resources as imaginatively as possible, but we may question what could be more far removed from an ordinary home.

Ultimately, discussion on the relative merits on the size of homes will still need to face up to a key question posed by Ryan and Thomas (1987) in a challenging and influential book *The Politics of Mental Handicap*. 'Why do we assume that, whatever the nature of a living unit, mentally handicapped people should live with each other at all?'

Smaller 'group homes', effectively ordinary houses in residential areas, will often be found operating as part of a larger network, with differing staffing levels that reflect the needs of the residents. For Local Authorities, the flexibility afforded by such a model is attractive, as it facilitates the shifting of resources as needs change rather than having to move the residents.

Practice example
Following its closure, three former residents of a long-stay hospital moved back to the town they came from. They shared an ordinary semi-detached Local Authority house and significantly increased their daily living skills beyond the level indicated by their initial assessment.

On reviewing the progress made it was suggested that the three could move on to a more independent setting with fewer staff, giving an opportunity for others to move into the group home from the local hostel. Recognizing that although this might make sense in resource management terms, it represented an unwelcome and unnecessary move for the three residents, the homes manager successfully fought for an alternative development involving the three staying in the house with the staff hours reduced allowing redeployment to other projects.

Day services

Day care remains at the foundation of Local Authority community care provision. This continues to be based in purpose-built or converted buildings often exceeding 100 daily attenders from school leavers to people of retirement age and beyond.

Like the hostels, they were initially established in the early 1970s, and likewise are also considered outmoded. Although the earlier industrial/occupational model of Adult Training Centres has largely been overtaken by a more developmental, social-educational model, their essentially segregated environment with large groups remains difficult to align with an ethos of an ordinary life.

Fieldwork services

The prevailing model of community-based social work support is found within multi-disciplinary teams. Community Learning Disability Teams vary in their composition. Brown (1990) reported that research into 303 teams found 94% included community nurses. Variations exist in the inclusion of other professions such as psychologists, occupational therapists, physiotherapists and speech and language therapists. The role of the social worker will also vary, with some holding a case management brief and others maintaining a more traditional casework approach.

In addition to the respective individual role, the community teams can also be found with a strong developmental function within their localities.

Control and Influences

The nature of the relationship between Local and Central Government will be influenced by a number of factors including the compatibility of the majority political parties. Building upon the work of Stanyer (1976), Butcher (1995) suggests that methods of control 'presume a confrontation between central government and the delivery agencies', while methods of influence intend to prevent conflict occurring. Butcher goes on to identify the key control methods as legislation and judicial control. Methods of influence, he adds, are departmental circulars, finance and an inspection.

The Social Services Inspectorate (SSI) Established in 1983 the SSI is part of the Department of Health's Social Care Group and monitors the efficiency and effectiveness of SSDs. Exercising statutory powers on behalf of the Secretary of State for Health and its functions include:

- The provision of professional advice on Government policy and the quality of social services provision.
- Carry out a national inspection of Social Services Departments.
- Assisting Government Ministers responsible for social services.

The Audit Commission
Responsible for the external auditing of Health and Local Authority accounts. Undertakes studies to promote economy, efficiency and effectiveness of services, producing statistical data comparing authorities. More specialist studies aim at identifying and promoting examples of best practice.

In addition to Governmental agencies, an enormous contribution to the knowledge base of learning disability has been made by a range of independent organizations (Box 4).

Box 3 Key bodies

- British Institute of Learning Disabilities
- Hester Adrian Research Centre
- Joseph Rowntree Foundation
- Kings Fund College
- National Development Team
- Norah Fry Research Centre
- Tizzard Centre
- Values into Action
- Welsh Centre for Learning Disabilities- Applied Research Unit

Box 4 Key bodies (non-Governmental)

Training and Qualifications

The principal qualification for social work is the Diploma in Social Work (DipSW), a college- or university-based course accredited by the Central Council for Education and Training in Social Work.

Prior to the DipSW two qualifications were in operation, the Certificate of Qualification in Social Work (CQSW), and the Certificate in Social Services (CSS). Although students may have the opportunity to opt for specialist practice placements, professional qualification is generic in nature. Despite the presence of these qualifications the vast majority of personnel in social care settings for people with learning disabilities are unqualified.

One specialist qualification that did exist, mainly for staff working in day care, was the comparatively short-lived Diploma in Teaching and Training Adults with Mental Handicap. A significant gap therefore exists, and the development of National Vocational Qualifications (NVQs) represents a major opportunity to fill the gap between qualification training for the few and what may be offered to the rest.

Routes Through the Services

In common with the NHS, services provided by Local Authorities are from 'the cradle to the grave', therefore adults with learning disabilities are likely to have previously been known to SSDs as children. This will not always be the case, as people tend to move house, and information systems are rarely comprehensive, for even though registers are in operation families may chose not to be included. Two key processes in routes into and through the services are Referrals and Transitions.

Referrals – the route into service provision

The initial referral to the Social Services could be made by a number of sources, such as the family or other agencies. The purpose of the referral may be for a specific service request, such as residential or day care, or a more general request for information. Social work involvement for some may be instigated soon after birth through joint-agency working involving an automatic referral by the hospital medical team.

The prioritizing and targeting of services, and the availability of resources result in not every person with a learning disability being allocated a social worker.

Transitions – routes through the services

The principal milestones of service change for a person with a learning disability can be identified as:

- infant to school-age
- childhood to adulthood
- adulthood to old age.

These stages are identified more through

transitions in services rather than characteristics of the individual. SSDs have traditionally split, in organization terms, into Children and Adult Services and it therefore becomes as important for the two sections of the same department to communicate, plan and work together as it is for different agencies.

Transitions provide continuing challenges. Where services are static with more routes in than out their capacity to provide for school-leavers becomes restricted. Likewise, with the older population now living longer, local authorities are grappling with issues of retirement policies in day centres (begging the question of retiring to and from what?) and the desirability and capability of generic services for older people responding to the needs of the increasing number of older people with learning disabilities.

The Future: Proposals

Local Authorities have taken the lead responsibility for services for people with learning disabilities in a period which saw dramatic growth in the private and voluntary care provision. At the same time a number of NHS Trusts have branched into social as well as health care provision. Community care has presented new challenges, some of which are without precedent with more older people and people with complex needs such as challenging behaviour living in the community and using Social Services than before.

The future agenda has already been set in what Wright *et al.* (1994) call the 'brave new world'. They describe it as a number of puzzles in 'purchasing and providing services, financial planning and control, and the development of user and carer involvement in service management and delivery'. Desirable off-the-shelf solutions remain elu-

sive, for as Tyne (1996, p. 21) observes 'If it were easy to support vulnerable or distressed people in their own homes in dignified and thoughtful ways we would be doing it instead of running a dozen different variations on the residential institution'.

Whatever the developments of the final years of the 1990s, the prospects for the medium-term are unlikely to be radically different to Towell and Beardshaw's (1991) view of the last decade of the twentieth century when they suggested that 'whatever the political scenario it seems safe to predict that people who depend on publicly financed services, and those who work in them, face a continuing struggle to achieve worthwhile objectives'. The reasons for this may continue to be seated in a lack of vision, and political will to provide truly integrated services as much as any resource deficiency. Where progressive, appropriate services are not being developed it cannot always be attributed to lack of funds, rather a decision to tie up the funding to existing models of care. It is safe to predict that funding will remain an issue, for quite simply there are not enough funds available, but there never has been and there never will be.

The outstanding contribution of research, information and ideas from institutions and bodies noted above has helped establish an unprecedented knowledge-base for planners, managers and practitioners in the field of learning disability. Lack of knowledge or examples of good practice models can rarely be found as an excuse for static, inappropriate services from any sector or agency. In an age of information technology, access to material that can inform practice development has become significantly less of a problem than professionals' capacity to learn from, and effectively use it.

Historically the transition towards comprehensive, integrated services has been conservative, slow and incremental and

Local Authorities must strive to make an 'ordinary life' a reality. The field of learning disabilities has undoubtedly attracted outstanding individuals of commitment, flair and imagination. It remains a test of large organizations, such as SSDs, of how they nurture, encourage and support the architects of the next generation of services.

For the thousands who remain in institutions the social welfare reforms of the 1990s have largely passed them by, and along with people with learning disabilities within the community it remains of central importance that the politics and administration of care do not lose sight of the individual. How is the quality of his or her life improved and maintained, and how would we know?

Discussion Questions

- Is it appropriate that an agency, such as a Social Services Department, has the combined role of purchasing, providing and inspecting services?
- In the development of a comprehensive range of services, is there still a role for large group settings such as residential hostels or day centres?
- Even where integrated services are achievable, do you consider that there will always be a need for some form of specialist services for people with learning disabilities? If so who would they be for and what would they look like?
- If the aim of legislation was to 'clarify responsibility and distinguish between health and social care', are you clear as to what these responsibilities and

differences are in the area you work or live in?
- Should there be a specialist qualification in learning disability for staff working in social care?

References

Audit Commission (1989). *Developing Community Care for Adults with a Mental Handicap*. HMSO, London.

Audit Commission (1996). *All Change: Managing Local Government Reorganisation and Beyond*. HMSO, London.

Booth, T. (1988). *Developing Policy Research*. Gower, Aldershot.

Bradley, G. and Manthorpe, J. (1997). The price of care: charging for services. *Journal of Learning Disability for Health and Social Care* 1(2): 84–89.

Brown, S. (1990). *Variations on a Theme*. Community Mental Handicap Teams Practice Paper No. 1. HMSO, London.

Butcher, T. (1995). *Delivering Welfare*. Open University Press, Buckingham.

Chartered Institute of Public Finance and Accountancy (1994). *Personal Social Services Statistics 1993–4*. CIPFA, London.

DOH (1992). *Equipped for Independence? Meeting the 1992 Equipment Needs of Disabled*. Department of Health, London.

Hudson, B. (1995). A seamless service? Developing better relationships between National Health Services and Social Services Departments. In *Values and Visions* (eds. T. Philpott and L. Ward), pp. 106–122. Butterworth Heineman, Oxford.

Jones, K. (1991). *The Making of Social Policy in Britain 1830–1990*. Athlone, London.

Kings Fund Centre (1980). *An Ordinary Life: Comprehensive Locally Based Residential Services for Mentally Handicapped People*. King Edwards Hospital Fund, London.

Langan, M. and Clarke, J. (1994). Managing in the mixed economy of care. In *Managing Social Policy* (eds J. Clarke, A. Cochrane, and E. McLaughlin). Sage, London.

Lewis, J. and Glennerster, H. (1996). *Implementing the New Community Care*. Open University Press, Buckingham.

Mandelstam, M. with Schwehr, B. (1995). *Community Care Practice and the Law*. Jessica Kingsly, London.

Ryan, J. and Thomas, F. (1987). *The Politics of Mental Handicap*. Free Association Books, London.

Stanyer, J. (1976). *Understanding Local Government*. Fontana, London.

Towell, D. and Beardshaw, V. (1991). *Enabling Community Education*. King's Fund College, London.

Tyne, A. (1996). Five values for every care plan. *Care Plan*. March 1996.

Wistow, G., Knapp, M., Hardy, B. and Allen, C. (1994). *Social Care in a Mixed Economy*. Open University Press, Buckingham.

Wright, K., Haycox, A. and Leedham, I. (1994). *Evaluating Community Care Services for People with Learning Disabilities*. Open University Press, Buckingham.

Further Reading

Local authorities

Butcher, T. (1995). *Delivering Welfare*. Open University Press, Buckingham.

Tossell, D. and Webb, R. (1994). *Inside the Caring Services*. Edward Arnold, London.

Policy

Mittler, P. and Sinason, V. (Eds). (1996). *Changing Policy and Practice for People with Learning Disabilities*. Cassell, London.

Ryan, J. and Thomas, F. (1987 – Revised edition). *The Politics of Mental Handicap*. Free Association Books, London.

Wistow, G., Knapp, M., Hardy, B. and Allen, C. (1994). *Social Care in a Mixed Economy*. Open University Press, Buckingham.

Services

Booth, T. (ed.) (1990). *Better Lives; Changing Services for People with Learning Disabilities*. Community Care/Joint Unit for Social Services Research, Sheffield.

National Development Team (1990). *Promises to Keep*. National Development Team, London.

Walker, C., Ryan, T. and Walker, A. (1996). *Fair Shares for All*. Pavillion/Joseph Rowntree, Brighton.

Philpot, T. and Ward, L. (1995). *Values and Visions*. Butterworth Heinemann, Oxford.

Towell, D. (1988). *An Ordinary Life in Practice*. King Edward Hospital Fund, London.

Wolfensberger, W. (ed.) (1972). *The Principle of Normalization in Human Services*. Toronto, National Institute of Mental Retardation.

O'Brien, J. (1987). A guide to personal futures planning. In *A Comprehensive Guide to the Activities Catalog: An Alternative Curriculum for Youth and Adults with Severe Disabilities* (eds G.T. Bellamy and B. Willcox). Bathmore, Paul H. Brookes.

Chapter 5

Education

Leslie Hall

Key Issues

- Background to educational provision and statementing procedure
- Educational options
- Provision in a severe learning difficulty (SLD) school and some factors affecting it
- Approaching work in a special school
- Roles, responsibilities and collaborative approaches
- Working with the disabled child

Introduction

Recent legislation has strengthened established approaches to the education of children with severe learning difficulties (SLD) but changes such as the introduction of the National Curriculum have also affected provision. This chapter outlines educational options and provision for SLD children and discusses the need for collaboration between professionals within the school setting.

Background to Educational Provision and the Statementing Procedure

Schools for children with severe learning difficulties were created in 1971 as a result of the 1970 Education Act to provide education for a group of children who had been considered ineducable. Originally for pupils aged 5–16 years, the service has expanded to provide nursery and post-16 education and a range of opportunities more comparable to those available to pupils in the mainstream.

The terminology has also changed to reflect the changing climate of opinion relating to educational approaches. Once referred to as schools for educationally subnormal (ESN) children, they are now termed SLD schools as emphasis moves away from the child's disability to the child's needs. Such schools form part of a variety of educational provision as opportunities in other parts of the educational system are explored by parents, relatives and teachers.

SLD children needing early intervention may be recognized at birth, for example children presenting the physical characteristics of conditions such as Down's syndrome, microcephaly or cerebral palsy. Furthermore, the majority of children will be diagnosed by the time they are 3 years because of marked failure to reach developmental milestones at the appropriate age. Only a minority of children will fail to be diagnosed before they reach the age of compulsory school attendance at 5 years. Quite exceptionally, a few children develop severe learning difficulties after that age as a result of severe illness or accident.

The 1981 Education Act, reinforced by the 1993 Education Act, laid down the rights of such children to an education which meets their individual needs and set out formal procedures for the admission or transfer of children to special schools. The Health Authorities are legally obliged to refer such children to the Local Education Authority (LEA) as soon as their needs are recognized. The LEA then appoints an educational psychologist (EP) to work with parents and to make an educational assessment of the child. Statutory assessment can, but will not normally, begin before the age of 2 years. Placement within a special school or unit should only occur if provision within a mainstream setting cannot meet those needs. The procedures are common to all children whose disabilities (e.g. physical, sensory, emotional or learning) are severe enough to require specialist teaching not available in most mainstream settings.

Both the 1981 and 1993 Acts adopt a broad definition of special needs to include the needs of pupils who might require 'additional or supplementary provision' at any stage in their school education. All schools are required to name a Special Needs Co-ordinator and maintain and update a register of pupils with special needs. Each governing body must review its special educational needs (SEN) policy annually. It is estimated that about 20% of pupils fall into this category at any one time and all but 2% can be educated in mainstream schools. The child's difficulties must be viewed in context so that two children with largely similar needs may require different provision.

The 1994 Code of Practice formalizes best practice in the assessment of special needs. Five stages are identified in the statementing procedure, so-called because it may lead to a written statement of educational needs which the LEA is legally required to meet (Figure 5.1).

The statementing procedure

Stages 1–3
The first three stages take place within the mainstream school and identify remedial steps which can be taken within the school's existing resources or with some external support such as that of an EP. Parents will be informed and consulted at all stages. Where these steps do not meet the child's needs, the school's EP will recommend stage 4, formal assessment.

Stage 4
Once the LEA informs parents and professionals that it proposes to start statutory assessment the whole process must be completed within 26 weeks (Figure 5.1). Those closely involved with the child are requested to submit a written assessment of the child's abilities and needs, plus their advice as to the kind of provision which should be made but without naming a school or unit. Advice is requested from the child's parents/carers, teachers, therapists, school medical officer or paediatrician, the EP and others working with the child. A suggested check-list, drawn from the Code of Practice, provides guidance for those completing advice.

The parents' advice is crucial to the

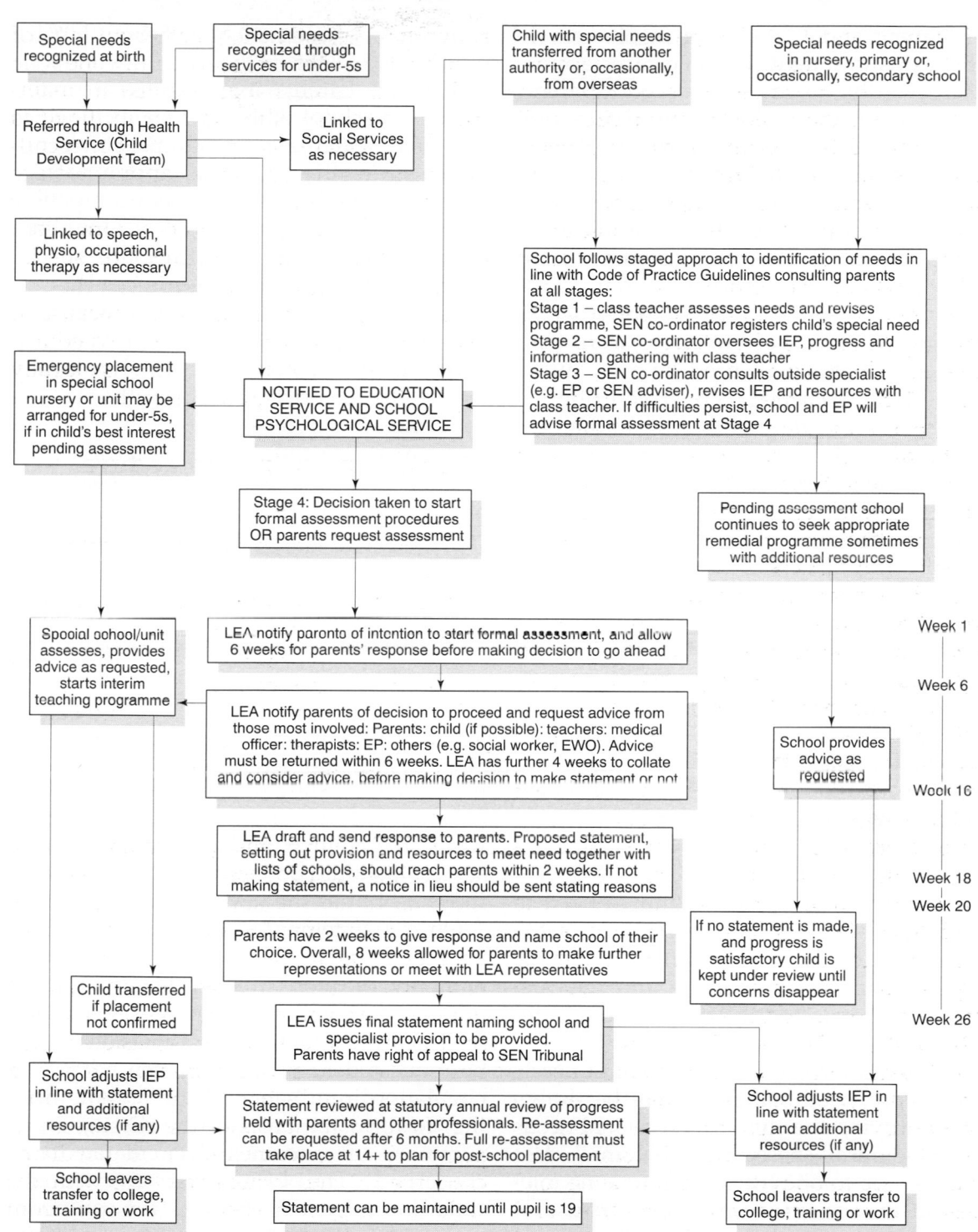

Figure 5.1 Route through the educational system for a child with special needs. EP, educational psychologist; EWO, education welfare officer; IEP, individual education programme; LEA, Local Education Authority; SEN, special educational needs

assessment and LEAs differ in the way in which this is sought. In some cases a more 'user-friendly' form encourages parents to express their opinion of the child's progress and needs in their own words. Parents may have an opportunity to give their views verbally. In many cases the professionals (including the psychologist) make their assessment after discussion with the parent(s) and after observation of the child in a familiar setting. Even so, parents may be unaware of the need to put forward their own advice and may need help to understand the importance of their contribution to the statementing process within the time limitations.

Parents can also nominate an independent Named Person who could support them, for example at meetings or reviews.

There may be urgent educational or social reasons for these children to be admitted to school at the age of 3 years pending assessment. The placement, whether in a special school or mainstream nursery, will be provisional pending the final statement and will only be arranged with the agreement of the parents/carers.

Upon completion of stage 4 the LEA considers whether to issue a statement.

Stage 5

The advice will be collated and referred to the LEA statementing panel (probably including a senior representative of the School Psychological Service and the Special Needs Inspector or Adviser) to consider action to meet the child's needs.

If it is decided that a statement is necessary, a proposed statement will be drawn up identifying the child's educational needs and resources. These might be small class groups, one-to-one teaching, part-time integration in a mainstream class, the use of sign language, a developmental/modified curriculum, and support needs from other services (e.g. speech or physiotherapy). A copy of this statement together with a list of schools is sent to the parents/carers for agreement. Parents may express a preference for a school which will be included in the final statement unless the LEA can demonstrate that it is not appropriate to the child's needs or that it is not compatible with the 'efficient education' of other children or the 'efficient use of resources'.

The process is completed once the LEA issues a final statement which will bind the LEA to make the stated provision. It will also specify non-educational provision which the District Health Authority has confirmed it will make.

If parents disagree with the terms of the statement they have a right of appeal to an SEN Tribunal, but LEAs try to resolve difficulties before the issue of a formal statement by consulting with parents at every stage of the assessment.

The statementing process causes anxiety and distress because it highlights the child's difficulties in relation to the school curriculum and creates fears about the quality of alternative provision. However, it should be in the interests of the child to have such a statement because it makes available additional specialist resources to which the child would not otherwise have access. It should be viewed not as 'labelling' the child but as the key to services.

Once a statement is in place, the child's progress must be formally reviewed annually or more frequently for children under 5 years. Under the 1994 Code of Practice, parents and professionals will be requested to prepare written advice for circulation in advance of the review meeting, to form the basis of the discussion. A summary of outcomes is circulated to all concerned. The LEA must give parents time to respond either to the proposed action (e.g. a child remaining in a mainstream nursery until age 7 years may need to transfer to other provision) or the decision not to make an amendment to the statement.

If there are significant changes, the annual review may give rise to a request for reassessment.

Confidentiality

The statement and annual review reports are confidential, as are records, notes and case conference reports kept on the child's educational file. They are available to parents, teachers and other professionals on a 'need to know' basis. Parents may give permission for others to have the information.

Educational Options

For the SLD child, what are the educational options? As a result of the Warnock report on Special Education Needs and the subsequent 1981 and 1993 Education Acts, there is an expectation that LEAs will make provision in a mainstream setting wherever possible, if compatible with the child's needs but a range of options may be available.

Most SLD children and their families benefit from early intervention. Local initiatives differ. They may include a portage service in which workers help parents and families to undertake a limited home teaching programme based around one or two carefully selected objectives. Alternatively, a home–school liason teacher will undertake this task. Some children will be placed in nursery classes pending assessment. Even when placement is in the nursery class of a special school, the final statement may recommend an alternative placement or package to meet the child's individual need.

Amin, a 4-year-old boy with Down's syndrome, was placed in our nursery class for assessment, though similar children of comparable ability were supported in mainstream nurseries. Amin had specific behaviour problems such as pinching, scratching and kicking which made it doubtful that he would succeed in a mainstream nursery. During the assessment period with particular attention given to the behaviour, it became clear that Amin responded very well to a behaviour management programme allied to an appropriate learning programme. The class teacher advised that, provided such a programme could be carried out and adequately supported in the mainstream, Amin should transfer to a mainstream nursery. The statement recommended that he attend a nursery class within his own neighbourhood with appropriate support and he was transferred just before his fifth birthday.

Box 1 Case example

The 1993 Education Act (s 161(4)) lays a duty on those providing for a child's special educational needs in a mainstream school to ensure that the child engages in activities of the school together with children who do not have special needs 'as far as is practicable'. Ideally, teaching by means of an adapted curriculum and individual lesson plans should encourage the pupil to operate independently whilst remaining socially integrated, but a variety of approaches exist.

In some cases this has resulted in the establishment of special units within mainstream schools. Elsewhere, special services support individual pupils or groups of pupils within mainstream classes. The support may take the form of direct teaching by specialist teachers or of an advisory service helping the mainstream teacher to adapt programmes, methods and resources to the individual needs of pupils. Integration may be part-time or full-time.

For SLD pupils additional support is needed from classroom assistants working under the guidance of the teacher, to increase the attention span of the pupil or to assist the pupil with self-help skills which other pupils manage for themselves. Extra cover may be needed during staff breaks at dinner-time or in the playground.

Policies which seek to integrate pupils always require a high level of resources. It is rarely possible to make a straightforward financial comparison between the allocation of resources to a centralized special school and the dispersal of resources across a number of mainstream schools, since there may need to be duplication of provision.

The arguments for integrated provision are strong in that they stress the rights of children with special needs to have access to as near normal an education as possible alongside their contemporaries and within their own community. It is also right that disabled children should have access to opportunities available to their contemporaries wherever possible. With improved training and understanding of the teacher's role in the support of pupils with special needs, there is greater willingness to accept pupils with severe disabilities in mainstream schools. Additional funding attached to such placements helps to provide extra resources. However, many of the child's individual needs resulting from the disability may not be best met within an integrated setting. Where support is needed from speech, occupational or physiotherapist or from peripatetic teachers, there may be a strong argument for a central educational provision so that children can receive greater input and time from specialists. Hydrotherapy pools, soft-play equipment, specialist computer switches and software

for children with profound and severe disabilities are increasingly available to special schools but are not so easily acquired within a budget which has to meet the needs of all pupils within the mainstream schools.

Widely differing views are held by groups of parents and professionals alike. Although the parents of pupils with the highest level of disability may be those most concerned about the effect of integration on services available to their children, parents of more able pupils often express anxiety about the way their child may cope with large numbers coupled with less adult time and assistance. Parents also worry about the time and information about their child's progress they can expect to receive from a classroom teacher responsible for 25–30 pupils.

Professionals who counsel and advise parents about schools should have appropriate information and be realistic about the kind of education which each setting can offer to children with lifelong disabilities. This will help parents to judge advantages and disadvantages in the light of their knowledge of their own child's difficulties. Parents have changed and have the power to change attitudes towards the provision of education for children with special needs, and authorities will try to meet their wishes, but the child may not meet the parents' expectations for progress if placed in an inappropriate setting. It is a dilemma to which there are no easy answers.

Aspects of school ethos, organization and provision must also be considered. Children need a carefully structured environment if they are to make sense of what is provided, but the kind of structure appropriate to a child without learning problems may provide a degree of choice and stimulation which overwhelms the learning disabled child. A very formal setting may require an attention span or degree of participation of which the child is not yet capable. Developmentally, the child may not be able to share and co-operate and may become frustrated, disruptive or withdrawn. Is the physical access and toilet accommodation adequate? Is the environment safe for a child with limited understanding of danger? Constant supervision and separate teaching may increase the child's dependence on one or two adults and reinforce a perception of disability and difference in his/her mind and in the minds of contemporaries.

George was admitted to a Social Services nursery at the age of 3 years. A boy with Down's syndrome, he was socially well adapted and physically able but as he approached the age of 5 years it became apparent that his attention span and speech were not sufficiently well developed to enable him to cope in a mainstream reception class. However, he needed models of play and speech which were not available in the special school class to which he would transfer. The advice submitted stressed this aspect of learning, which was included in George's statement of special needs. As a result, he now spends five mornings in the special needs school and five afternoons in the mainstream nursery class close to his home, with the support of a classroom assistant. The special school provides specialized teaching, individual work and access to speech therapy in the morning. In the mainstream nursery he is able to observe and join in with the play and group activities set out for all the children. In addition, his mother is able to collect him from school and meets up with local parents at the school gate.

This placement will need to be reviewed as George gets older and physically outgrows the nursery-aged children, though he may still need models of speech and play at that developmental stage.

Box 2 Case example

Because SLD children learn more slowly than their contemporaries, it may be necessary to consider different forms of provision at different stages of the child's education, so that the child does not lose confidence or become socially isolated.

Muhammad, aged 8 years, links with a reception class for three afternoons a week. He needs support to join in some of the activities and considerable adaptation of the curriculum. For example, while others practise writing skills, he will use a crayon to scribble. However, he continues to be socially integrated, to hear good models of speech and to be with children from his local community. As the other children get more involved in formal literacy and numeracy skills, he will have more difficulty being part of the class. His parents will feel heartbreak and anxiety if he can no longer attend the mainstream school, but the question now arises as to whether Muhammad continues to gain educationally. Other links may need to be formed.

Box 3 Case example

It is erroneous to assume that integrated provision is necessarily a preferable option since the concentration of expertise within a special school and the acquisition and development of good practice, related to knowledge of disabilities and appropriate teaching methods, often produces a quality of education for special needs which mainstream schools cannot match.

There is a danger that all agencies, and particularly parents, regard the special school as a last resort rather than as a specialized resource that can meet the needs of children with particular difficulties. All involved need to be flexible in their attitude to placement. Provision must allow for a variety of placement needs but funding to provide one form of service, for example units within mainstream schools, may mean that alternative options such as individual placement with support in mainstream classes are not available.

Very occasionally, parents wish to exercise their right to educate their child at home or privately. Parents may wish to put their child through a particular programme of training or therapy not available within the LEA. Conductive education or Doman–Delacato programming require highly intensive staffing ratios not available in schools. Provided that parents can make suitable arrangements which the LEA agrees are satisfactory, the Education Act 1993 (5) (a) supports the right of parents to remove their children from school.

Provision within a SLD School

SLD schools normally follow a pattern of organization similar to that found in mainstream schools. Teachers will have a normal teaching qualification. Some will have an additional specialist qualification. The school day is of normal length and follows a pattern not dissimilar to an infant school.

As a result of the policy of integration into mainstream schools the disability and needs of those remaining in SLD schools are more complex with additional physical, emotional, sensory and language problems which require increased levels of input and care. In particular, those with profound and multiple handicaps and those with difficult or bizarre behavioural patterns cannot easily be integrated into mainstream classes.

In the past decade special schools have also had to adjust to legislation which reduced the power of Local Authorities and transferred to schools many of the duties of the LEA, whilst restricting the school's control over curriculum and other aspects of school organization.

The curriculum

The 1988 Education Reform Act lays a responsibility on headteachers and governors to ensure that all pupils aged 5–16 years in maintained schools, including those in special schools, should have access to the National Curriculum and should receive a 'broad and balanced' education.

The advent of the National Curriculum has created considerable challenge for teachers within special schools and provided an opportunity to review the content and structure of the curriculum already established during the 1970s and 1980s.

Since 1971 the SLD curriculum has been the subject of much discussion and research leading to wide agreement that these pupils need a developmental curriculum which is planned individually, using age-related experiences and methods appropriate to the child and the task. The individual education programme (IEP) was not planned against national criteria for a balanced curriculum, but against the school's own guidelines. Terminology related more to child development (e.g. perceptual development) than to the normal curriculum (e.g. maths).

By contrast, the National Curriculum is subject based and divided into three core subjects (English, Maths, Science) and seven foundation subjects (PE, Art, Geography, Modern Language (for ages 11–16 years), Technology, History, Music), each divided into four Key Stages and 10 Levels of Attainment. Religious Education is also compulsory. Pupils in SLD schools are generally deemed to be working *within* Key Stage 1, Level 1 of the National Curriculum and most will not achieve even Level 1 outcomes.

The 1988 legislation allows for time-limited disapplication from the National Curriculum for individual pupils with special needs pending the completion of an assessment. Statements may recommend the modification or disapplication of any or all of the requirements of the National Curriculum for individual pupils, but only the Secretary of State can authorize general disapplication for pupils.

Although National Curriculum documents recognize the need to adapt approaches for students with disabilities, schools must decide how this should be done. Some teachers drew up their own recommendations for a revised curriculum. Others rejected this approach as having no relevance to pupils, particularly pupils with profound and multiple learning difficulties (PMLD), and wasteful of a valuable resource – teachers' time. They decided to continue with their established curriculum.

Subsequently, the Office for Standards in Education (OFSTED) Inspectors have made clear that they expect special schools to work within the requirements of the National Curriculum as far as possible and have judged as failing schools that did not adapt their curriculum.

Colleagues working within the mainstream have also had difficulties with the introduction of aspects of the National Curriculum and expressed concerns that teaching to targets that are narrowly focused will restrict the breadth of the curriculum. However, there is widespread acceptance that agreement over programmes of study and the content and assessment of subjects eases the task of the teacher and provides for smoother progression for pupils from class to class and school to school. Parents also become familiar with the terminology and may be better able to understand their child's progress.

The introduction of the National Curriculum has not brought similar advantages to SLD schools. Although the Programmes of Study provide guidance on opportunities which could be offered to pupils, National Curriculum targets do not meet the needs of most SLD pupils. Sadly, there has been no centralized support to co-ordinate the many valuable initiatives in schools and colleges to provide guidance on the core content of a mainly pre-Level 1 curriculum. An opportunity to bring special schools more fully into an education system which offers a continuum of curriculum to meet the needs of all children has been lost. SLD schools continue to struggle individually to describe pre-Level 1 progress and targets and to provide a 'broad and balanced' curriculum for its pupils. In my view this is evidence that the education of these children has still not gained an equal footing with other areas of education.

In devising IEPs class teachers will continue to draw on their knowledge of pupils' needs but will have to consider carefully whether a broad and balanced curriculum with a range of experiences is being offered. There will continue to be differences between schools in this respect and even between teachers in individual schools. The lack of a common language to describe the curriculum will emphasize the differences that exist between mainstream and special schools and may make it harder for some parents to understand what their child is learning.

The IEP

The IEP remains the basis of day-to-day teaching. Based on the detailed observation and assessment of the child's skills, abilities and motivation it seeks to produce progress by means of very small steps broken down to the level appropriate for the child for whom it is written, and to establish consistency in methods and identification of success.

In order to achieve one-to-one teaching, staffing levels are high with additional support from classroom assistants. Both within classes and across classes a team approach is necessary if pupils are to learn and make sense of their experience. Those working with the child need to share their knowledge by means of accurate recording of progress and by sharing information which enables others to understand the child's background, personality and motivation.

Achievement will be recorded either following the school's own procedure or against a series of published assessment schedules widely used within schools (e.g. Derbyshire Language Assessment, Pre-Verbal Communication Schedule) and relevant National Curriculum Targets. The assessments form the basis for future teaching and for the report provided at the annual review meeting. Although the IEP enables the teacher to plan work at the appropriate level, much of the teaching takes place within group settings and age-appropriate contexts. At nursery level children will be encouraged to explore a variety of materials and equipment in much the same way as their contemporaries, though more time needs to be devoted to helping each child use and share equipment appropriately and to develop communication and independence. Efforts are made to link with home and cultural background.

At a later stage, even though progress through the basic curriculum has been very slow, more adult equipment and experiences will be provided. Libraries, swimming pools and sports facilities available to their contemporaries may also be used if funding allows.

By supporting different approaches to special education, LEAs influence opportunities and experiences available to SLD pupils. Similarly, within the wider community there are numerous competing priorities and demands which affect opportunities to link into community services. The degree to which they do so depends both on the level to which equal opportunity policies have been developed within the community, and on financial restraints.

The first annual review after the pupils' 14th birthday must follow procedures set out in the Education (Special Education) Regulations 1994 and the Code of Practice. Representatives from the Careers Service and Social Services must join parents and other professionals to draw up a transition plan for the young person and to establish links with future providers, for example colleges, training schemes or day centres. For one or two students, supervised work placements may be available. Even for those pupils with the greatest degree of disability, link programmes are important in ensuring that the student is prepared for change and that knowledge and understanding of the student is transferred to those responsible for adult provision.

In recent years teachers have come to realize that the emotional and sexual development of pupils needs to receive more attention as part of preparation for adult life. Sex education programmes have been developed which aim to teach SLD pupils about their rights and responsibilities as well as to help them recognize exploitation by others. Such programmes are not easy to put into practice. They require considerable planning at an individual level and may benefit from collaboration from other professionals with knowledge or interest in this field. The school nurse or social worker may work directly with young people or parents. Other groups may have a role.

A group of teenaged SLD students took part in regular drama sessions as part of a Drama-In-Education initiative. Several of the group were demonstrating emotional involvement and sexual awareness. In planning a forthcoming series of sessions actors and teachers decided that drama could provide a vehicle for sex education which would help the young people learn about their own bodies and understand their sexual and emotional feelings.

Actors and staff agreed that the team involved should remain the same for each session because of the sensitivity of some of the issues to be addressed. The team leader was a former SLD teacher of senior pupils who had joined the external drama group. Very detailed preplanning was necessary to allow students to explore relationships, individual rights and responsibilities within the context of the group. Single-sex sessions and individual support for students were included as the sessions progressed.

Parents were involved from the start as, without their support, the project might founder. A meeting was held to which governors, school nurse and social worker were also invited. With encouragement, all parents attended. Plans were outlined in detail, setting out clearly the issues to be tackled — issues such as knowing the name of body parts, appropriate and inappropriate attitudes and touching, recognizing the feelings of others and, by the end of the year, learning about sexual intercourse and pregnancy. Parents revealed that it was an area where they felt very uncertain how to help their child because of the learning difficulty. They and governors were very supportive.

Once the sessions had begun, team-planning and review became the key to the success of the project. The team needed regular opportunities to discuss outcomes and explore their own feelings about difficulties which arose. The school had to make a commitment to release staff for planning and follow-up sessions in addition to timetabled drama sessions for at least a year. The role of the team leader and actors was crucial as they had time to take away the plans drawn up each week and transform them into a detailed drama session.

In the light of student reactions expectations were revised. It became clear that the students needed to spend more time than planned on some issues, so that the course was not completed within the year. The drama group could not make the same commitment for the following year but agreed to give support if one of the school's teachers could take over as team-leader. A new development plan was drawn up for the existing group of pupils and for other, less able students who had moved into the age group. The initiative became the blueprint for a sex education programme throughout the school.

Box 4 Case example

Teacher training

One beneficial outcome of the 1970 Education Act was the establishment of graduate teacher training courses for those wishing to specialize in the teaching of SLD pupils, to ensure that those who had taught SLD children in Junior Training Centres could become fully qualified teachers and that teaching became a graduate profession regardless of the type of pupil being taught. At first-degree level the courses also attracted young, enthusiastic, aspiring teachers keen to make a career in special education. These graduates started teaching with a good grounding in current research and methods and an understanding of SLD pupils' needs.

LEA budgets also had funds earmarked

for additional training which supported the secondment of existing teachers on specialist postgraduate courses or allowed schools to assist teachers wishing to attend in-service short courses.

By 1985, most teachers in the SLD sector were well qualified and SLD pupils benefited from a high level of understanding of their needs, skills in planning IEPs and appropriate teaching methods.

Post-1985 and coinciding with the increase in integrated places for special needs pupils, initial teacher training courses specializing in the teaching of SLD pupils were discontinued. By 1991 the last course had been phased out. Initial training courses now contain a special needs component intended to meet the needs of all teachers but which may be more relevant to the needs of the mainstream. At the same time, funding restrictions within LEAs and demographic changes in the general school population created a need to relocate redundant teachers to other phases of education, including special schools.

As these changes took place it became more difficult to recruit new staff with experience of SLD needs. Whilst secondary teachers brought welcome expectations of age-appropriate experiences and environment for secondary-aged pupils, they needed considerable support from experienced colleagues in planning for pupils with multiple and complex needs. They also needed opportunities for specialist training.

Secondments have largely been replaced by part-time distance-learning courses as teachers have become increasingly responsible for the cost of their own postgraduate study. Schools now receive delegated funding for training, but most is likely to be school-based. The lack of opportunity to meet others working in the SLD field outside the school makes it more difficult to share ideas and SLD schools in small LEAs may be quite isolated.

There is cause for concern that unless funding initiatives directly support specific SLD training and encourage teachers to enter SLD schools, it will be difficult to provide skilled teaching to meet the specialized needs of these pupils in the future.

Other changes affecting provision

Delegated funding
Since 1994, governing bodies of special schools receive a delegated budget to meet day-to-day running costs. Only capital costs and the costs of some services such as educational psychology are met centrally.

Schools have considerable freedom in the expenditure of the budget and delegation has created opportunities for development. Staff costs are large but governors can now appoint more flexibly according to the current needs of the school. Savings in one area can meet urgent needs in another. Classroom resources, often underfunded in the past, can be replaced or the refurbishment of a classroom can take place without endless negotiation with the LEA.

On the other hand, much of the administrative work undertaken at LEA level is now devolved to schools and centrally based resources (e.g. for curriculum support) may no longer exist. It remains to be seen whether the level of funding is maintained or whether the ability to allocate the budget according to the perceived needs of the school will create greater diversity between SLD schools and maintain opportunities for pupils.

OFSTED inspections
The Education (Schools) Act 1992, 1992) set up procedures for regular independent

inspection of maintained schools to replace systems established by LEAs and HMIs.

Teams of inspectors report on all aspects of the school's organization and teaching, after observation of the day-to-day work of the school and examination of relevant documents on policy, curriculum and financial management. Governors and parents are invited to meetings with the inspectors and, at the end of the inspection, the governing body must circulate the inspectors' report on the school to each parent. This report is brief and formal and judges performance in the light of pupil capabilities and national standards. It highlights strengths and areas for improvement which schools are required to remedy.

It is too early to judge how well a scheme with the National Curriculum at its core will serve the needs of SLD pupils, but inspection will undoubtedly influence the way schools plan their approach.

Approaching Work in a Special School

The team approach

The Warnock Report in 1978 identified the importance of partnership between the three major statutory services involved in the provision and care of children with special needs. More recently, the 1993 Education Act and the Code of Practice have imposed a statutory duty on LEAs, Health and Social Services to co-operate in 'effective action' on behalf of the child with special needs, recognizing the contribution which they can make to the provision of appropriate support to both child and parents.

The nurse and social worker appointed to a special school are valued members of the school community which has high expecta-

tions of what they can achieve. The ability to support children and families in areas of which school staff may have limited knowledge and experience can, by itself, provide the basis for a satisfactory partnership. More interesting and rewarding partnerships may also result through the exploration and development of team work.

The school views the child as an individual with the potential to learn but for whom the disability is a complicating factor in the learning process. It seeks to enable the child to operate in society with increasing autonomy and, through recognition of individuality and personal strengths, to encourage the child's sense of identity, ability to make choices and social awareness.

To achieve these aims the school is very dependent on the co-operation and goodwill of parents and upon other services to support and supplement the work. For example, the amount of speech, occupational or physiotherapy provided by the local Health Authority is governed by factors outside the influence of the Education Service and varies considerably from school to school.

Organizational structures and communication

Anyone working within a school setting has to be sensitive to the structures within which they are working. Ethos, organization, staff ratios, class groupings, staff training and expertise vary from school to school and can change over time within one school. Differences between one part of a service and another are not unique to education but they do demand a degree of flexibility from anyone working within or with the organization if co-operative working patterns are to be established. Many schools will be equally willing to consider new patterns of working if it can be made clear how their pupils will benefit.

In a hierarchical organization, the channels of communication may be very tightly established so that all information is passed through the head or deputy head. At the other extreme may be organizations where access to any member of staff is acceptable but there is no guarantee that information will be transmitted to others who need to know. Most schools have a system which lies between the two. It is always helpful to identify someone on the staff who will be the point of contact and liaise reliably between school staff and the peripatetic worker.

Since the hours and conditions of service vary so considerably between workers in Education, Health and Social Services, it is important to have a good job description that is understood by the service within which one is operating. For instance, the role of a social worker is considerably affected by the numbers of hours worked and the school needs to understand how the time can be deployed. A post that is jointly funded across services may create quite different working relationships and responsibilities. Hopefully, the job description has been jointly negotiated and will allow for future development to meet the needs identified both by the school and the worker. This flexibility is much more likely to produce a dynamic and rewarding partnership for all involved.

Getting to know the school

Schools should have a statement of aims and this could be a starting point to understanding where the school's priorities lie (see Appendix). It would be naive to believe that every individual within the organization will keep in mind or share these aims and it is difficult initially to understand how these aims are translated into the general work of the school and programmes for children.

In my view, the best way to get to know the school is to spend time observing and helping in classrooms. Knowledge of individuals – staff, children, parents and regular visitors – can be built into a clearer picture of the school. Insight can be gained into the varying needs of children and into differing styles of teaching and organization. It can also provide an opportunity for closer contact between the new member of the 'team' and other staff members forming the basis of future working relationships. Schools might find it difficult to introduce new members in this way or the demands of the post may not allow time, but it is often the quickest way to get a feel for the school.

It can also be helpful to attend staff meetings, sit in on educational reviews of children and attend staff training sessions. Some of these activities may become integral to the normal working pattern.

To understand fully the child's capabilities, the child needs to be observed in a number of settings of which the school is only one. Children may reveal strengths and weaknesses at school which are not demonstrated elsewhere and vice versa.

By focusing on the child, the school nurse and social worker can also arrive at a better understanding of the full range of needs. The needs of most children (particularly as they get older) cannot be fully met within a school day or within the family setting. Most need after-school clubs, holiday play schemes, experiences away from home. Some need a range of equipment or services in their own home and many families need assistance with the management of the child. These may be areas requiring close liaison with other services through links made and supported by the nurse and social worker (Figure 5.2).

Roles and responsibilities

Many aspects of the work undertaken by the school social worker or nurse (whether

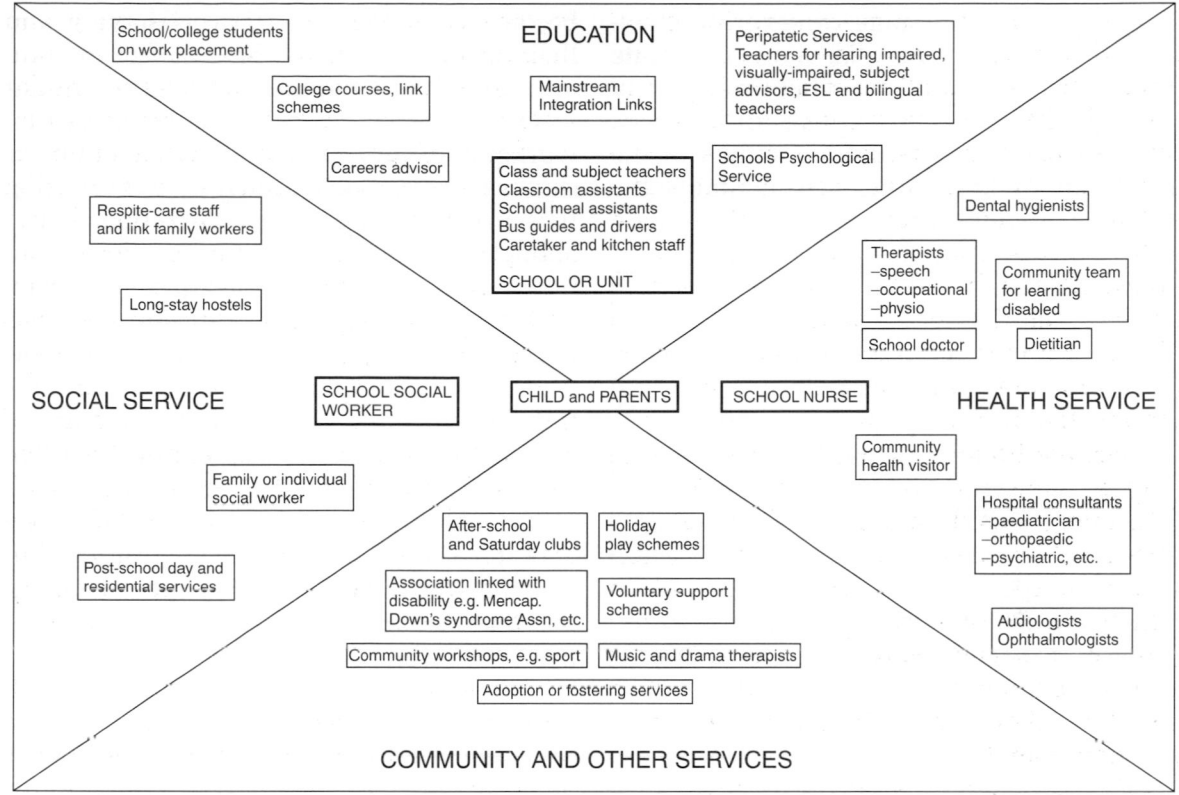

Figure 5.2 Outline of the involvement of services with each child. ESL, English second language

with a general or specialist training) will be those expected from any member of that profession and will be clearly understood by all those working in the school setting.

The social worker will receive referrals from the parents or the school when difficulties arise about benefits, respite care and other services available to disabled children, and will be called upon when family emergencies arise. However, because of the severity of the disability, the social worker needs to have as much information as possible about a variety of solutions and situations since each child may present a new set of problems. For example, respite-care hostels cannot always take the most profoundly disabled or behaviourally disturbed children either as an emergency or for long-term care. Doctors, making an assessment for the attendance allowance, may interpret the regulations with regard to the child's mobility to the disadvantage of some families. Appropriate advice to the parent at the time of the assessment or support during the appeal procedure can influence the outcome to the advantage of the disabled child and family.

There will be referrals where the problems are far from clear. Occasionally, children coming into school each morning are poorly or inadequately dressed. Incontinent children may be dirty or dishevelled when they arrive. The class teacher or headteacher will usually contact the parents in the first instance to try to resolve the problem, but where it persists there will be concern about the family situation. This may centre upon parental attitudes towards the child or upon fear that the carer is entering a stage of severe depression. The answers may be more mundane or more complex but the school staff rarely have time either to explore or to seek solutions to family situations which in the long term could be quite detrimental to the child's well-being and progress.

Two children with profound disabilities attended the school regularly but over time the bus guide reported that the children were rarely ready when the bus arrived. Their attendance became less regular and they showed signs of physical neglect, being less clean and well-dressed. It was known that the mother was pregnant. Previous contacts had shown her to be caring and concerned. The family were recent immigrants and non-English speaking. When the social worker visited she discovered that the problems of washing, feeding and dressing two totally dependent children were overwhelming the mother in the last stages of pregnancy. The problem was compounded by the attitudes towards disability within her own community which left her feeling guilty and unsupported even by her own husband and family. The social worker arranged for help to get the children up and ready for school and took on the role of befriending and counselling the mother. It was more difficult to find appropriate support systems within the community so that the parents felt less isolated.

Box 5 Case example

Because of the additional dimension resulting from the disability it is extremely difficult to judge whether sudden changes in children's behaviour result from changes in the school or home situation or from changes within the child. Some children become very distressed at certain stages in their school life, developing self-mutilating or aggressive behaviour. The school might discuss the changes with the school social worker and nurse, to decide whether action can or need be taken jointly or individually. It is important to keep a very open mind about what is happening because investigations into the family background which destroy trust between professionals and family are rarely beneficial to the child. Actions which appear critical of the family's handling of the child may create great bitterness in parents struggling to cope with problems quite outside most people's experience.

Both social worker and nurse can become the repository of much confidential knowledge. The greater the degree of trust the more both parents and teachers will divulge in their regular discussions about individual children. Their fears and concerns about how the other works with the child may be stated. This requires great sensitivity on the part of the social worker or nurse, so that school and home can still work in harmony.

The nurse will have a considerable role in dealing with attitudes and feelings around major conditions such as epilepsy, heart conditions and self-mutilation, and will be expected to be a source of information on the lesser known conditions and syndromes. These expectations may be unreasonable (and a good medical dictionary may help to solve the problem) but both parents and staff within schools sometimes feel inadequate in dealing with the child if they do not understand the underlying cause. Where fits are severe, or a child has a severe accident, breathing difficulties or a heart attack, the immediate attention given to the child (such as taking the child to hospital) often needs to be followed up with staff training either as a whole or in the classroom as part of the day-to-day work. As these situations occur, the school nurse may take on these responsibilities but the responsibility can become overwhelming. Sometimes, even nurse managers and headteachers need to be reminded that the school nurse needs support.

Other aspects of the nurse's work – arranging appointments, giving medication, monitoring the weight and general health of children, liaising with other parts of the school health service, dealing with cuts and bruises and minor injuries, encouraging parents to attend appointments both at school and at hospital, maintaining the medical records – also provide opportunities for liaison and joint support of the child.

Opportunities for collaborative working

For parents of children with special needs, the first contact with the special school and the child's subsequent admission may be the moment at which they realize the true extent of their child's disability. Some cannot accept the degree of disability or the assessment made of their child's needs. Others may be overwhelmed and show resignation/acceptance which is not necessarily to the child's advantage. This is a time when collaborative working between professionals can have a significant effect upon the child's future progress. School social worker and nurse have an important role to play in helping parents understand the degree of disability, in offering opportunities for discussion and counselling, in developing support services for carers, in providing and supporting channels of communication between family and school in their initial contacts. By being slightly apart from the school and school structure, the social worker and nurse can enable the parent to reveal anxieties, problems and even anger. As the child settles into school more

specific problems can often be dealt with best by collaborative working.

Naomi, an only child, was admitted to school at age 4 years with a severe feeding problem. She resolutely refused to take food by mouth and at age 2 years, because of severe weight loss, had been recommended a special diet which was given by tube. Settling Naomi into school was the priority but the 4-hourly tube feeds required her to leave the group or interrupt other parts of her programme during the morning and afternoon sessions.

It was suggested that the school start a programme to introduce her to feeding by mouth using a spoonful of baby food. Naomi's mother became extremely anxious at the suggestion, so feeding by mouth was not pursued. Naomi was given opportunities to put her hands into food in the hope that she would take them to her mouth and begin to taste foods. She was not keen!

The school nurse (who works very closely with parents of nursery-aged children) began to monitor Naomi's weight regularly and tried to support the mother by helping her to understand that apart from the weight loss there were no medical reasons for Naomi to feed entirely by tube. She confirmed with the community health visitor and the hospital which Naomi attended that Naomi could be fed normally if we could establish a programme and maintain her weight.

After giving Naomi her special feed by cup on one or two occasions when she pulled the tube away, it was decided to try feeding by mouth again. This time a certain amount of the special feed was to be given by mouth at one feeding session a day. Her mother was willing for school to try but
Continued overleaf

continued
was not willing to do so at home. She remained anxious but had been reassured by the weighing programme and the willingness of school staff to co-operate with her.

About this time a school social worker was appointed and began to support Naomi's mother at home in a very general way. Everyone involved was kept informed about progress (and sometimes regression). When Naomi changed class the system of mutual support and collaborative working was transferred to the new class.

Naomi is not yet totally fed by mouth. At age 6 years she regularly takes one whole feed by cup, she occasionally takes a spoonful of other food, but is not always co-operative. The programme is likely to take a number of years but there is every possibility that it will eventually succeed if the different professionals continue to support Naomi's mother and each other.

Box 6 Case example

The school invariably seeks to work closely with the parents or carers of the child. However, the emphasis of their work with parents will be to help them to understand the child's abilities and needs, to help them work constructively with their own child and to explain the work of the school.

Parents need support over and beyond the support given by the school and a range of initiatives needs to be developed to support them at different stages of their child's school life and in their understanding of the disability. School nurses and social workers often find themselves in a unique position of trust with parents and families. For example, the school nurse may be thought to understand the problems of the most difficult children because the medical aspects of the disability may pose the great-

est problems or are believed to be the cause of all subsequent difficulties. The nurse or social worker may be seen as more sympathetic and less judgemental than the teacher who suggests management techniques!

In such cases the trust established can be wholly beneficial, providing working relations between all professionals within the school are positive and channels of communication to share information function well.

The possibilities for joint working are varied and may range from the support of an individual child as illustrated to supporting parents as a group and in different contexts. The amount of support that parents or carers need to pursue a programme that they may well understand to be in the child's best interest, but which creates additional stress and anxiety or which disrupts their own lifestyle, should not be underestimated. Joint home visiting by professionals is one way in which more realistic aims can be set and the need for support from the different services can be identified.

A child's need may appear more complex than it really is because it requires two or more services to collaborate in resolving the problem (see Box 7 for an example).

Attendance at annual education reviews and discussion of future needs with the parent has to be part of joint professional working. Apart from the evident advantage of sharing information first-hand, it can overcome some of the disadvantages which arise when several agencies are involved with a child (Figure 5.2 outlines agencies involved).

Reciting their child's life history again and again can be a difficult experience. If parents can hear from all involved at the same meeting they can avoid unnecessary repetition and obtain a fuller picture of their child's progress. Life changes, such as the need for respite care or post-school placements, can be discussed more fully if all agencies are represented. Furthermore, the parent can hear what is being said by all agencies.

A traveller's child was unable to get into school regularly because the family caravan was pitched in the centre of the site and the school bus could not reach it. The mother could not get the child to the site entrance because she could not leave two other disabled children. After working for several weeks in isolation, a case conference was called to resolve the problem jointly. The education transport manager could not justify over-spending his budget for an individual taxi and escort since transport was already provided. However, a bid for additional funding (allowed for the education of travellers) could go forward for the new financial year. The parent offered to find an unpaid escort from the site so that the cost of transport was reduced and social services agreed to look at short-term joint funding of the taxi if part of the cost could be met by the education service. Social services arranged for the installation of a phone in the caravan to enable the parent to cancel the taxi if it was not needed. The taxi was arranged and the child returned to school a week later maintaining good attendance thereafter.

Box 7 Case example

Responding jointly to individual need is one way forward but there are other initiatives which can be launched between services such as joint training to enable better joint planning and to increase co-operation and understanding of roles at all levels of operation – from managers of services through to field workers.

In my own school, workshops for parents were jointly planned at field-worker level by the parent liaison teacher and social worker. The initial coffee morning was used to identify how parents would like to use the regular meetings. Visits to the local respite-care hostel and Makaton signing workshops were identified. The latter led on to a video being made for the parents' use and expanded to the production of further videos of other curriculum areas, workshops in areas such as sex education which involved the school nurse and a parents' support group aiming to empower parents to meet their own needs.

Joint working is likely to be beneficial in working with children from ethnic minorities. Within my own LEA the range of countries and backgrounds represented is so numerous that workers with knowledge of one particular culture or language are not always available for advice and help. In addition, the range of needs of child and family might require sensitive and co-operative approaches to create a better understanding of the child's disability or of resources within the community. The school social worker or nurse may become the most trusted ally in making links into that community.

Working with the disabled child

Most initiatives involve work with parents and carers but opportunities also exist for work with pupils. The school nurse often has a vital role to play in dietary, health and sex education and may work very closely with groups of children. Much depends on the nurse's experience and willingness but it can provide opportunities to develop new skills and expertise.

The social worker too may have a role in support groups for older teenagers about to leave school or in the counselling of individual children. Support groups for siblings provide an extension of the role if opportunities and resources can be found.

Within the partnership which parents and professionals try to establish, there may well be misunderstandings as to the nature and extent of respective roles and of how far each professional can achieve the outcomes desired by other partners.

Parents and carers may have expectations that the teacher will succeed with the child and advise them on aspects of the child's functioning, but the child remains an individual whose progress may be impeded for any number of reasons. The child's disability may be such that normal developmental progress is not possible and the way forward is very difficult to determine. Organizational difficulties within a school, such as staff changes, absences or even pressure from other students, may affect the progress of children.

Similarly teachers may well expect social workers or nurses to have access to resources or additional services that are not necessarily available or operate to different time schedules from that expected by the school. Such misunderstandings may require considerable discussion in order to reach a more realistic appreciation of the way each service works.

Working within a school may mean adapting to new routines and structures. Hopefully, all involved will demonstrate flexibility and understanding, an ability to take and share responsibilities, and will share a commitment to partnership and team working.

Conclusions

Legislation during the past 10 years has supported and strengthened the rights of SLD children to receive education in an integrated or special setting to meet their needs. Parents' right to choice and partnership in the education of their children is formalized in the new Code of Practice, as are the duties of the education, health and social services to collaborate in the provision of resources.

The effect of other legislation on the role of special education and the special school is not yet clear. How will the delegation of funds from central LEA to individual school and the results of OFSTED inspection affect resources and the pattern of provision in the future? Will the flexibility funding brings to schools outweigh any disadvantages or, coupled with the parents' right to choice, will some schools gain reputation at the expense of others or become more selective of pupils if they can easily fill places? Will the statutory duties laid on health and social services ensure they fulfil their commitments to statemented pupils despite funding shortages?

Similarly, will work within the National Curriculum offer a more balanced curriculum to SLD pupils despite lack of support for its development in relation to these pupils? The IEP remains the accepted way to tailor the curriculum to individual need and work within the National Curriculum may occur in name rather than in reality.

Concerns about the future of specialized teacher training have already been raised. With the integration of more pupils into other types of provision, the needs of pupils within SLD schools become more complex. If teachers are to be fully effective they require specialized training if special needs pupils are to be given the opportunities that are their right.

Collaboration between professionals remains essential to ensure that SLD children and their parents benefit from team working whilst offering professionals mutually rewarding opportunities to develop new initiatives and extend their own skills.

Discussion Questions

- With increasing emphasis on the achievement of nationally recognized standards within a National Curriculum, is it realistic to suppose that integrated educational provision can meet the needs of children with severe learning difficulties?

- Do national funding and policy decisions, rather than the needs of children with special and severe needs, lead developments in the provision made for such children?
- How far might pressures at local level within each service limit the possibilities of collaborative approaches to the support of children with special needs?

Appendix

Some questions to consider in order to facilitate work in a school setting (see Figure 5.2).

- Is the post funded by one service or jointly by more than one (e g Social Services and Education)?
- Who is the line manager? To whom do I report and who will support me?
- Who are the key people with whom I should liaise?
- What kind of information should I share and what is confidential to my service?
- Are members of other services with whom I liaise aware that certain kinds of information are confidential to my service?
- Is the school clear about what my job description entails?
- How can I gain and share information with teachers closely involved with the children?
- Is there a teacher with whom I might develop work with parents?

- What written information about the school and pupils is available to me?
  school brochure
  school aims, policies and priorities
  staff and class lists
  parental involvement and support
  dates of terms and times of school day
  dates and times of staff meetings
  children's reports and programmes
  dates of annual reviews
  key people other than school staff
  working within the school setting
- Are there LEA policies with regard to special educational needs which I should know about?
- How can I observe children within the school setting and acquire greater understanding of the various disabilities?
- Can I (within my job description) take an informed and active part in school life? How can I support the work of the school to benefit individual children?
- Which other support services are most closely involved with the school/child? Are there opportunities for joint or collaborative working?
- How can I help school staff to understand my role and provide information about support available to children and families from my own service?
- What forms of parental support operate within the school and can I take part in them?
- How can I work within my own service to highlight the needs of children or young adults with severe learning difficulties?

References

1970. *Education Act (Handicapped Children)*. HMSO, London.
1978. *Report of the Committee of Enquiry into the Education of Handicapped Children and Young People.*

Special Education Needs (Warnock Report). Cmnd. 7212. HMSO, London.

1981. *Education Act 1981. Special Educational Needs.* HMSO, London.

1988. *The Education Reform Act, 1988.* HMSO, London.

1992. *Education (Schools) Act 1992*. HMSO, London.

1993. *Education Act 1993*. HMSO, London.

1994. *Code of Practice on the Identification and Assessment of Special Educational Needs.* HMSO, London.

1994. *Education (Special Education Needs) Regulations 1994*. Statutory Instrument No 1047. HMSO, London.

Chapter 6

The Community as an Arena for Shared Learning and Practice

Stephen J.G. Clarke

Key Issues

- Shared training and learning
- Understanding and defining community
- The development gap
- A model of practice: community social work

Introduction

It is during practice training that students come face to face with some of the contradictions between the theory and practice of their courses. There, they are able, if given the space, to evaluate for themselves the validity of some of the high-minded ideals of the classroom. Moreover, they are put in a position to discover how actual practice exposes some of the more vaunted claims of public policy. The results can breed uncertainty, which may undermine a qualifying student's confidence. The priority, then, will be to find a secure frame of reference on which to base future professional behaviour. Seldom are these factors more clearly felt than in the field of interdisciplinary collaboration. This is a concept about which most professionals express positive opinions in theory and yet few, if any, training programmes offer any provision to explore them.

Students who are qualifying today find themselves in the midst of the establishment of a new era for their professions. There has been massive restructuring in the thinking behind the provision of services for people with learning difficulties. This manifests itself most pointedly in Government policies about care in the community (DOH, 1989) and they have already had considerable effects on services for health and social work (UKCC, 1986; CCETSW, 1989). Today, few can predict just how it will all work out. This is especially so because many of the statements about new policies do not exactly 'fit' the earlier descriptions and expectations. There are still open questions concerning the value framework, the funding levels, the channels of communication and accountability. There are so many unknowns and they need to be resolved in practice at the workface, if effective services are to be provided. So, for today's student, there may be a desire to seek comfort in those aspects of practice training that offer the clearest picture and the most straightforward messages.

Not only are today's professionals expected to master their traditional skills and value systems, they must also be familiar with the potential of all other professionals in the field. They must be able to unlock that potential for the benefit of their service consumers by engaging in active co-operation across professional boundaries. Today, with the relocation of most major services out of the institution, the arena for professionals to practice together is in the community.

I hope to show here that, despite all the mixed messages and uncertainties, some of the risks attached to change are overstated. If the way forward for professionals in the field of learning difficulties is for interdisciplinary work, then students should actively seek out the opportunity for practice experience whilst in training. The opportunity to share supervised training with someone from another profession will prove to be the safest and most rewarding change to gain the necessary experience for the real challenges of post-qualifying/registration practice.

Deploying new-style services in the community will continue to have great impact on the way professionals work. For many decades, professionals have been working on perfecting 'professional' models of practice. While this has, to a certain extent, required that the facts of community life be taken on board, the self-image of most professionals has been more inward looking. At worst, the community has been taken for granted as a passive element in the exclusive process of professional minis-

try. At best, it has either been put on 'hold' or engaged in tokenistic ways. The development of professional practice was supported by statute. This increasingly dictated that the presenting problems of patients and clients should be best dealt with using the most efficient, 'clinical' skills or legal processes. Training programmes reinforced this. For example, since 1970 training for nursing and social work staff has become systematic, highly specialized and founded on progressive ethical principles; it can also be said that their ways are far better understood within the profession than outside them.

Now that the Government has clarified its ideas about the future of services, it has become apparent that the drive for excellence within the professions has not progressed along quite the same lines. To the extent that it has, it has not gone far enough (Audit Commission, 1992). This obviously reflects underlying differences in principle. However, it also reveals that in interdisciplinary work there is now a considerable gap between the needs of future services and the basic training that is being provided. Øvretveit (1993) describes in vivid detail the types of professional (multidisciplined) formation that are emerging as health and social welfare systems respond to the 'mixed economy of welfare'. The management of professionals through a wide variety of mechanisms, from integrated multidisciplinary structures, to arms-length, multisupplier contracts, points to the need for professionals to receive a thorough understanding, at the earliest possible opportunity, of the complexities of interdisciplinary co-operation and insight into the role, skills and expectations of complementary professional activity in their field. Stewart (1993) reports that there is considerable professional reluctance to implement these culture changes at the level of training. Nevertheless, despite these negative attitudes that have impeded any really fruitful developments to date, there are openings where qualifying students can obtain useful and demanding experience in interdisciplinary work. Shared training is possible at this level if the effort is made.

Shared Training

Policy-makers have been surprisingly coy in making positive recommendations about training across professional lines. In 1980, it was the Secretary of State for Social Services who invited the General Nursing Council (GNC) and the Council for Education and Training in Social Work (CCETSW) to look into the general training needs of staff caring for people with a mental handicap (GNC/CCETSW, 1982). Almost three decades later, these accreditation bodies have still done little to produce a framework for progress.

There has been some purposeful interest at the workplace and on the margins of official recognition (CETHV, 1979; England, 1979). Seminars and information exchanges have taken place. But the overriding attitude has been one of benign neglect. This is particularly regrettable as major changes have been taking place in the structure of both nursing and social work qualifying training (UKCC, 1986). These new approaches to training now formally recognize, and explicitly state, the need for inter-professional contact. Changes in public policy relating to the provision of Health and Welfare Services and also to the educational needs of the nation may prove to be much more persuasive and far less respectful of these established professional boundaries. For example, Sections 5 and 8 of *Working Together* (DHSS and Welsh Office, 1988; DHSS, 1989) spell out in great detail the degree of co-operation and training that is required. Today's training at qualifying level appears oblivious to these requirements.

The establishment of the National Council for Vocational Qualifications (NCVQ) in 1986 was to bring cohesion and purpose to the nation's vocational training mechanisms. The exact relationship between the 'professions' of nursing, social work and 'vocational training' has still to be finalized but the strong industrial outlook and links of the NCVQ have already forced many changes of attitude. The vocational training model is looking to create a framework of training for role flexibility, modular learning and the transferability of credits from one sector to another. National levels of competency in the skills of each occupation will be agreed.

In the White Paper *Caring for People* the following quotation underlines the trend:

It will be important to continue to develop multi-disciplinary training for staff in all caring professions, including the provision of joint training at both the qualifying and post-qualifying stages.

(DHSS, 1989)

Developments such as the accreditation by the NCVQ in 1996 of NVQs at levels 2, 3 and 4 in community work may assist this process, but so much is down to the managerial preferences of the service purchasers within the 'mixed economy' (Mayo, 1994; Wistow *et al.*, 1994) that it may in the end depend on individual professionals taking time out themselves in order to upgrade their skills and understanding.

The GNC/CCETSW Joint Working Group's Reports (GNC/CCETSW, 1982, 1983) specifically ruled out shared training for certain qualifying programmes. At the time, the college-based CQSW qualifying route for social workers was thought to be unsuitable owing mainly to the lack of a specific knowledge base. They did, nevertheless, suggest that further work be done, especially for the in-service qualifying route for social workers (Certificate in Social Service).

CCETSW and the English National Board for Nursing (ENB) produced a fresh report in 1987. This projected six possible models, three of which could be integrated into the emerging restructured proposals for qualifying training for nurses and social workers (ENB and CCETSW, 1987). The report also suggested that renewed public discussion takes place.

It is obvious that the priorities for the accreditation bodies in nursing and social work should be directed each towards their own new qualifying programmes. The proposals for the Diploma in Social Work (DipSW) (CCETSW, 1989, Revised edn 1991, pp. 20, 27) makes explicit the requirements that in future social workers should be trained to provide them with interdisciplinary skills. At a national level, CCETSW established a working group to investigate the requirements and needs of practice teachers if they work across professional boundaries. And so, as Project 2000 and DipSW training programmes take shape and learn from the experience of their early crop of graduates, there is interest to discover whether or not there are signs that things are gradually moving. Weinstein (1994, p. 32) concludes that 'initiatives from below', may be the only answer in the short term, and that they may not be adopted as models for concerted professional training.

An earlier discussion paper issued in conjunction with CCETSW states that it is *impossible* to train social workers

... for a multi-disciplinary approach in isolation from other professional groups or service users ... training methods must themselves be multi-disciplinary.
 (Inter-Disciplinary Assn and CCETSW, 1989, p. 5)

It goes on to outline what it calls the social worker's 'distinctive contribution' (*ibid,*

p. 11). This includes the abilities to instigate 'community action' and to undertake networking activities with the voluntary sector and thus to increase the range of effectiveness and resources of the team's work. These statements introduce some controversial questions which are dealt with in more detail below, but this seems to bear out Weinstein's predictions (above). Suffice it to say that the fruits of a pioneering experiment in Wales in the early 1990s were not capitalized upon (Clarke, 1991). Here, groups of students from social work and nursing (learning difficulties specialists) undertook practice learning together, under the supervision of qualified workers from both professions. When working together, each group spontaneously adopted a similar model of social intervention (a socially developmental approach) instead of a more individualistic, or clinical, form (Clarke and Lile, 1990). This is discussed below in 'A model for practice'.

The Community as an Arena

One area where there has been prolonged public discussion and debate is the concept of 'community'. The term itself is an emotive one – from within academic disciplines such as sociology (Stacey, 1969) – between structuralists, functionalists and/or systems analysts; and Social Policy with Community Care, Community Health, Community Enterprise, European Community, to the practical level of service provision: community homes, community care, and the nature of the Welfare State itself. These are all issues of critical importance to us, but the terms themselves illustrate how mere possession of the term 'community' seems to create an image of added potency. If all are claiming that 'community' describes the essential ingredient of the issue or activity, then it follows that all those practising in the field must have a well-versed understanding of what it means. From this understanding will flow the necessary insight to create the most needed services and professional support. The difficulty arises when every slogan that lays claim to the word requires a new interpretation and decoding. Few captors of the idea demonstrate any desire to subscribe to commonly held definitions. Many are patently avoiding too precise a message as to what they mean. This has been called the 'Community Prefix Syndrome' (Barr, 1989):

'When I use a word,' Humpty Dumpty said in a rather scornful tone, 'it means just what I choose it to mean – neither more nor less.'

The Government has designed its whole strategy for Health and Social Services with care in the community in mind. Even people with acute needs, who are dependent on institutional care, are being assessed against the feasibility of an appropriate service being available in the community. The trend away from institutionalization appears to be irreversibly set. But, whereas the trend may now be clear, the form of the replacement services has still to be worked out. Likewise, the relationship of these services to the community is left vague, as is the definition of the sort of community within which they operate. The battle over the definition of community care has begun. It is in the climate of this debate that the next generation of trainees will have its skills assessed.

The move towards a form of community care began in the late 1950s with the Report of the Royal Commission on Mental Illness (Royal Commission, 1957) and the subsequent Mental Health Act, 1959. The framework envisaged was for the *site* of service and care to be moved. This implied some changes in the form of care (e.g. from in-patient drug therapy to out-patient treat-

ment) but it did not necessarily imply any changes in the *nature* of care. Eleven years after the passing of this Act, the Seebohm Report stated:

. . . the widespread belief that we have 'community care' of the mentally disordered is, for many parts of the country, still a sad illusion and . . . will remain so for many years ahead.

(Seebohm, 1970)

It went on to say that the 'promise of community care is considerable' (*ibid*, para 340). This is a promise that Governments are still legislating for in the 1990s. Because of the delays in implementation described above (Audit Commission, 1992), the Department of Health has published a Green Paper (DOH, 1997) which will force greater co-operation amongst fundholders and the creation of a more unified service for people with a mental health difficulty. This may force the issue for service planners and purchasers. It would, if implemented, reduce professional reliance on the elusive and unspecified 'community', but it will create more intensified pressures elsewhere. 'Care in the community' by more highly integrated health and professional services will not work just because it has been decreed. Lack of integrated training and the burden on the community of the 'residual needs gap' between service resources and the actual level of need in the community will make the plight of those excluded all the more acute (Clarke, 1996).

Changes in the location of services have been shadowed by changes in the thinking about the nature of service as well. The thinking of those providing the services, and others directly involved, have made huge contributions to changes in the value system at work (All Wales Working Party, 1982). In society at large, questions about the nature and quality of services became bound up in the debate about the role of the citizen and the *control* of those services.

It had become painfully obvious to large sections of our society that technocratic solutions often did not work and, if they did, they did not bring the benefits to the direct consumer in the way in which they had been promoted (IDC, 1982, 1984; Kings Fund, 1980, 1984). The wholesale destruction of many inner-city communities under the powers of the Housing Act 1957 is a good example. The conflicting interests of community and 'urban renewal' could not be reconciled, even with designer mechanisms to achieve consensus (Skeffington, 1969). In that case, the slogan was 'participation'. Today they are 'community' and 'community care'.

All who work in, or plan services for, Health or Social Services have a vested interest in the existence of 'community' and yet it is one of those abstract social phenomena which defies precise identification. As we have seen, the term is being bandied about and we can discern very interesting shifts in meaning as the process develops.

We may understand 'community' in a number of ways. Each definition has implications for the conception and planning of subsequent actions. All contain implicit value judgements which must be carried along through any subsequent developments.

The most common definition of community concerns the geographical location of human settlement. A non-geographical use of this description can easily lead to assumptions which have not been validated. For example, to imply that all those who live within particular boundaries are both aware of, and value that association may be suggesting far too much.

The idea that in a complex industrial society the notion of community could provide a basis for shared values (and hence for consistent social policies) is erroneous.
(Pinker, 1982, p. 241)

Here, Professor Pinker was making a statement about the form in which social care should be organized. If he is right, then he raises the question about that other definition of community, the 'community of interest'. This definition draws upon the ties and relationships which people make for themselves out of common cause or circumstances.

Willmott (1986) considers this aspect of social life in great detail. He investigates the complexity of relationships that can and do exist between people – relationships of family, work, common talent and self-help, etc. In a later work, Willmott covers a wider scenario and includes case studies to illustrate the extent to which relationships can extend beyond the immediate network of every day life (Willmott, 1989). He draws out what distinguishes those associations to which people are attached: the degree to which they feel a sense of identity with either a place and/or group. He describes how these relationships are dependent on the particular priorities and circumstances of the individual. He endorses Professor Pinker when he states that these distinctions

put us on our guard against the almost mythical feelings that can be stirred by the work community.
(Willmott, 1989, p. 4)

In extending the analysis in this way, Willmott opens up the question of power relationships within systems. He draws particular attention to the power implications behind the definitions of community care. Those with power have the freedom to define the community and to allocate resources/services to it. Such is the explicit intention of the White Paper *Caring for People* when it states as its first 'key change' for funding arrangement that it will be ' . . . within available resources' that collaborative care assessment, service design and delivery will be carried out (DHSS, 1989).

In May, 1990, the BBC 'File on Four' (BBC transcript, 15th May, 1990) programmes studied the implementation of this policy in Kent. They discovered that clients of the pilot home care service who no longer fell within the priority category (DHSS, 1989) could not afford the alternative services in the private sector to which they were directed. This was despite the bridging payments which they received in lieu of home care. For these people, community care is no care!

Community care also provides the clearest example of the gap between promise and performance.

(Willmott, 1989, p. 64)

If the people who are in this situation are to obtain assistance, they must rely on other mechanisms. These may be family, friends or voluntary organizations. They may offer their contribution out of loyalty, love or sense of duty. Their wish or ability to make their contribution may change with their own circumstances. Some of them may be bound into a caring or dependent relationship by forces over which they have little or no control. Is this the 'community' that must fill in the gaps in the community care tapestry?

It is also obvious from our social experience that there are a multitude of social and care networks within our society. Many of them link people who have little direct contact with each other – family ties, members of extended associations such as sporting bodies or, of interest to us, disability or professional associations. And yet all these relationships make their contribution to the quality of life of their members and also the other members of society.

Thus, any individual may be 'attached' in sentiment or by tangible links to a complex web of groupings and networks. But, at the same time, that contact is highly individual and dependent on the will of all concerned to sustain it. If this is the ground on which the basis of community care is founded then intensive effort is needed to consolidate it into something more stable and reliable.

Abrams et al. (1986) conducted research into the nature of neighbourhood care schemes. They concluded that this form of care 'did not just happen' (ibid, p. 73). Neither did people generally look to their immediate community for care and support. They also showed that the physical, economic and social conditions in each neighbourhood would all go into producing very different local capacities and forms of care. Anyone concerned with planning and developing locally run services must indeed have a very thorough and sensitive understanding of these local conditions and capacities (ibid, p. 67). Attempts to standardize these forms of care may be doomed to fail.

Heginbotham (1990) suggests conditions under which these factors can be both encouraged and enhanced. He outlines the present relationship between the voluntary sector and the funding agencies of Government and emphasizes the problems of the unequal power relationship and the leverage that that can exert (ibid, p. 60). The exploitation of voluntary effort and the corruption of its goals must be one of the largest issues facing non-state services in the dawning era of the 'contract culture'.

Griffiths developed his proposals for a 'mixed economy' (Griffiths, 1988, p. 82) of welfare in his paragraphs on the voluntary sector. He makes explicit the need to supply organizations drawn into care in this way with stability of funding and clear planning guidelines (ibid, p. 26). These sentiments are endorsed in the White Paper (DHSS, 1989) but in less strenuous terms than Griffiths'. The only specific attention that is given to creating sympathetic conditions for voluntary or self-help organizations is for services being planned for ethnic minorities (Griffiths, 1988, p. 26).

If community life is as complex as Abrams claims, it is interesting, to say the least, that this question should be approached as an isolated issue. Does this imply that minorities are normally excluded from services, or that they will/may be excluded in some future state of community care? There is certainly no mention of the racism that besets our community and the differential way in which services are delivered (Williams, 1994). The problem of planning and delivering sensitive and responsible services to multicultural and diverse communities requires a deal more attention to detail than the framers of these policies concede.

The entanglement of strategies for community care and the lack of clarity about their value base, ride heavily over what we know of the nature and facility of community life. If the undoubted goodwill of carers, voluntary groups and the neighbourhood at large is to be retained and enlisted for the benefit of the less able amongst us, then policy-makers must engage actively in the question instead of hiding behind assumptions and prescriptions.

To counter this, Heginbotham (1990, p. 10) calls for a communitarian approach by self-help and voluntary bodies. We are then left with the question 'how?'. Etzioni (1993, 1995) and Atkinson (1995) describe how suitably resourced communities (i.e. the middle class suburbs) can well provide for themselves in this way through the exploitation of commonly understood values and easily accessed networks. Their investment is in the strengthened community with resilient and capable organizations and the proper social care provisions to meet people's needs. Communities with the greatest levels of unmet need, often predicated on poverty, will not find this a panacea. If one of the objectives of community care should be an empowered consumer, not an encapsulated dependant, then professionals will have to become receptive to values and practices that maximize their resource pool, despite the institutionalized administrative structures which are still powerfully resisting change in this direction.

The Development Gap

We have described how service providers are attempting to explore some of the unknown frontiers of professional care through the framework of interdisciplinary training and activity. We have heard from the experts on 'community' and the cautionary approach that they would take towards implementing community care without considerable changes in attitude. Nevertheless, we are faced with the continuing implementation of these policies from now on, regardless of party political leadership. Now that they have begun to take effect, it will not be possible to turn the clock back. Our purpose, therefore, must be to seek the best way forward to try to avoid as many of the pitfalls as we can.

The Government's proposals contained no apologies. They made no concessions towards the wider community for the de-institutionalization of some of its most needy members and the total re-organization of the care services for everyone. In fact, the White Paper (DHSS, 1989) goes so far as to state that, for the voluntary sector, some of their activities are not suitable for contractual funding (i.e. not considered to be part of community care).

Foremost in this list is 'development work' (DHSS, 1989, p. 24) but they do allow that Local Authorities may wish to grant aid voluntary organizations towards their 'administrative expenses'.

The initial failure of the Government to 'ring-fence' community care funds against re-allocation by Local Authorities (*The Times*, 29 June, 1990), later gave way to the 'ring fencing' of most specialist budgets. This produced service rigidities, some career stability, but yet more frustration for those seeking more community, and in particular, consumer participation (Beresford and Croft, 1993). The Court of Appeal's decision to uphold the right of the Minister of the Environment to poll-tax cap Local Authorities (*The Times*, 28 June, 1990), did not create a favourable outlook – especially for agencies which had hoped to engage in more diverse activities. Earlier, the 1989 White Paper stated that, in order to take on the responsibilities of contractual funding, they (the voluntary organizations) may need to make major changes into the way they work. Perhaps some activities may have to go altogether. The rest may be tied in so closely through contracts and financial conditions that they allow no flexibility, development or criticism of the system.

There is no mention in the revised regulations for the training of social workers or nurses (CCETSW, 1989; ENB, 1989; WNB, 1989) of training for development work. Nurses had been specifically identified as 'community workers' in the White Paper (DHSS, 1989, p. 39) and so it is sad that they are not going to receiving any preparation at pre-registration level. For social workers, the marginalization of community development has all but run its course. Since the re-organization of training which began in 1975, programmes which offered specialisms in community development have all but been eliminated. By 1982, only one dedicated diploma remained and that, too, now survives only in a disguised form (CCETSW, 1977). Either the accreditation bodies are in collusion with the sentiments expressed by Mrs Thatcher to the Church of Scotland in 1988 'I don't believe in Society – just in people and their families' (*Guardian*, 17 June, 1988) or they are terribly adrift

from reality. Their constituency, the nurses and social workers, and those bound into relationships with them, their clients, will fall into the huge gap between need and the capacity to respond. Some branch of Health or Social Service must commit itself to the wider interests of the communities into which community care is to be precipitated. To ignore this need is to ignore all the advice that social work has been giving itself since 1968.

The Seebohm Report (Seebohm, 1970) devoted a chapter to the needs of the community as a whole. It drew attention to the then current diagnosis of the declining inner cities. The report highlighted the benefits that accrue to citizens and service-providers alike when the general quality of social interaction is improved. The report drew attention to the positive influence that community development interventions could bring (pp. 148–52). Despite the negative response of government to the 7-year Community Development Project (Loney, 1983) and its suggestions that the problems of society were rooted in structural causes rather than in the pathology of individuals, there have been less confrontational attempts to introduce the concept of development into the networks. Most notable amongst these are the Gulbenkian Foundation (Calouste Gulbenkian, 1968) and the Working Party set up by the Secretary of State for Social Services in 1980) – the Barclay Committee (Barclay, 1982). In parallel with the deliberations of CCETSW to devise new training guidelines for social work, The National Institute for Social Work has been sponsoring a steadily developing stream of theoretical and practical guides to a new methodology – 'community social work'.

Community social work is discussed below, but it is worth recording at this stage that it represents a complete break with the traditional *casework* approach to social work. It builds its own model for 'good practice' around the structures in the community (Smale *et al.*, 1988) but there is evidently still much uncertainty about its credentials. Bamford, in his book on a possible future role for social work (Bamford, 1990), offers some descriptions of the contenders in this discussion. In the final account, however, he redefines the future for social workers without any reference to a developmental role. Counselling, case management and service planning are the order of the day. These priorities are in stark contrast to the representatives of the *consumer* in one specified priority area in the White Paper – people with learning difficulties.

The IDC (IDC, 1986) defines quality in terms of the following: the degree to which a service empowers the users; the level to which the consultation and participation process involves the widest possible constellation of 'stakeholders', including the local community; and the extent to which the service user can be assisted to live 'an ordinary life' (Kings Fund, 1980). It is sad to report that, even in the *All Wales Strategy for the Development of Services for People with a Mental Handicap* (Welsh Office, 1983), the pressure on service providers has not been to build up the consumer and advocate dimension of the strategy (Hawker, 1988).

In 1989, the Government reconstituted the entire membership of CCETSW. This defused any reaction to the Government's refusal to accept the proposed 3-year training scheme (QDSW). The new Council meekly accepted a 2-year qualifying model. One is not aware of how interested the community at large is in these developments in social work. The problem is that the profession does not seem to be in any shape to make a stand for itself – not even on issues which are of the greatest possible importance to their service consumers. However, the case for 3-year training is still being pressed by CCETSW, which also lends its voice to the creation of a General Social Services Council (the brainchild of the newly founded British Association of Social Workers, in the early 1970s). It seems that they have a limited amount of influence over professional matters with the responsible Minister. When the implications of community care are felt in the community, *by the community*, they will have to lodge their own protest if they want to find an effective champion for their cause.

A Model for Practice

We have seen how there is now pressure on professionals to work closely together – in the community – and that training at qualifying/registration level must be restructured to assist this development. The current structure of social service teams placed the vast majority of qualified staff in 'fieldwork' (Local Government Training Board, 1986) and working in a community setting of one kind or another. This is still true despite the 'mixed economy of welfare' (Wistow *et al.*, 1994), and the necessity for many to find themselves either in a social planning role (conceptualizing and managing contracts), or on the fringes of this as assessors of need for the purchasing authority. Contemporary reviews of nursing services have underlined the same trend. Words like 'proactive' and 'prevention' abound and one can readily discern the pressure towards creating autonomy of spirit as well as autonomy of role in the culture of community nurses: whether as practice nurses in primary health care teams or in specialist deployments (DHSS, 1986). This process was underlined in the citation of 'community workers' given to community nurses which was referred to earlier. The homeless and local community groups are seen as target areas, and the development of new services is seen as the logical extension of the role (DHSS, 1986). The other heavily emphasized aspect of skill requirements is the development of team-work.

In many instances, these trends mark new departures in nursing as they move part of their function away from a purely 'curative' role. For social workers, in theory at least, they represent a significant part of their current repertoire. In practice, this claim may prove to be rather hollow. In addition, they have claimed to be providing the resources for empowerment, networking, promoting participation and understanding the processes of oppression (CCETSW, 1989). For social work, at a time of great change in the provision of care and social support services, it would appear that these are the attributes that should be given the highest profile. We suspect that these attributes are those which are being submerged under a tide of new priorities due to restructuring, new legislation and lack of professional will. If they are to be employed to their greatest effect, a great deal of re-orientation will have to take place in the minds of workers and also in the policies of employers. Other, more highly specialized, skills of community-based professionals can then be much better utilized if there is a common base of competence and understanding. Training will have to be completely revamped to meet this need.

The crucial question now, is how best to deploy these resources so that they can meet the often conflicting demands: professional values, employer's policies and resource allocations, workers' skill levels, etc. It will be important to establish some common understanding, in certain settings, of the best way to get the most out of specialized professional skills and which of those resources can be made generally available by professionals in their less specific caring and supporting role. An appropriate model of social intervention currently exists on the margins of social work. It is a model that is

seeking credibility within social work as a 'model of good practice' (Clarke, 1996). The re-emergence of this dialogue about what constitutes 'good practice' in social work may revive some of the old tensions and conflicts which are *old hat* for social workers, but which may appear novel to nurses in their new community roles. This model is called *community social work*.

The term 'community social work' received prominence with the publication of the Barclay Report (Barclay, 1982). In trying to bring some systematic analysis to the contemporary role of social workers the report located community social work in the community, intervening with a combination of community development skills and statutory responsibility to:

. . . tap into, support, enable and underpin the local networks of formal relationships which constitute our basic definition of community, and also the strengths of a client's communities of interest.

Generally, the Barclay Report was overlooked by the policy makers but it did highlight the confusion that existed in social workers at the time. There was considerable lack of clarity even within the ranks of those who wished to set aside completely the cold clinical model. The Barclay Report re-introduced a contentious issue when it stated:

The community approach we are advocating seeks to *share* more fully with citizens the satisfaction and the burdens of providing social care.

(Barclay, 1982, p. 199)

It was the word 'share' that revived the old debates.

Three works (Brown, *et al.*, 1982; Hadley, *et al.*, 1987; Payne, 1986) brought special prominence to the *professional* social work perspective on this new practice model. They sought not to challenge the context within which Social Services are offered to the community. They also chose not to question the unequal power relationships which professional, service providers create. Statutory power, socially controlling agendas and public resources cannot be shared – or not, at least, without considerable modification (Hadley and McGrath, 1984). Payne deliberately sets out his stall by precluding the involvement of social works in the context of:

> . . . promoting a political, social and service context in which the client's needs can best be met. . . . Such work is not directly concerned with a client's needs or those of a defined group of clients, nor necessarily with social provision at all. It is concerned with creating a more just and equal society . . ..
>
> (Payne, 1986, pp. 4–5)

Thus, the limit of a social worker's responsibility, according to Payne, is the provision of Social Services alone, albeit, with and by the community. He baulks at confronting the issue of who defines social service, or whether its aims should extend beyond the horizons of the centralized policy-makers. Willmott (1989, p. 36) notes with alarm the dangers to the established Welfare State through restricted funding. He points out the weakness of a limited view of the problem and may be in danger of succumbing to ' . . . rhetoric, myths and under-resourcing'.

Barr (1989, p. 165) agrees with much of this but extends his criticism to include the plight of consumers whose:

> . . . structural intractability of their situation becomes ever more apparent . . . but who are, nevertheless, bound in through their . . . goodwill to supplement the resources of an increasingly stretched Social Work Service.
>
> (Barr, 1989, p. 166)

The National Institute of Social Work team has now developed sufficient resources for us to explore some of the deeper theoretical issues behind this method (Smale et al., 1988). They have succeeded in a number of important areas, including the production of a theoretical text. There are handbooks for training and implementation, and now a series of commentaries has been released on the field experiences of using this framework. They have done this in the face of a number of pressures, the most daunting of which must be the apparent denial of their existence by all those who were in on the process of restructuring training for social work (Smale and Bennett, 1989; Darville and Smale, 1990).

Smale and colleagues approach the problem from an 'agnostic' perspective (Smale et al., 1988, p. 20). Their *Paradigm for Change* can best be described as a 'spiral' of action, learning, re-appraisal, planning and renewed intervention – in partnership with the client community in all its dimensions. They assume a holistic view of social phenomena and yet they recognize that the values of the workers themselves are the key to discovering just how far action initiatives will be oriented towards continuing social change – change in the individual, the organization and the social system. This is a team process and it also involved interdisciplinary work at every level (Smale et al., 1988, pp. 37–52).

The primary task of community social work 'to engage with the people in the community in setting aims and objectives' (*ibid*, p. 37) immediately pits this theory against the structuralist views of the Community Development Project (see above). Furthermore, it fails to address some of the more pressing issues which rate high priority even within the establishment approach to professional practice: issues such as *gender* and *racism*. Ballinger (1988, pp. 50–1) suggests that community social work is merely a myth which has been created to allow social work to avoid facing up to some of the more difficult questions relating to their craft. Dependence can be transferred from the worker onto the community group, anger can be dissipated and social control can be reimposed under a new guise. More dangerously, this new definition of practice will allow employers to do away with the 'thorns in their side': community development workers.

Nevertheless, there have been some very positive outcomes from this dynamic intrusion into the debate. It highlights the reluctance of CCETSW to consider the challenge of including 'development' within the ambit of the DipSW. This shows the influence of the traditionalists within the Council and the degree to which employers prefer direct line-management control over their staff.

Further, within the community social work 'tendency', a body of internal criticism is emerging which drives home the importance of making values explicit. It calls attention to the potential value divide within social work at the point where 'partnership' and unequal power relationships collide. It challenges workers to confront their own allocation of resources between service provision and preventative strategies. It taxes them to examine how they actually define, in practice, terms which have by now become widespread: 'normalization', choice, participation and empowerment.

The emergence of this approach to fieldwork has demonstrated again for the 1990s, that community development, at the natural end of the practice theory continuum, provides the necessary values, insights and skill requirements for effective intervention at community level. The implication of this for the purveyors of community care from this must be obvious. The move towards decentralization in Local Government forces more and more reliance on creative and mutually supportive measures from the planners and providers of services. This creates fresh openings for interdisciplinary team work and collaboration with local service users. In Scotland, this is an established tradition, but it is one that those south of the border are slow (or reluctant) to exploit (Barr, 1997).

Not least, it highlights the fact that community development practitioners have accepted the inevitable, and that they are now at the centre of the 'community care' debate, instead of being left anguishing on the wings.

The Future

The charity, Opportunities for Women, conducted a survey of 3000 carers in 1990. Their report presents a graphic picture of at least one target group for community care. The respondents reported many significant features in their lives – stress, unsympathetic social and working environment (for the 2000 employed women in the sample), intractable problems and an apparently indefinite commitment. These citizens are currently living in our community and they are one target for the Government's community care proposals. New services will be designed which will help to alleviate the burden which so many assume so willingly (DHSS, 1989, p. 9).

We have to judge from the evidence whether we consider that our public and voluntary services are now prepared and able to meet these challenges. They have entailed changes and adaptation. In addition, we must consider how best we have prepared both the communities and the consumers for the changing face of social care. Whereas it is proving much more time-consuming for the whole edifice of the community care system to become fully operational, we are still some way off agreeing an appropriate mechanism of achieving many of its goals.

We have attempted to outline the scenario that confronts students of nursing and social work, and it is a problem for all professionals engaged in this field. Professionals are being asked to consider demands upon their loyalty which have been suppressed by much stronger restraints in the past. The further they are asked to come out from under the protective mantle of their own professional base, the less security there will be. Professionals must be secure in their own identity and also secure when working with others. For this new form of integrity, they must be properly trained.

'Properly trained' must mean trained to work together and to understand each other's contribution:

. . . the most effective setting for learning about multi-disciplinary teamwork is in the placement in a multi-disciplinary team.

(Inter-Disciplinary Assn and CCETSW, 1989)

It may be anticipated that the professions will respond positively to the pressure to implement inter-disciplinary training. This will produce some interesting tension as the dynamics of the team situation place strains on the system.

Placements in the community entail students taking on wider responsibilities for designing their own learning. This mirrors the task of the qualified professionals as they strive to make their skills available to the consumers.

In the community, the worker seeks the freedom and responsibility to respond, sometimes without delay or further consultation, to a larger number of unpredictable and non-uniform events in his (sic) dealings with local people and groups.

(Thomas and Warburton, 1977, p. 67)

Students will, and must, experience the tensions that emerge as the community's response to need runs into the professional's organizational constraints: different priorities, lack of resources or sensitive political issues. The test for community-based professionals working together is how they sustain their joint effort under these pressures.

Their collective, professional response to the community's needs can only be maximized if it is designed as a partnership effort with the community. This is illustrated in the discussion about community social work. The experience of introducing partnerships, of responding to need and opening up choices, results in a value-shift from service-led to *development-led* practice. The nature of skill required to achieve this task is that which has been omitted from the latest training proposals.

Students in the field of learning difficulties today are facing challenging times. In some quarters, community-based services for people with learning disablities have been the only ones of their kind. The community care policies see these services competing for resources with all other special needs groups. This competition is not confined to public funds but to community resources as well. As those who have already qualified have little experience of what is in store, it may be up to the students themselves to design the training that they need.

Discussion Questions

■ What insight into community dynamics is expected of students being trained by you and your colleagues at the end of their period of practice training in your agency/ team?

- What experience of training with other professionals, or other professional students-in-training, do social work students get while on practice placements in your agency/team?

- What model of capacity building could be used to consolidate networks or small community groups around your social work clients who are in significant need, in their community setting?

- How does your agency/team rate its knowledge of the local community and how is this knowledge verified and updated?

- How are issues such as gender, race, age, etc. positively engaged within your work setting? Does your agency/team engage in routine practices which may reinforce discrimination in these fields? What steps are taken to empower people who may experience disadvantage through the operation of discrimination through these factors? Had you thought of a capacity-building approach for this purpose?

References

Abrams, P., Abrams, S., Humphrey, R. and Snaith, R. (1986). *Creating Care in the Neighbourhood*. Advance, London.

All Wales Working Party on Services for Mentally Handicapped People (1982). Welsh Office, Cardiff.

Atkinson, D. (ed.) (1995). *Cities of Pride: Rebuilding Community, Refocusing Government*. Cassell, London.

Audit Commission (1992). *Community Care: Managing the Cascade of Change*. HMSO, London.

Ballinger, F. (1988). Community Social Work – myth or reality. In *The Quest for Community* (ed. F. Ballinger), pp. 50–51. Leicester Board for Social Responsibility, Leicester.

Bamford, T. (1990). *The Future of Social Work*. Macmillan, London.

Barclay, P.M. (Chair of Working Party) (1982). *Social Workers: Their Role and Tasks*. National Institute for Social Work/Bedford Square Press, London.

Barr, A. (1997). Editorial. *The Scottish Journal of Community Work and Development*, **1**, 3–4.

Barr, A. (1989). A new dog – new tricks. In *Pictures of Practice. Vol. 1, Community Social Work in Scotland* (eds G. Smale and W. Bennett), pp. 163–184. NISW, London.

Beresford, P. and Croft, S. (1993). *Citizen Involvement: A Practical Guide for Change*, London, Macmillan.

Brown, P., Hadley, R. and White, K.J. (1982). A case for neighbourhood-based social work and Social Services. In *Social Workers: Their Role and Tasks* (Chair of Working Party, P.M. Barclay), appendix A, pp. 218–235. National Institute for Social Work/Bedford Square Press, London.

Calouste Gulbenkian Foundation (1968). *Community Work and Social Change*. CGF, London.

CCETSW (1977). *Guidelines for Courses Leading to the Certificate of Qualification in Social Work, Paper 15.1 (as amended)*. CCETSW, London.

CCETSW (1989). *Requirements and Regulations for the Diploma in Social Work*. CCETSW, London.

CETHV (1979). *Inter-professional Co-operation – Training for the Primary Health Team*. CETHV, London.

Clarke, S. (1991). *Shared Training Project for RMNH & CQSW Students 1988/89. Occasional Paper No. 25*. School of Social Studies, University of Swansea.

Clarke, S. (1996). *Social Work as Community Development: A Management Model for Social Change*. Avebury, Aldershot.

Clarke, S. and Lile, J. (1990). *Shared Competencies of Professionals in Mental Handicap*. CCETSW, London and Welsh National Board.

Darville, G. and Smale, G. (eds) (1990). *Partners in Empowerment: Networks of Innovation in Social Work*. NISW, London.

Department of Health (1989). *Working for Patients*. HMSO, London.

Department of Health (1997). *Developing Partnerships in Mental Health*. HMSO, London.

Department of Health and Social Security (1986). *Neighbourhood Nursing – A Focus for Care*. (The Cumberlege Report). HMSO, London.

Department of Health and Social Security (1989). *Caring for People*. HMSO, London.

DHSS and Welsh Office (1988). *Working Together: A Guide to Arrangements for Inter-agency Co-operation for the Protection of Children from Abuse*. HMSO, London.

ENB (January 1989). *Project 2000 – A New Preparation for Practice: Guidelines and Criteria for Course Development and the Formation of Collaborative Links Between Training Institutions within the National Health Service and Centres of Higher Education*. ENB, London.

ENB and CCETSW Working Group (1987). *Co-operation in Training and Post-Qualifying Training: Mental Handicap*. ENB and CCETSW, London.

England, H. (1979). Education for co-operation in health and social work. *Journal of the Royal College of General Practitioners*, Occasional Paper 14.

Etzioni, A. (1993). *The Spirit of Community: The Reinvention of American Society*. Simon and Schuster, New York.

Etzioni, A. (1995). Nation in need of community values. *The Times*, February 20th, 1995.

GNC for ESc and NI and CCETSW (1982). *Co-operation in Training Part 1 – Qualifying Training*; & (1983), *Part 2*. GNC and CCETSW, London.

Griffiths, Sir Roy (1988). *Community Care: Agenda for Action. A Report to the Secretary of State for Social Services*. HMSO, London.

Hadley, R. and McGrath, M. (1984). *When Social Services are Local*. London, Allen & Unwin.

Hadley, R., Cooper, M., Dale, P. and Stacey, G. (1987). *A Community Social Worker's Handbook*, London, Tavistock.

Hawker, C. (1988). *Unpublished Report into Participation Schemes*. Dept. of Applied Social Studies, Swansea.

Heginbotham, C. (1990). *Return to Community*. Bedford Square Press, London.

Independent Development Council for People with Mental Handicap (1982). *Elements of a Comprehensive Service for People with Mental Handicap*. IDC, London.

Independent Development Council for People with Mental Handicap (1984). *Next Steps*. IDC, London.

Independent Development Council for People with Mental Handicap (1986). *Pursuing Quality*. IDC, London.

Inter-Disciplinary Association of Mental Health Workers and CCETSW (1989). *Multi-Disciplinary Team Work*. CCETSW, London.

King's Fund (1980). *An Ordinary Life*. King's Fund, London.

King's Fund (1984). *An Ordinary Working Life*. King's Fund, London.

Local Government Training Board (1986). *Survey of Manpower and Qualifications within Social Service Departments in England and Wales & Social Work Departments in Scotland*. HMSO, London.

Loney, M. (1983). *Community Against Government*. Heinemann, London.

Mayo, M. (1994). *Communities and Caring: The Mixed Economy of Welfare*. Macmillan, London.

Opportunities for Women (1990). *Carers at Work*. Opportunities for Women, London.

Øvretveit, J. (1993). *Coordinating Community Care: Multidisciplinary Teams and Care Management*. Open University Press, Buckingham.

Payne, M. (1986). *Social Care in the Community*. Macmillan, London.

Pinker, R.A. (1982). An alternative view. In *Social Workers: Their Role and Tasks* (Chair of Working Party, P.M. Barclay), appendix B, pp. 236–262. National Institute for Social Work/Bedford Square Press, London.

Royal Commission on the Law Relating to Mental Health 1954–57 (1957). Cmnd 169. HMSO, London.

Seebohm, F. (1970). *Report of the Committee on Local Authority and Allied Personal Social Services*. Cmnd 3703. HMSO, London.

Skeffington, A.M. (1969). *People and Planning (Committee on Public Participation in Planning)*. HMSO, London.

Smale, G. and Bennett, W. (eds) (1989). *Pictures of Practice, Vol. 1. Community Social Work in Scotland*. NISW, London.

Smale, G., Tuson, G., Cooper, M., Wardle, M. and Crosbie, D. (1988). *Community Social Work: A Paradigm for Change*. NISW, London.

Stacey, M. (1969). The myth of community studies. *British Journal of Sociology* **20**, 134–47.

Stewart, M.J. (1993). *Integrating Social Support in Nursing*. Sage, Newbury Park, CA.

Thomas, D.N. and Warburton, R.W. (1977). *Community Workers in a Social Services Department: A Case Study*. NISW/Personal Social Services Council, London.

UKCC (1986). *Project 2000 – A New Preparation for Practice*. UKCC, London.

Welsh National Board (1989). *General Guidelines for Curriculum Development for Project 2000 Programmes*. WNB, Cardiff.

Welsh Office (1983). *All Wales Strategy for the Development of Services for People with a Mental Handicap*. Welsh Office, Cardiff.

Weinstein, J. (1994). *Sewing the Seams for a Seamless Service: A Review of Developments in Interprofessional Education and Training*. CCETSW, London.

Williams, F. (1994). 'Race', welfare and community care: a historical perspective. In *'Race' and Community Care* (eds W.I.U. Ahmad and K. Atkin), pp. 15–28. Open University Press, Buckingham.

Willmott, P. (1986). *Social Networks, Informal Care and Public Policy*. Policy Studies Institute, London.

Willmott, P. (1989). *Community Initiatives*. Policy Studies Institute, London.

Wistow, G., Knapp, M., Hardy, B. and Allen, C. (1994). *Social Care in a Mixed Economy*. Open University Press, Buckingham.

Chapter 7

Commissioning and Providing Services

Jan Gilbert and Steven Rose

Key Issues

- The commissioners
- The providers
- Care management
- Joint commissioning
- GP fundholding
- Service brokerage
- Housing grants and Social Security benefits
- Principles & methods of commissioning
- Setting standards and measuring quality
- The involvement of service users

The Needs of People with Learning Disabilities

Service delivery for people with learning disability is now based on the belief that people with learning disability should lead an ordinary life in community settings. This is also based on the belief that people with learning disability have essentially the same needs as anyone else to seek to enhance their way of life, the main components of which may be described as the need for:

- a place to live
- financial security
- work opportunities
- access to opportunities for personal development
- access to leisure
- access to and involvement in local community life
- primary and specialist health care
- opportunities to develop relationships.

Having the same needs does not mean that they can always be met in the same way as other people. Additional help may need to be provided for many conditions that are associated with learning disability such as:

- epilepsy
- hearing and visual problems
- communication problems
- obesity

- cardiovascular and gastro-intestinal abnormalities
- respiratory problems
- impaired mobility
- Alzheimer's disease (in people with Down's syndrome)
- Mental health problems.

(Kay *et al.*, 1995)

Introduction

Since 1990 a revolution has been taking place in the way services are delivered to people with learning disabilities. The cause of this revolution is, of course, the NHS and Community Care Act (Department of Health, 1990). One of the main aims of the Act was to improve the way in which peoples' needs are met. The Act has been implemented over several years; parts came into effect in 1991, whilst the implementation of other parts of the Act was delayed until 1993. It has brought about a number of key changes to the way that services are provided to people with learning disabilities and their families. All of these changes were designed to ensure that people's needs were better met. Amongst these are the lead role for Social Services in the purchasing of social care; contracts and the 'purchaser/provider divide'; changed funding arrangements for community care; disincentives and restrictions on the statutory agencies continuing to be the direct providers of services; and the introduction of care management and new quality monitoring processes.

The most fundamental change the Act brought about was the introduction of the purchaser/provider split. This affected both Health Authorities and Local Authorities, but in different ways. Local Authorities were identified as lead purchasers for learning disability services. General practitioners (GPs) and primary health care were also potentially affected with GPs being given the opportunity to become fundholders.

At the same time other Government initiatives have had significant influence. The Health of the Nation (Department of Health, 1992a) identified five target areas for health gain for the whole nation. This was followed up by a specific publication aimed at the health of people with learning disabilities (Department of Health, 1995a). These initiatives, together with a move towards locality based commissioning and GP fundholding, have all begun to impact upon how learning disability services are commissioned and provided.

In spite of early opposition to the Act from some professionals, statutory and voluntary agencies, it is now largely implemented and has brought sweeping changes to just about every aspect of service delivery.

The guidance upon which the purchasing of Health and Social Services is currently based was issued in the form of two circulars (Department of Health, 1992b, NHSME 1992), published following the NHS and Community Care Act (1990). The aim of this guidance is the creation of comprehensive, locally based services planned on an individual basis. For the first time a number of key issues are addressed in Government guidance. The importance of choice is recognized by acknowledging that differences between the person and his or her relatives over services will exist but that 'in general, the views of the person with learning disabilities should be respected' (Department of Health, 1992b). This circular also reinforces the importance of advocacy.

However, in spite of the helpful manner in which the guidance addresses a number of key areas, there is a significant omission. Nowhere is guidance offered on what course of action should be taken where the person cannot express his or her preferences.

The Commissioners

Local Authorities

Under the Community Care legislation Local Authorities have been given the lead responsibility for commissioning services for people with learning disabilities. They are also responsible for the production of a local Community Care Plan each year. The Local Authority Social Services Department co-ordinates the input of other agencies into the plan. Others inputting into the production of the Community Care Plan would usually include the Health Authority, NHS Trusts, voluntary sector organizations, the Housing Department, parents and carers and service users themselves.

The extent to which service users are meaningfully involved in the planning and management of the services that they receive varies enormously across the country. In some areas users are beginning to be involved, in others 'lip service' is paid to user involvement, whilst in others there is little or no user involvement (Flynn, 1995). Throughout this chapter the theme of user involvement will be examined and examples of best practice will be used, to illustrate how user involvement can be achieved.

The care management and assessment process

The care management process is intended to provide an effective method of targeting resources and planning services to meet the specific needs of individual clients. The elements of care management are:

- identification of people in need (including referral systems)
- assessment of care needs
- planning and securing the delivery of care

- quality monitoring the service
- review of client needs.

In reality many care managers also fulfil a social worker provider role and are thus unable to fully express an objectivity that is necessary for the purchasing/commissioning role of care management.

Additionally, although a care manager may have the authority to 'spend' up to a specified level on an individual package of care, she/he does not have a budget as such. They usually have limited financial information about the organization as a whole and will make purchasing decisions independently from other care managers. Thus there is often little evidence of strategic planning and co-ordinated use of funds.

The money available is so limited and the demands of clients are so great, that it could be said that care management is a process of denial, based upon prioritization of the risk of not securing a service for an individual.

Health Authorities

Traditionally, Health Authorities were responsible for significant levels of resources that were expended on services for people with learning disabilities. As hospitals have retracted and closed, the role of Health Authorities in commissioning services for people with learning disabilities has changed and diminished. In some ares where large resettlement programmes have taken place, the local Health Authority still retains a significant commissioning role. However, this role is increasingly being passed to Social Service Departments, either directly or through joint commissioning.

In a few instances, NHS specialist learning disability trusts exist. This has occurred where previously there was a large hospital or cluster of hospitals. In these instances the Health Authority retains a significant commissioning role for learning disability services. However, this role will largely diminish as the remaining hospitals close over the next few years.

The health role in commissioning services for people with learning disabilities has become more focused and specialized. It now tends to concentrate on, and be limited to, services for people who in addition to learning disabilities have challenging behaviours or mental health problems or other complex health needs. The health care purchased is often not direct provision of care, but input from specialists who usually work in teams. These specialists include psychologists, dietitians, physiotherapists, community learning disability nurses, psychiatrists, speech and language therapists, and occupational therapists.

One of the problems that was experienced immediately after the purchaser/provider split was that all of the specialism and expertise relating to learning disability was lodged within providers. This made it very difficult for some commissioners to make informed operational or strategic purchasing decisions. Additionally, some commissioners were unclear regarding the role of some professionals and future workforce requirements. This made workforce planning very difficult, and had a 'knock-on' effect on the training colleges and universities.

The most notable group to be affected were learning disability nurses and by 1994 serious concerns were being expressed that the profession was no longer viable. A report was commissioned by the Chief Nursing Officer for England. Part of this report was 'A guide to learning disability nursing for health and social care commissioners, GP fundholders, NHS Trusts and the independent sector' (Department of Health, 1995b). The problem of health commissioners having a lack of expertise in learning disability has lessened in recent years as the commissioning process has matured.

Joint commissioning

The Department of Health guidance on joint commissioning (Department of Health, 1995c) defines joint commissioning as 'the process in which two or more commissioning agencies act together to co-ordinate their commissioning, taking joint responsibility for translating strategy into action'.

Health and Social Services joint commissioning for people with learning disabilities is well advanced in parts of the country, with Social Services as the lead agency. There are a number of perceived benefits for service users:

- jointly agreed assessment procedures ensure a more holistic approach to service provision;
- scarce resources are used more effectively as duplication of effort and activity is reduced;
- a single point of entry means a service that is more streamlined and seamless;
- the holistic approach enables more innovative service solutions;
- the development of the care market is stimulated, fostering co-ordination between service agencies.

Key issues in the process of joint commissioning are:

- local history of joint working
- involvement of key stakeholders
- geography
- local financial position.

Lewisham Partnership: a case study in joint commissioning
The Lewisham Partnership (see Figure 7.1) was formed in April 1994, when services previously purchased by Health and Social Services became purchased through a single commissioning agency. The main features of the Partnership are:

- a joint agency team (part of management structures of both organizations) reporting to joint member level committee;
- complete commissioning budgets from both authorities;
- complete strategic and operational integration – joint strategy, project development, contracting, consultation, information systems, monitoring, quality assurance and individual care planning.

The main advantages of the Partnership are:

- it ensures a full breadth of resources available for everyone, therefore better care plans;
- integration ensures reduced overlap of services and gaps, also equity of access;
- significantly improved strategic perspective – can see whole service and develop as system;

- access to both authorities' resources gives greater potential for development via a wide range of opportunities.

GP fundholders

Initially, it was predicted that GP fundholding would have a widespread impact on the purchasing of learning disability services (RCN, 1994). In reality, this has not been the case. Generally, learning disability services have been included in fundholding, albeit on a fairly simple basis, and a widely varying approach has been adopted in different parts of the country. In some areas learning disability services have been fully included in GP fundholding, whilst in others, particularly deprived inner city areas where there are few fundholders, there has been little or no impact.

GP fundholding was launched under the

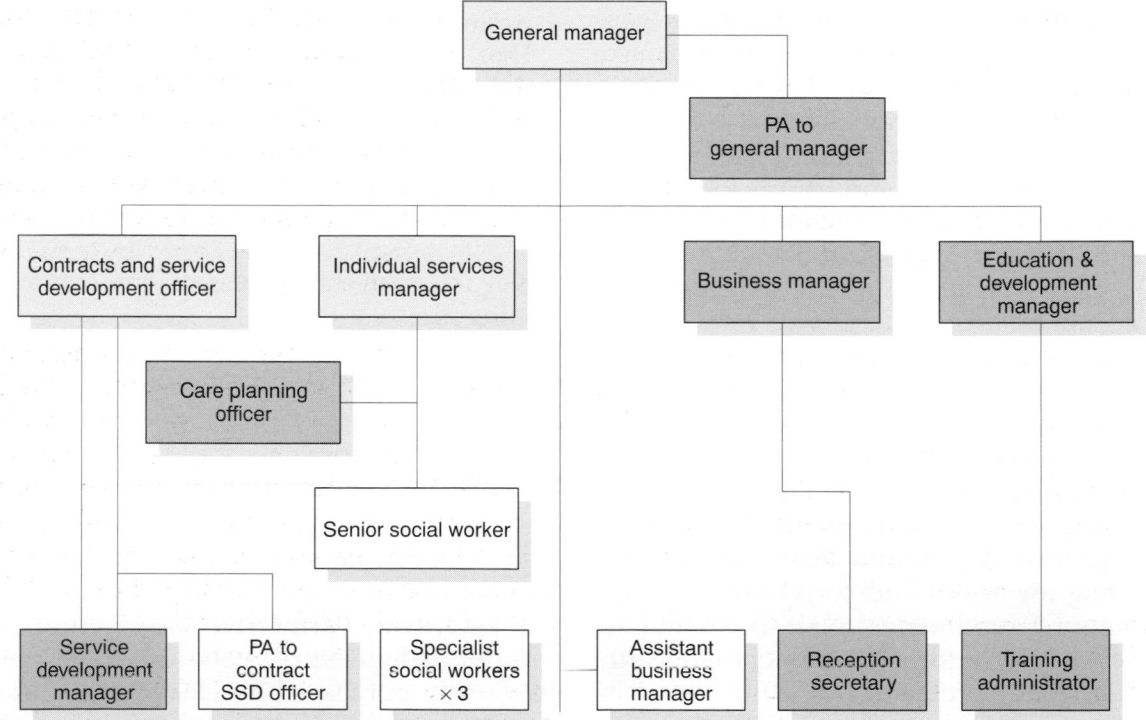

Figure 7.1 Lewisham Partnership. ☐, Joint officers; ☐, Social Services Employees; ■, Health Service employees. SSD, Social Service Department

Table 7.1 Differences between acute and learning disability services

Acute services	Learning disability services
Attributable to individuals	Often block contracts – not attributable
Specified time span of treatment	May be lifelong and linked to family
Often a choice of provider	Usually only one provider
Clear information about services from provider	Lack of clarity about actual service provided

NHS Community Care Act 1990. By 1995/96 53% of the population was registered with a fundholding practice (Flynn *et al.*, 1996). Funding for each practice is determined by patient population size.

The purpose of GP fundholding was to offer GP practices an opportunity to enhance the development of primary care through the identification of local health needs and the provision of a needs-led, high quality service. The reality for people with learning disabilities has been somewhat different.

GPs often have concerns about purchasing health care for people with learning disabilities as it is so different from the acute services with which they are familiar (Table 7.1).

A number of key issues have been raised in the transition of funding from health purchasers to GP fundholders:

- Many GPs have a limited knowledge and understanding of learning disability and often fail to distinguish between people with learning disability and those with mental health support needs.
- Some GPs may question the need for specialist services that appear to be more expensive or unattainable than current generic services.
- Some community teams are multidisciplinary with staff from both Social and Health Services. At times there may be lack of clarity whether a client is receiving 'health' or 'social' input, or both. Clearly GPs do not wish to purchase

social care which, for them, is free at the point of delivery.

- The information need of GPs is often very different from the information that is currently collected. There needs to be a mutually agreed format of data collection that not only meets the GPs' information requirements but is also manageable for those providing the service.
- In some localities modifications to the standard rules of GP fundholding have been agreed in the short term to allow self-referral and referral by a family member. This has been to facilitate the transfer into fundholding without major disruption to services that already exist.
- A few GPs exercise a form of gate-keeping by refusing to take on patients with learning disabilities. They are anxious that having a number of dependent people as patients may be costly in terms of time and other resources.

The key issue is, perhaps, that when GP fundholding is fully operational the GP will be in the position of purchaser who, while open to professional advice, has the power to make the purchasing decision. This may mean that staff will have to work in a different way to ensure that the GP has relevant, accurate and timely data and is kept informed and 'on board'.

However, whatever the influence on commissioning of GP fundholding so far, announcements made following the election of the new government, in May 1997, indicate that the current GP fundholding arrangements will diminish and change over the course of the next two years.

Direct payments: service brokerage and individualized funding

The first service brokerage project was set up in Vancouver, British Columbia, in the 1970s, by a group of parents of people with learning disabilities. The two key components of service brokerage are handing over the control of individualized funding to people with disabilities and their circles

Joe is a 65-year-old man who was living in a large residential home. Because of its size, it wasn't meeting his individual needs and wishes. Joe wanted to move nearer to his family. His family were also unhappy with the situation and regretted not being able to see more of Joe.

Joe was put in touch with a service broker who listened to what he and his family had to say. With this information the service broker was able to find out about all the suitable and available services in the area to which Joe wanted to move, and to present the information to Joe and his family. Joe and his family then arranged to visit one of the places on the list to see if Joe liked it.

Meanwhile the service broker negotiated financial details with the agency responsible for funding Joe's placement. Joe and his family liked the place he had seen, it met all of his support needs and it was even less expensive to live there!

Joe was delighted to move to a place which was smaller and more homely and where he could see his family more often. (Dook et al., 1997)

Box 1 Case study – Joe's story

of supports, and using service brokers (Rose, 1994). One of the first service brokerage projects to be set up in the UK was established in Southwark, South London, in 1992 (Dook et al., 1997). The Southwark project has three aims:

- to increase the choices available to the people of Southwark who have a learning disability, and to make sure that they have the support and power to make those choices;
- to support people with a learning disability to make the changes that they need and want in their support and accommodation;
- to move control and decisions closer to individuals with learning disabilities and their networks.

In spite of the enormous potential for empowerment offered by service brokerage, and the evident success of projects such as the Southwark project (Holman, 1994), the practice has not become widespread in the UK. There are several possible reasons for this. The word brokerage itself may have changed or lost some meaning when it crossed the Atlantic. There are subtle differences in the meanings of some North American English words to their English (UK) counterparts. Also, almost predictably, service brokerage has met with a certain amount of hostility from professionals. An effective service brokerage service can be seen to challenge the care management process, social work and other professional inputs.

Furthermore, the law in Britain was restrictive in terms of giving money directly to clients, and in all but a few very rare cases, which usually involved innovative voluntary organizations, money had to be channelled through services. The direct payments legislation (Department of Health, 1996a), which became effective on 1 April

1997, has the potential to change all of this (see below). Current guidance on interpreting the Act (Department of Health, 1996b) still potentially places restrictions on people with learning disabilities accessing direct payments. Even if the problems around accessing direct payments are surmounted, most people will not be in a position to take advantage of such payments without the support of a service advocate or service broker. This is where service brokerage may finally find its niche in the UK market.

Housing-related grants and Social Security benefits

Whilst the majority of funding for support and care comes from one or other of the statutory funding agencies, there are other sources of funding that often come into the equation, and a chapter on purchasing and providing would be incomplete without offering the reader an understanding of these. Comprehensive advice on housing-related grants and benefits is well beyond the scope of this chapter; however, set out below are the main sources of other funding that is available at the time of going to print.

Transitional Special Needs Management Allowance (TSNMA)

TSNMA is a grant paid by the Housing Corporation to special needs properties (projects) and replaced a former grant, Hostel Deficit Grant (HDG), in 1991.

The main elements of TSNMA are:

- it is paid on a per bed basis;
- the amount paid was originally based on the property's historical HDG element;
- thus, the final HDG claim formed the basis of the first TSNMA claim;
- the amount paid has been brought into line with SNMA (see below);
- TSNMA is gradually being phased out to be replaced by SNMA.

Special Needs Management Allowance (SNMA)

SNMA replaced HDG as the revenue grant paid to special needs housing schemes developed and approved for funding after 1 April 1991.

The main elements of SNMA are:

- it is paid to schemes originally capital funded by Housing Association Grant (HAG);
- it is paid at a flat rate per bed space, calculated on a staff to tenant ratio basis, i.e. *c.* £2500 per bed space for a staff ratio of up to 1 per 5 residents, or *c.* £1500 per bed space for a staff ratio of 1 per 10 to 15 residents.

Income Support

Income Support is the basic means-tested benefit for people who do not have to be 'available for work'. It is calculated as follows: (i) add up the applicable amount; (ii) subtract means (e.g. other benefits which count as income, or wages, or assumed income from savings); and (iii) result is the amount payable. Income Support stops completely if money which is counted as the person's capital is over £8000 (£16 000 if the person lives in a residential care home). Applicable amounts usually consist of a personal allowance and any premiums which the individual qualifies for because of individual circumstances. However, other amounts may be included or substituted, for example if the person is in residential care.

Registered Homes Act – as it affects benefits

Local Authority owned or managed homes are not subject to registration. Income Support is normally only payable at a restricted rate of £61.15 per week (1996/97 rates). Housing Benefit is only payable in restricted circumstances.

For private and voluntary sector homes,

the Income Support applicable amount will either be entirely according to 'Preserved Rights' rules, or it will include a 'Residential Allowance' on top of personal allowance and premiums. In either case individuals in registered homes cannot normally be paid Housing Benefit.

However, in the case of accommodation transferred from Local Authority management to be registered in the private or voluntary sector, Income Support may be limited to the restricted Local Authority home rate for as long as the claimant remains in the same accommodation. Whether this happens depends on the date of transfer and the particular circumstances.

Disabled Living Allowance (DLA)

DLA must be understood to consist of two distinct parts: payment towards mobility and payments towards care. Some people over 65 years are paid attendance allowance rather than DLA Care Component – the two are very similar. There are two rates of mobility award, and three rates of care award, according to needs. Attendance Allowance is paid only for the highest levels of care need.

In any of the above scenarios of residential care, DLA Care Component or Attendance Allowance should not be payable if the Local Authority is arranging the provision of residential care, for example by contracting with a voluntary organization. Even if the Local Authority is not involved, the claimant should not benefit financially if they receive income support according to the 'Preserved Rights' rules.

The change in DLA Mobility rules which took place in 1996 related to stays in hospital of more than 28 days.

'Preserved Rights'

Preserved Rights protect the level of Income Support applicable amount for residents of private or voluntary residential care homes who are counted as having been continuously resident in a registered care home or nursing home since 31 March 1993. The exact rate payable depends on the category of care, but the protection does not of itself depend on whether board is provided.

Residential Allowance

This is the amount (£60.00 per week at 1996/97 rates) included in the income support applicable amount for someone who moves into a private or voluntary residential care home from another form of accommodation, if the move is after 31 March 1993 (see above regarding transfers of Local Authority accommodation).

Housing Benefit

Housing Benefit is means-tested help towards your liability for rent on the place of your principal home. Payment of Housing Benefit is usually excluded for people in Local Authority accommodation (see above), and it is always excluded for people who qualify for the Income Support Residential Allowance because they moved to a private or voluntary care home after 31 March 1993, and for people with 'Preserved Rights'.

Direct Payments for Care

From the date when it is brought into force the Community Care Direct Payments Act 1996 allows (not requires) Local Authority Social Services to pay money to someone to buy their own care services. Payment can be for the person to buy a part of the services. The level of payment can be linked into the charging policy of the Local Authority. Money not used on the care that the Local Authority assesses as needed may be repayable. (NB: 'Direct Payments' of Income Support or Housing Benefit are something quite different: these are where part or all of the amount payable is paid direct to a landlord or other creditor, rather than to the claimant.)

The Providers

NHS Trusts

The advent of the purchaser/provider split in the National Health Service (NHS) reforms created changes that were initially slow to be recognized. Although the newly formed Trusts had to respond in very different ways in how they conducted themselves as organizations, the service delivery to clients remained largely unchanged in the early days.

The majority of learning disability services have combined or merged with mental health or primary care services over the past 5 years and there are now only 10 NHS Trusts in England dedicated to services for people with learning disabilities. Increasingly, as purchasers seek a mixed market economy of care, services for people that were originally provided in a Health or Social Services setting are now being delivered by independent providers. This has created a competitive market for the historic service providers who are having to change the way they deliver services.

A key issue for NHS Trusts is that they must meet statutory requirements as NHS bodies and many still deliver the traditional nursing model of care and support. However, this does not enable them to remain competitive in a market where other providers are less restricted in terms of employment and financial targets.

Local Authorities

The Community Care Act 1990 heralded the split between purchasers and providers in local authorities. Initially, the confusion and separation was greater than that experienced in the health service. People who had been working together in the same organization now had very different roles and expectations. The providers delivered residential and respite care and day services. The social worker/care manager role became part of the purchasing/commissioning function.

Most of the contracts were continued with 'in-house' providers on a 100% block purchase with a percentage reduction each year over a specified time. This was to encourage a mixed economy of care, although local authorities have always used a range of providers – particularly for domiciliary support services.

The trend with Local Authority purchasing for residential and day care is still highly geared to block contracts, with cost per case spot purchasing used for emergency or domiciliary intervention. The cost and volume contracts are mostly used by care managers to purchase individual packages of care.

The Audit Commission (1993) urged Local Authorities to set very tight eligibility criteria based on how many clients they could afford to manage – needs-led budgeting. Although this provides a clear model for rationing it raises the question of how needs are defined. Increased demand and limited resources make it inevitable that need is assessed upon dependency and risk and the ability and/or willingness of the carer to cope.

'Charging' was introduced in 1994 as a means of reconciling the gap between demand and resources. It remains an area of contention and raises issues about equity and access. A family of a child who uses a respite care bed in a Local Authority facility will be charged a specified amount for each overnight stay. The child who uses a respite care bed in a health facility uses the service free.

Local Authority commissioners of learning disability services have had to face tough purchasing decisions around who will/will not receive a service. In the process of prioritization those who score low on the matrix of risk and dependency are now having to manage with less, or often, no support. The preventative monies that were available only a few years ago have now dried up completely and care managers are rarely able to adopt a proactive mode of purchasing. In some extreme cases if a person's need is not urgent it is left unmet until it becomes urgent. It often then requires a level of spend on crisis intervention much greater than the cost would have been to meet the original need. Every time this happens the resources available for other clients are reduced and the care manager is trapped in a downward spiral of reactive decision-making.

Housing Associations

Traditionally, the role of Housing Associations focused on the development and management of special needs housing schemes. The management of the scheme was often carried out on behalf of the Association, by a management agency, which had special needs housing expertise relevant to the particular client group.

During the 1980s and early 1990s, there was an enormous growth of Housing Association special needs provision, as community care schemes developed and hospitals closed. Large amounts of capital finance were available from the Housing Corporation, via the Housing Associations, to provide special needs housing for people with learning disabilities. This source of capital finance has now largely dried up as funds have become more scarce and other client groups have been prioritized. Revenue funding to support schemes in the form of Hostel Deficit Grant, Transitional Special Needs Management Allowance and Special Needs Management Allowance have also

been available via Housing Associations; see above.

Increasingly now, Housing Associations that previously only provided housing are diversifying to become providers of social care. Some are also running nursing homes. This change is a direct result of the NHS and Community Care Act (1990), and the 'mixed economy' of care that has been encouraged. The growth of direct care provision by Housing Associations represents a major contribution to the increase in choice of service providers available to commissioners. On the other hand, some would argue that the move by the Housing Associations away from their area of core business and expertise could lead to poorer quality services. This could prove to be true in some cases, but should not be the case if effective monitoring systems exist.

The current move towards Housing Associations becoming providers of care as well as housing is contrary to what was seen as good practice just a few years ago, when the involvement of Associations in service for people with learning disabilities was being encouraged on a large scale. At that time a clear separation between housing/the individual's home, and all of the rights associated with a licence, tenancy or ownership, and care and support was seen as good practice.

Private sector

The private sector has mushroomed in recent years and the scope and range of service provision has greatly increased. There are large private companies with homes and services for people with learning disabilities across the country and there are small private providers who may be supporting only one or two individuals. The difficulty lies with small organizations that may be isolated and less easy to monitor.

Although registration requirements are

the same across the private and public sector, there is often a very different interpretation, across different localities, of the standards that have to be achieved. It is also clear that registration requirements focus largely upon service inputs (what is provided for a person), rather than outcomes for the individual (what changes/difference this makes in the person's life). So, while every bedroom in a registered service must have a sink, there is no requirement that other people must always knock on an individual's bedroom door before entering. The focus tends to be more on the environment than the philosophy of service.

There is often no common denominator between services in the private sector apart from the fact that they are all services for people with learning disabilities. There is also frequently prejudice from the public and voluntary sectors, largely because of a distrust of a care service organization that operates 'for profit'. 'Care' and 'profit' are perceived to be mutually exclusive terms. Yet there are many independent private providers who operate as effective businesses, turning the profit to further develop good services.

Perhaps the private sector would benefit from a regionally co-ordinated approach to technical support, information, training and quality monitoring. However, this may offend those with purist notions of how the 'market' should operate.

Traditional voluntary sector, new voluntary sector

The traditional voluntary sector has continued to grow at a steady pace, but a whole new voluntary sector has emerged over the past few years. In some areas care and housing consortia have been set up and supported by Health and Local Authorities to establish and develop an independent market sector. Many other small, 'not-for-profit' organizations have been developed as registered companies with charitable status.

The small, independent organization can benefit from a greater measure of autonomy that allows creative and innovative services to be developed for individuals. However, their smallness also means that they do not reach a critical mass that affords them the economies of scale the larger organizations enjoy. They are also vulnerable in that if one or two people move on from the service the money moves with them and it may leave the company financially not viable.

Families

Recent Government policy has placed greater emphasis on maintaining people in need, whether elderly or disabled, in their own home. In reality, this often means that people remain in the care of their relatives with other supports provided by statutory services. Relatives have, therefore, become more important in achieving policy aims. In one sense this represents a formal acceptance of what has been the position for years. Relatives and carers have always carried a large proportion of the burden of caring for a disabled member of the family, often with no recognition or help from statutory agencies. However, the policy has not clearly set out its expectations of relatives as carers. As we have seen, policy has also not specified the role of relatives in instances where an adult with learning disabilities cannot express a preference about services.

Hospitals and village communities vs. other models

There is currently a small, but vocal, lobby – mainly parents – who are putting forward the case for alternatives to care in the community; namely village communities (Cox and Pearson, 1995). There is no strict definition of what a village community is, and there are many different examples, ranging in size from a cluster of just a few houses to congregate care for over 300 disabled people. The attractiveness of the village community to its supporters rests with the alleged ability to maximize shelter and security for people, whilst avoiding the excesses of institutional living. It is also claimed that the cost of village community care is considerably less than care in the community, although this claim has been questioned by a recent Department of Health funded report (Department of Health and PSSRU, 1996c).

Principles and Methods of Commissioning

Negotiating and agreeing contracts

The developing contract culture has been seen by some in the voluntary sector as having the potential to stifle flexible and innovative practices. Indeed, many voluntary organizations have experienced a culture change as they have learned to adopt a more 'business-like' approach with a greater focus on planning, development and management control.

Types of contract

Block contract

The block contract usually specifies the quantity and quality of inputs. It is favourable to providers as the contract usually reflects a guaranteed annual purchase on a specified service. For example, 10 places may be block-purchased at a day centre and the provider will receive the income irrespective of the actual take-up of the service.

Cost and volume contract

A cost and volume contract specifies the volume of service to be provided and the total cost. Accurately costed units of care, for example in an individual's care and support package, enable the purchaser to make informed decisions about the affordability of service within given resources.

Cost by case contract

A cost by case contract allows a purchaser to 'spot purchase' individual units of care on a 'pay as you use' basis. This is often used to buy services in a crisis or unplanned situation.

It is important that the contract relationship between purchaser and provider is open, respectful and trusting. The negotiation process is one which aims to elicit the best deal possible for the client within resources available. If this remains the key focus of both purchaser and provider then contracts can be designed to be imaginative, flexible and responsive to the changing needs of the individual. Where the contract relationship breaks down, the person who stands to lose most is the service user.

Checklist for contract design

- *Introduction* – includes the names of the parties to the contract, dates, etc.
- *Common terminology* – language needs to be clear and comprehensive to both purchaser and provider.
- *Payment* – specifies the amount to be paid and the payment arrangements.
- *Terms agreed at outset* – the volume of service to be delivered, when and where.
- *Change clauses* – allows for contract variations as changing needs of individuals are reflected in funding changes.

- *Time-frame* – contracts are time-bound – most frequently annual.
- *Review process* – a mechanism for this is built into the contract to ensure ongoing review.
- *Cultural awareness* (Lewis, 1996) – demands that the service is delivered in a way that reflects the cultural, ethnic and religious lifestyles of the individual.
- *Termination* – states the circumstances in which the contract may be terminated and the process.
- *Monitoring standards* – the contract should specify measurable quality standards and state how frequently monitoring returns should be completed. Some contracts may include penalties for non-compliance with contract information requirements.
- *Complaints process* – the provider organization monitors and records all complaints and advises the purchaser on a regular and agreed basis of complaints received and resolutions.
- *Arbitration* – this identifies the procedure to follow in the case of non-agreement between purchaser and provider.
- *'Force majeur'* – this is an essential clause in a legal contract that indemnifies both parties for eventualities outside their control, for example flood, earthquake, etc.
- *User involvement* – the contract should specify how users will be consulted about their services.
- *Meeting health needs* – there must be clarity about how users will be supported to access generic health services wherever possible. Specialist health support needs should be clearly identified and costed according to individual need.
- *Equal opportunities* – many contracts make clear the expectation that the provider organization will be seen to practice equal opportunities – some may require ethnic monitoring statistics.
- *Staffing provision and support* – this

includes training and development opportunities for staff recruitment criteria, appraisal systems and supervision procedures.
- *Insurance* – the provider should reference its insurance details.
- *Signatures and dates.*

Ensuring User Involvement

Ensure purchaser knows and understands needs of people with learning disability
Purchasers commonly have responsibility for purchasing services for users across a range of sectors and disciplines. They need to be informed and encouraged to understand the distinct care and support needs of people with learning disability. This can be achieved through the care management process, service brokerage and/or the provider contracting relationship.

Make information accessible
Contracts can appear to be lengthy and laborious for most people to read. This is particularly so with service users and yet they are the people to whom the contracted service is being delivered. The use of pictures, symbols, signs and tapes can easily be incorporated into a contract, making it more accessible to the people it concerns (Moffat, 1996).

Systems that enable the needs and wishes of users should be included in the contract standards
This can be done through individual service contracts. The focus of the standards to be achieved is on the outcomes for individuals and the quality of the service is measured by how frequently these outcomes are achieved.

Mechanism by which users can understand and participate in monitoring

Service users are rarely consulted in this matter. Although they may be supported to understand the contract for their service, they do not see the contract monitoring information that the provider of their service makes to the purchaser. This could, again, be made accessible through use of pictures, symbols, etc. It would be interesting to see if a user's perception of the service he/she received matched what the provider claimed to have delivered.

Clear and explicit process through which users can give feedback and make complaint

Views of users need not only to be heard but to be sought. The complaints policy must be accessible in terms of being easily understood and readily available. People who do not easily make known their views can be supported to give feedback with the support of a family member, friend, service broker or advocate.

Opportunity for involvement of an advocate

Where users are unable to clearly express their wishes or participate fully in the contracting process it is important that they are offered the opportunity to be represented by an independent person acting in the role of advocate. This person acts purely in the interests of the individual.

Contracts Do Not Change Lives but People Can

Much of this chapter has focused on the purchaser/provider model of providing services with which we have all become familiar in recent years. The purchaser/provider model, contracts, or for that matter any other service system cannot change a thing without people. Those people are often par-

ents and carers, sometimes workers (we use the term workers to include managers, professional support workers/care staff, educationalists and academics), and sometimes volunteers.

Models of service delivery and service systems are essential when an organization is charged with meeting the needs of a large number of people with disabilities; without models and systems chaos would reign. However, some would argue that chaos already reigns in some areas, often the more deprived inner city areas. There are many examples of individuals having to wait for many months before a needs assessment is completed.

So, if models and systems alone cannot solve problems and ensure that need is met, what is the added ingredient required? The answer is simple, it is people; not just any people, but skilled people, people with vision, innovators, people with courage, and most importantly of all, leaders with the courage and commitment to empower others to continually strive to find new and better ways of meeting need.

Michael is 19 years old and has been given the label of having a moderate learning difficulty. Whilst he can read and write and has many good social skills, he has always found it hard to understand complex conversations. He does not like having a label of 'learning difficulty' and likes to be with people he can look up to. Unfortunately, some of the people he looks up to are not good role models and he has been in trouble with the police on more than one occasion. He seems to run a thin line between being easily led by people and doing things that he knows to be wrong to impress people.

Michael has a very committed family: his mother, stepfather and two brothers. A voluntary organization took on the respon-

continued opposite

sibility of co-ordinating Michael's support. The voluntary organization's contract manager, Michael and his family worked out a service that they thought might suit them. This would be for Michael's family to buy a property and split it into two flats with Michael and his elder brother Andrew living in one flat and the rest of the family living in the downstairs flat. The Social Services Department made a capital grant to the voluntary organization, which was passed on to the family, to enable them to purchase the property. (It would have been illegal for Social Services to make the grant directly.) The grant was equivalent to the full year cost of a private hospital placement, which was where it was feared Michael would end up. Had Michael been placed in a private hospital the commissioners would not have been faced with a once off payment, but the potential of revenue costs year after year. A small revenue budget was also made available to the family, to enable them to employ a support worker and someone to co-ordinate the planning of his service.

Like any 19 year old, Anthony does seem to find it difficult living so closely with his family, and it was agreed at a planning meeting that he would spend 1 day a week without support staff or family around. Unfortunately, Michael appears to have used this time to mix with some of his less desirable friends, and he took part in an extremely serious criminal incident which led to his arrest.

His family and supporters, Social Services and the voluntary organization met to prepare information for the court about the nature of his disability; the possible reasons for him offending; and proposals for how to tackle these issues within the home environment. The service promised to undertake the following:

- co-operation with probation;
- 24-hour supervision with a long-term aim to help Michael gain greater responsibility for himself, and therefore independence;

- training for support staff;
- therapeutic support from counsellors and psychologists to help Michael work through issues such as anger, self-esteem, and making appropriate friendships;
- attendance on a course for young offenders;
- the provision of positive role models and the chance to make supportive and appropriate friendships;
- working with local police to build up links and greater understanding of Michael's needs;
- to hold regular reviews.

The case came to the Old Bailey, and the contract manager and the chief executive of the voluntary organization feared that both they and their organization would attract severe criticism. Because the original charge had been kidnapping, by the time the case came to court the prosecution had dropped the charge to aggravated theft. The judge was very sceptical and needed a lot of persuading before granting the probation order, but eventually agreed to grant a year's probation because the service guaranteed 24-hour supervision.

The probation period was not without problems and Michael has committed other offences. The original package of support that was put to the court has had to be amended on several occasions. Michael's family and supporters and the contract manager from the voluntary organization have stuck with him. The way in which his support has been purchased has been flexible, and his family and supporters have been allowed to take control of purchasing. Three years on, the situation remains fragile. However, the longest previous period that Michael had lasted without residential care, due to the trouble that he gets himself in, was just 1 year.

Box 2 Case study – Michael's story

Lessons from Michael's story

Purchasing, the ability to use a range of providers, the close involvement of the family, contracts, innovation and courage all played their part in Michael's story, but there were other factors:

- The contract manager listened to what people wanted and responded to it.
- The contract manager, his manager and his organization, had the imagination, courage, commitment and conviction to make it happen. No one hid behind systems and structures.
- There was flexibility and responsiveness, an early recognition of problems and ability to make changes.
- There was a willingness to break away from more traditional models of support, in spite of the potential difficulties.
- Community integration and inclusion were at the heart of all plans and proposals.
- There was a recognition that everyone is different and that peoples' needs change over time.
- The contract was used as the tool upon which to base the relationship; the relationship is central.

Setting Standard and Monitoring Quality

It is vital that in agreeing processes for quality assurance both the provider and the purchaser are able to distinguish between: doing a good job and doing the right job.

(Duffy, 1996)

During the 1990s there has been a much sharper focus on quality, and especially the quality of public services. The purchaser/provider split and the move of services from the public to the independent sector, described in this chapter, are both results of the Government's efforts to improve the quality of services. Opinion remains divided as to the effectiveness of this strategy. As part of these changes most services have developed service standards, against which quality and performance can be measured. Examples include charters for rail users, setting out standards for the punctuality of trains and the publication of the Patients' Charter. Local Authority registration units are playing an increasing role in monitoring services, as more and more services move to the private and voluntary sectors. Set out below are some basic principles of quality monitoring, and an example of Service Standards for a learning disability service (Table 7.2).

Monitoring of services should ensure:

- the involvement of people at all levels in the service and service users, parents, carers and relatives;
- a system that ensures that information gathered is useful in planning service change and development;
- that the process of monitoring and gathering information should be made comprehensible to staff at all levels and to as many clients as possible;
- that the process is two-way, with regular feedback that can be used to improve the service;
- that key decision-makers are alerted to services that may be of poor quality or at risk of breaking down;
- the production of accurate and relevant information to funders;
- that information is collected from as close to the individual level as possible.

Table 7.2 Specimen service standards (From Hill, 1997, reproduced with kind permission of Southwark Consortium, London.)

Requirement	Indicator	Monitoring mechanism	Reported by	Frequency
(a) Customer focus and feedback				
Complaints procedure	(i) Complaints procedure will be written in a way so that as many service users as possible can understand it	(i) Complaints procedure availability and accessibility	Complaints officer	Quarterly
	(ii) Complaints are dealt with within the time limits stated in the complaints procedure	(ii) Information/statistics compiled from complaints returns	Complaints officer	Quarterly
	(iii) Number of complaints received	(iii) Information/statistics compiled from complaints received	Complaints officer	Quarterly
User consultation	A consultation strategy will be developed in partnership with user groups such as Southwark Unity and the Black Users' Group	Reports from consultation meetings	Chief executive	Annually
Carer consultation	Southwark Consortium will continue to support carers groups and involve carers in planning and decision making. Carers will continue to be encouraged to monitor an individual's service	Reports from consultation meetings	Chief executive	Annually
		Individual contracts	Contract manager	Annually
Services should demonstrate the development of appropriate strategies for decision making by clients, including client involvement in the recruitment of staff	The development of appropriate strategies including development of communication strategies, individualized IPP processes, house meetings, the use of citizen advocacy, professional advocacy and service brokerage, facilitating access to self-advocacy groups	Descriptive reporting	Team manager	Annually

Table 7.2 *continued*

Requirement	Indicator	Monitoring mechanism	Reported by	Frequency
As many clients as possible should have a key to their house door	Number of clients with key to door	Numbers on house returns	Team manager	Annually
Individualizing contracts	(i) All clients should have an individual contract (ii) There should be a progressive increase in the number of contracts that describe the aims of services offered to the individual and how these aims will be met and monitored (iii) There should be an increase in the number of individual contracts that have been adapted to the ability of the client to understand them	(i), (ii) and (iii) numbers on house returns	(i), (ii) and (iii) Team manager Contract manager	Annually
Relationships	(i) Number of personal visitors to the home, i.e. friends or family (ii) Number of visits by clients to other people's homes	(i) and (ii) numbers on house returns	Team manager	Monthly
(b) Communication with GPs/ primary healthcare issues				
Health profiles	Each individual will be assessed by support staff and a health profile produced recording incidents of ill health and highlighting areas that require further investigation or referral to a relevant health-care provider	Annual audit	Audit team	Annually
Each individual to have access to the services of a GP	Each client to be registered with a GP	Annual audit	Audit team	Annually

Psychotropic medication should only be used appropriately	Recorded usage of psychotropic medication	House returns	Team manager	Annually
	Consultation with clinicians on appropriate strategies towards this aim across the services	Descriptive reporting	Named individual	Annually

(c) Discharge/resettlement/move-on

Co-ordinated discharge from hospital	Southwark Consortium will ensure that a named individual is responsible for facilitating and co-ordinating discharge of a client from hospital	Descriptive reporting	Named individual	Annually
Moving from Southwark Consortium's services	Moving from Southwark Consortium services will be co-ordinated by a named individual in consultation with the user, carer, provider and appropriate professionals	Individual contracts	Contract manager	Annually
	Information on moves will be reported to the Health Commission in a descriptive reporting format	Number of moves per year and length of time taken to move will be recorded to produce a baseline	Contract manager	Annually
		Descriptive and quantitative reporting	Named individual	Annually

Table 7.2 *continued*

Requirement	Indicator	Monitoring mechanism	Reported by	Frequency
(d) Activities Developing individual occupational and recreational skills through planned programmes of activities and accessing local educational, community and leisure activities in response to individual needs	(i) Development of the use of New Moves, Integrate, EDAS, Options, Toucan, Bede, Surrey Docks Farm, and improvement of relationships with Adult Education (ii) Number of times client leaves the home for activity/contact outside their home (iii) Level of activities within the home (iv) House visit descriptive reports, describing range, suitability and frequency of activities	(i) Individual and block contracts House returns Monitoring of contracts for day activity and employment services (ii) House returns and annual audit (iii) Annual audit (iv) Descriptive reporting	(i) Contract manager Team manager Contract manager (ii) Team manager and audit team (iii) Audit team (iv) House visitor (annual audit by audit team if not a registered home)	Quarterly Quarterly Quarterly Quarterly/ annually Annually Monthly (annually)
Holidays	Each client should be offered at least a total of 1 week holiday per year	House returns	Team manager	Annually
(e) Staffing Reducing number of temporary staff	Monitoring use of agency/bank staff across each service and house Promotion of strategies to reduce numbers taking into account seasonal variations Ensuring teams use named bank staff wherever possible	House returns	Team manager	Quarterly
Reduce sickness and staff turnover levels	Reduced levels on a house to house basis	House returns	Team manager	Quarterly
Staff training	To identify key staff needs and identify new areas, and types and amount of training undertaken	House returns Service manager reports	Team manager Service manager	Monthly Annually
Team meetings	Staff teams to meet on a regular basis	Annual audit	Audit team	Annually

Standard	Method	Measure	By whom	Frequency
Staff supervision	Staff members receive regular supervision with the appropriate line manager	Annual audit	Audit team	Annually
(f) Supported living Service provision for people with challenging behaviour	Specialist training for team leaders and support staff	Training returns	Team manager	Monthly
	Audit of what should be in a service, e.g. planning for length of shift, regular reviews of medication, systems to debrief staff, etc.	Annual audit	Audit team	Annually
Involvement of users and carers in changes of service for individuals	Person centred planning	Individual and block contracts	Contract manager	Annually
	Service brokerage	Descriptive reporting and number of service users in receipt of service	Service broker	Annually
	User consultation	Descriptive reporting	Reports from consultation meetings	Annually
Reducing service breakdown	Define and record on a house to house and agency basis	House and agency returns	Team manager	Quarterly
			Agency manager	Quarterly
	Development of an alert system	Alert system 'triggers'	Contract manager	Quarterly
Accident and incident reporting (including contact with police)	Number of accidents/incidents and instances of contact with police/criminal justice system	House returns	Team manager	Quarterly
	Health and safety training for staff	Training returns	Team manager	Quarterly
Personal care and support offered in ways that are ethnically and culturally appropriate, and that there is an appropriate match of staff to clients	Southwark Consortium will ensure clients are supported appropriately, recognizing the needs for care, food, language, religious practices, contact with family and community, training	Annual audit	Audit team	Annually

Table 7.2 *continued*

Requirement	Indicator	Monitoring mechanism	Reported by	Frequency
(g) *Housing*				
Repairs	Repairs are carried out within the timescales set out in Charter	Housing Dept returns	Housing manager	Annually
Visits by housing officer	Visits are made by housing officer as stated in Charter	Housing Dept returns	Housing manager	Annually
Benefit entitlements	Users are assisted in claiming full entitlement to benefits	Housing Dept returns	Housing manager	Annually
Housing audit	Environment furnished and equipped and maintained which conforms to recognized standards of safety and supervision	Annual audit by chief executive	Chief executive	Annually

Examples of alert indicators: absences of first line manager; staff turnover; low activity; previous service breakdown – for individuals or the service (within last 6 months); high number / repeated complaints. IPP, Individual Programme Plan; EDAS, Employment and Day Activities Service.

Discussion Questions

- What practical steps can be taken to ensure that the information in contracts is accessible to service users?

- How can service users be more meaningfully involved in the commissioning of their services? Consider the practical steps that you would have to take to achieve this.

- In the light of the new 'Direct Payments' legislation, how can direct payments and service brokerage empower users to take more control over the purchasing of their services?

- Joint commissioning was heralded as the new, effective way of purchasing seamless services; in reality there are still very few examples of truly successful joint commissioning. Consider how closer interagency commissioning in your locality might improve services for people with a learning disability

- Contracts alone will do very little to change people's lives. The true ingredient for change is a person-centred contracting process in which the professional listens to what people want and finds a way to make it happen. Consider how this approach may be implemented for people whom you support.

REFERENCES

Audit Commission (1993). *Taking Care*. HMSO, London.

Cox, C. and Pearson, M. (1995). *Made to Care. The Case for Residential and Village Communities for People with a Mental Handicap*. The Rannoch Trust, London.

Department of Health (1990). *National Health Service and Community Care Act*. HMSO, London.

Department of Health (1992a). *The Health of the Nation, a Summary of the Strategy for Health in England*. HMSO, London.

Department of Health (1992b). *Social Care for Adults with Learning Disabilities (Mental Handicap). LAC (92) 15*. Department of Health Circular, London.

Department of Health (1995a). *Health of the Nation: A Strategy for People with Learning Disabilities*. HMSO, London.

Department of Health (1995b). *Learning Disability: Meeting Needs Through Targeting Skills*. Department of Health, London.

Department of Health (1995c). *Practical Guidance on Joint Commissioning for Project Leaders*. HMSO, London.

Department of Health (1996a). *Community Care (Direct Payments) Act*. HMSO, London.

Department of Health (1996b). *Community Care Direct Payments Act (1996): Draft Policy Guidance*. HMSO, London.

Department of Health and PSSRU (1996c). *Residential Provision for People with Learning Disabilities: A Report of a Research Study into the Cost of Village Communities*. DOH and PSSRU, London.

Dook, J., Honess, J. and Senker, J. (1997). *Making Changes: Service Brokerage*. Choice Press, Choice Consultancy Services, London.

Duffy, S. (1996). *Unlocking the Imagination. Strategies for Purchasing Services for People with Learning Difficulties*. Choice Press, Choice Consultancy Services, London.

Flynn, C. (1995). *User involvement in community care planning: a study of the London Borough of Southwark*. Unpublished MA dissertation, Goldsmiths College, University of London.

Flynn, M., Howard, J. and Pursey, A. (1996). *GP Fundholding and the Health Care of People with Learning Disabilities*. National Development Team, Manchester.

Hill, R. (1997). *Service Standards*. Southwark Consortium, London.

Holman, A. (1994). *The Southwark Consortium Evaluation: How Services Change to Meet the Needs and Wishes of People Who Use Them*. Values into Action, London.

Kay, B., Rose, S. and Turnbull, J. (1995). *Continuing The Commitment: the report of the Learning Disability Nursing Project*. Department of Health, London.

Lewis, J. (1996). *Give Us a Voice: Towards Equality for Black and Minority Ethnic People with Learning Difficulties*. Choice Press, Choice Consultancy Services, London.

Moffatt, V. (1996). *Life without Jargon: How to Help People with Learning Difficulties Understand What you are Saying*. Choice Press, Choice Consultancy Services, London.

National Health Service Executive (1992). *Health Services for People with Learning Disabilities (Mental Handicap) HSG (92) 42*. NHSE Circular, London.

Rose, S.J. (1994). *Canadian specific. Community Care*, **1010**, 30–1.

Royal College of Nursing (1994). *Learning Disability Nursing in the Contract Culture: A Royal College of Nursing Guide for Purchasers*. RCN, London.

Part Two

Effective Care Delivery

Chapter 8

Care Management in Community Care – Advantages, Disadvantages and Developments

Simon Biggs

Key Issues

- Case management in the USA
- Care management in the UK
- Criticisms
- Advantages and disadvantages of case management

Introduction

This chapter examines some issues surrounding a method of social work called case or care management; with care management emerging as the favoured term in UK contexts. In particular, implications for relationships between helping professionals and the users of services are explored.

Case management in the USA

Case management is a method of social work that arose in the USA as a means of reducing inadequacies of caring that resulted from fragmented services and partial funding by insurance companies (Sevick 1990). By pooling resources and linking them to assessed need, rather than strictly adhering to those responses for which a client would be covered by insurance (e.g. a company might pay for antidiabetic drugs, but not equipment), the method has been effective in developing a holistic approach which clearly defines objectives (Pantel, 1990). Once objectives are agreed it is easier for the user to discriminate between options, whilst the pooling of resources allows chronic problems to be addressed more easily. Recent summaries of case management in the USA indicate that a variety of forms of practice can be accommodated within this general framework (Beardshaw & Towell, 1990; Hollingberry, 1990; Phillipson, 1990). Austin and O'Connor (1989) in an extensive review of the US literature suggest a continuum of case management activities exists whereby any one approach can be placed on a point between orientations primarily based on either services or systems. At the service pole, case management is oriented toward work with individual clients, is integrated with other services, functions as a broker for care plans with an emphasis on advocacy and co-ordinates services with other community service organizations. At the system pole, the focus is on service delivery systems as well as individuals. Case management is provided by an autonomous service which functions as a gatekeeper with an emphasis in cost containment, the purchasing and termination of services and the monitoring of providers.

Although many of these qualities could prove a valuable addition to existing UK practice, there are also elements that make advantages less clear as they have been interpreted.

Care management in the UK

Many of the initiatives started in the UK have been derived from studies of Kent Social Services (Challis and Davies, 1986) and were based upon the transfer of older people from hospital back into the community. The work was long term, and rarely crisis-based, was specific to that service user group and was not primarily concerned with the co-ordination of multidisciplinary services. The social policy response, as outlined in the White Paper *Caring for People* (Department of Health, 1989) emphasized certain elements of the method.

Government sees considerable merit in nominating a 'case manager' to take responsibility for ensuring that individual's needs are regularly reviewed, resources

managed effectively and that each service user has a single point of contact.

(para. 3.3.2)

Case management provides an effective method of targeting resources and planning services to meet specific needs of individual clients.

(para. 3.3.3)

To be effective, care management should include:

- identification of people in need, including systems of referral;
- assessment of care needs;
- planning and securing the delivery of care;
- monitoring the quality of care provided;
- review of client needs.

Two powerful influences on government policy have made it clear that a cultural shift was needed to implement the new plans. Sir Roy Griffiths (1989) pointed out that:

A key challenge for social workers in community care will be to set priorities within available resources (currently) social workers tend to equate their work with an objective assessment of need, rather than setting it in a resource context.

(p. 7)

Howard Davies, Controller of the Audit Commission, had said that:

The main role of councils will be to assess what services are needed of what quality, then arrange other people to provide them . . . new budgetary responsibilities, turning them into clear rationers resources, will completely transform their role.

(Davies, 1989, pp. 8–9)

An indication of favoured mechanisms for implementing change can be found in the Department of Health report on public sector residential care (Dott, 1989). It recommends three ways of improving the 'quality of care and life for elderly service users, namely: improving management training including use of delegation, budgets, assessing care standards and point-of-entry strategies and monitoring systems to check quality, evaluate performance and set goals.

The findings reflect the importance of marketing and thus choice at the 'point of sale' and the view that the solution to quality assurance within limited resources lies in a more directive management initiative. These in turn require increased skills in boundary management as roles shift from provision within a service to transaction between services. When seen in the light of US models, it would seem that their decisions reflect the 'system' end of a continuum of care management approaches.

Criticisms of the Model

Proposals to adopt care management have been justified in terms of the increased flexibility of services that might result, increased choice on the part of the consumer (most notably the wish of many older people to stay in their own homes), and as an attempt to reduce Central Government funds paid to private proprietors of care via welfare benefits for service users' accommodation costs.

The method has not gone without criticism. Chris Phillipson (1990) has shown that many service users wish to reduce the 'burden' of care upon their relatives and it is unclear how the reverse would not happen. Ritchie (1990) points out that care managers working within multidisciplinary teams can become insulated from direct contact with service users and their expressed needs. Julia Phillipson (1991), in a feminist critique of community care policy points out that the majority of informal carers are daughters or female spouses or mothers whose unpaid labour has been exploited to alleviate Government expenditure. Whilst Biggs (1990) questions the notions of 'choice' and 'flexibility' in the context of a mixed welfare economy and points to trends that marginalize users.

Biggs has argued elsewhere that care management assumes a marketplace model of interpersonal relationships; that is to say, a meeting of two equals who come together to agree a bargain on an exchange of goods or services.

It [case management] proposes a vision of single persons, rationally in possession of relevant information and a cool grasp of their own motivation, finding an agreeable solution to a mutually agreed definition of need, both then returning to their private activities.

(Biggs, 1991, p. 10)

Care management therefore leaves out much of the detail of interpersonal thought, feeling and action. Guidelines from the US National Association of Social Workers for 'case management of the functionally impaired' would tend to confirm such a view (NASW, 1984). This document refers to the case management function as 'shared by the social worker, the client and the client's family and other professionals and agencies' (p. 10) as if relations between these groups were unproblematic. Problems, it assumes can be addressed by a correct delineation of tasks, plus adequate information given to the user.

Family members who have the time, a personal interest in a client and an extensive knowledge of and trusting relationship with a client can be in an advantageous position to schedule, supervise, monitor, adjust and interpret services.

(NASW, 1984, p. 12)

There is no discussion here of situations where the informal carer and service user disagree, have different interests or are working through conflicts arising from their life history together (of child and parent or husband and wife). Rather, emphasis would be on the efficient management of the service system itself, co-opting one party in the informal caring relationship into the rational care-providing world of the professional co-ordinator.

Advantages and Disadvantages of Case Management

So far a summary of US models and the particular one most prevalent in the UK have given rise to certain criticisms of case management. Some advantages and disadvantages are now taken up in more detail under four headings: focus on the individual, focus on transaction, rationalism, and the negotiating arena.

Focus on the individual

British care management emphasizes the individualization of care at different levels. At the level of professional intervention, an 'individual responsible worker' is expected to take and be held responsible for each case. In terms of provision, an 'individual package of care' has to be created based on an 'individual assessment of need'. An advantage of this approach is that it makes it less likely that the special needs of any one service user are lost in the system. By constructing a 'package' (leaving aside the question of whether a variety of options is concretely available) rather than relying on placement within certain existing services, the model allows more creative thinking about how those needs which fall within the remit of resources available can be

addressed. Concentration on a package can shift emphasis from fitting people into services to co-ordinating options around that person.

Disadvantages centre on the problem of a 'nominated client' or user of services, and the attendant danger of locating the problem with, and in some cases, within an individual. As noted earlier, interpersonal power relations which might include family conflict, professional versus user preferences, or cultural and ethnic allegiances are not seen as problematic. Neither is it clear how far the context of caring and the effect of environmental factors such as social disadvantage are added to the equation.

If a package fails, the individualizing trend of the model would make it more likely that the locus of failure would be perceived to reside either in the responsible worker or the individual user, rather than in the complex web of relations surrounding the caring endeavour.

Focus on transaction

The model tends to focus on the point at which goods and services are exchanged, which may then be monitored to ensure that contractual agreements made at that point in time are met.

An advantage of the transaction approach is that both sides to an agreement have a clear idea of what they should provide and receive. It thus becomes possible to examine objectives and their fulfilment. The identification of requirements that are addressed by a package becomes more clear and so, by comparison, those needs that will not be met. Limits are set, then, both for what is possible to achieve and for the circumference of the problem identified.

Disadvantages of this focus on transaction are closely associated with its rationalistic assumptions (to be examined in more detail). The point of transaction has also been associated in conservative ideology with the concept of consumer choice (Higgins, 1985). This has resulted in a narrowing of conceptions of choice to those 'at the point of sale'. This may be fine when buying breakfast cereal (if you do not like it, do not buy it next time) but when dealing with the whole environment within which a person receives care, it is more difficult to undo decisions and their consequences. It would be difficult for an older service user, for example, to put an incorrect move to residential care down to experience when it is widely recognized that changes of abode deleteriously affect them.

Similarly, monitoring of provider compliance would tend to be from the point at which a contract was agreed, referring back to requirements at that point in time. It is unclear how changes in need that have occurred since that time can be easily accommodated.

There are also perceptional difficulties that can follow from this focus. If one concentrates on this crucial point in time from a purchasing point of view, it would (in addition to assuming that the service user remains relatively unchanged by a move or 'improves by the provision of other services) tend to under-emphasize past history both in terms of personal life and in terms of attitudes to service systems that users may have. These previous experiences would be expected to influence significantly the success or failure of a package over time (Kanter, 1988).

Rationalism

Care management can be said to be rationalistic in so far as it attempts to simplify problems to those that can be solved by defining clearly achievable objectives.

Advantages would stem from the consequence that both worker and user have access to overt reference to the problems to be solved and the resources available to meet requirements. Problems are thus made manageable, broken down into understandable parts, whilst not losing sight of the fact that limited resources cannot be expected to fulfil unlimited needs. Unrealistic expectations by both parties may thus be brought down to earth. Role-modelling by helping agencies of coping with problems in this way may also be of value to certain service users.

The disadvantage lies in limits to the vision of the approach which arise, in part, from the market model of human behaviour outlined earlier. First, the possiblity of irrational choice is difficult to accommodate within this model (Kanter, 1988; Biggs, 1991). For example, questions about the effectiveness of a package of care would tend to crystallize around the quality of concrete parts. 'Will it do what he says it will do' or 'What might she do if the service is faulty'? If one starts from an assumption that motivation is often irrational, a number of alternative questions are also raised. 'Is what he asks going to fulfil needs of which he is currently unaware' or 'Is she going to use the service in a way that helps solve or adds to her expressed problem'? These last questions do not easily lend themselves to single, controllable answers.

Second, it is not at all clear that as problems arise they can be 'solved', however much both users and workers wish that this were the case. There is a paradoxical tendency in care management methods arising from the study of long-term care to adopt a view that 'cases' can be 'opened' and 'closed' and are then 'solved'. Although this view has much to merit it in terms of resource management for otherwise chronic problems and in keeping workers optimistic that problems can be cured, its relation to the actual amelioration of continuing social deprivation would require further critical study.

The negotiating arena

Care management has been seen as part of a wider project, continuing a trend in British welfare toward a mixed economy of care. A key element in such plans is a distinction between those who purchase and those who provide care. Purchasers, here, would be Local Authorities acting on behalf of service users, whilst providers constitute the private and voluntary contexts of care. The roles of welfare workers change, at least in the public sector, from being located within a particular caring milieu to those points of negotiation about services on the boundaries between caring contexts.

The advantages of this boundary management position (Bridger, 1980) have been said to include a move to open agency systems. That is to say, agencies become more flexible in their dealings with the outside world and are more able to adapt to changing external environments.

However, workers placed at the boundaries of caring systems also experience changes in terms of who they come in contact with, and the reasons why exchanges take place.

Emphasis changes from what happens on either side of the boundary, or the actual caring context, to negotiation and exchange across it, and ways of finding an acceptable compromise between those present. Success is gauged in terms of mutually agreed conclusions. There is thus a subtle change in the focus of the professional task toward interactions within that negotiating space. Agreement there, rather than direct intervention in the arena of care itself becomes a guiding criterion for effective provision. A focus upon transition across boundaries also reinforces assertions that the commodity (or person in the case of welfare services)

being moved is both inert and relatively unaffected by movement. Monitoring provision can inform parties of change over time; however, this would still be in terms defined within the negotiating space. Both of these trends would tend to protect the negotiating manager from the expressed needs of the user when balanced against the required agreement with a provider.

An additional consequence of the move to boundary negotiation has been noted by Phillips *et al.* (1986). This study found that providers themselves were often seen as clients in need of support and may effectively replace consumers as the recipients of the traditional social work skills of listening and helping, a position reinforced by many small providers' financial insecurity and the marital tension involved in 24-hour residential care. This slippage in perception finds justification in policy statements that private and voluntary provision should be fostered and 'enabled' to provide services. The purchaser and provider also often have more life circumstances in common than exist between the purchaser and service user (Biggs, 1989). A factor of empathic compatability may confirm a bond between harassed provider and case manager which itself reflects upon boundary negotiation. Meanwhile, the focus has slipped from client welfare to provider welfare.

Summary

So, what is all this saying? It seems that case management has qualities that are needed to clarify objectives and problem-solving within limited resources. As such it makes explicit the ground on which relationships between service users and welfare workers figure. Thus, the social policy context of its introduction has led to the promotion of a particular model that tends to focus on service systems rather than direct consumer involvement, the simplification of problems and a limiting of definitions of social deprivation.

Since the implementation of the 1990 NHS and Community Care Act, a number of tensions have emerged in the use of care management by helping professionals. These can be summarized in the following manner:

- Care management has shifted the balance between resource administration and contact with service users. The method would appear to be reliant on administrative procedure much more than originally envisaged (Lewis, 1997). The practice of skills concerned with direct care, such as counselling and family work, has been reduced as a consequence and may be in danger of being lost.
- Care management has largely been interpreted as a means of assessment and monitoring of services provided by others and by informal care. With the advent of community supervision orders in mental health (Atkinson, 1996), and the discovery of adult abuse as a 'new' social problem (Biggs, 1996), care management may increasingly play a surveillance role in community settings.
- An increasingly unfavourable policy and economic climate has had the consequence of focusing the role of care managers on rationing and targeting services only to those in most need. This, among other factors noted in the body of the text, has reduced the service flexibility and choice originally associated with the approach (Hadley and Clough, 1996).

Discussion Questions

- What are the key features of the care management approach?
- Can you identify advantages and disadvantages?
- What skills and knowledge are required of the care manager?
- Do you have or could you acquire this knowledge and skill?

References

Atkinson, J. (1996). The community of strangers. *Health & Social Care in the Community*, 4(2), 122–5.

Austin, C. and O'Connor, K. (1989). Case management: components and programme contexts. In *Health Care of the Elderly* (eds M. Peterson and D. White), pp. 280–304. Saga, New York.

Beardshaw, V. and Towell, D. (1990). *Assessment and Case Management*. Briefing Paper 10. Kings Fund Institute, London.

Biggs, S.J. (1989). Professional helpers and resistances to work with older people. *Ageing and Society*, 9, 43–60.

Biggs, S.J. (1990) Consumers, case management and inspection: obscuring deprivation and need? *Critical Social Policy*, **Dec.**, 30 pp.

Biggs, S.J. (1991). Community care, case management and the psychodynamic perspective. *Journal of Social Work Practice*, **May**, 26 pp.

Biggs, S. (1996). Elder abuse and the policing of community care. *Generations Review* 6(2), 2–4.

Bridger, H. (1980). *Consultative Work with Communities and Organisations*. AVP Monograph, Aberdeen, 31 pp.

Challis, D. and Davies, B. (1986). *Case Management and Community Care*. Gomer: Newbury Park.

Davies, H. (1989). Community Care. *Social Work Today*, **Jan.** 8–9.

Department of Health (1989). *Caring for People: Community care in the Next Decade and Beyond*. Making a reality of community care. Cmnd. 849. HMSO, London.

Dott, A. (1989). *Getting the Best Out of Life*. HMSO, London.

Griffiths, R. (1989). *Community Care*. **Nov** 7.

Hadley, R. and Clough, R. (1996). *Care in Chaos*. Cassell, London.

Higgins, J. (1985). *A Consultation on the Accreditation of Residential Care Homes*. Paper No. 6. Kings Fund Project, London.

Hollingberry, T. (1990). *Elderly Peoples Integrated Care Systems*. Helen Hamlyn Foundation, London.

Kanter, J. (1988). Clinical issues in the care management relations. In *Clinical Case Management* (eds M. Harris and L. Bacharach), pp. 361–368. Jossey-Bass, San Francisco.

Lewis, J. (1997). Our collective responsibilities. *Community Care*, **9–15 Jan.**, 2–6.

National Association of Social Workers (1984). *Standards and Guidelines for Case Management of the Functionally Impaired*. Standards No 12. NASW, New York.

Pantel, E. (1990). Systems designed for people. *SYSTED '90 Conference*, Bologna.

Phillips, D., Vincent, J. and Blackwell, S. (1986). Petit bourgeoise care. *Policy and Politics*, **14**(2), 189–208.

Phillipson, C. (1990). *Delivering Community Care Services for Older People*. Working Paper No. 3. University of Keele.

Phillipson, J. (1991). Education and training for community care. Paper to *CCETSW Conference*, March.

Richie, P. (1990). Case management and mental health. Paper to *CCETSW Conference*, Sept.

Sevick, M. (1990). *Case management in Pittsborough*. Unpublished PhD dissertation. University of Pittsborough.

Chapter 9

Care Management and Key Working

Gwen Swire

KEY ISSUES

- Tasks of the key-worker
- Identifying needs
- Protection of children and adults at risk
- Planning care to meet identified needs
- Managing care
- Key-worker skills

Introduction

The importance of different professional contributions to the care of people with severe learning difficulties is well accepted and there has been continued growth in interdisciplinary teams serving local areas and a continued search for better ways to integrate different perspectives into integrated programmes of care. Although the different skills and knowledge of each profession are recognized as important by families and people with learning disabilities, it is not easy to relate to an amorphous group of professional people whose interventions may seem to lack a co-ordinated approach. To make full use of the service provided, people need a worker who is recognized as theirs; whom they can trust and to whom they can turn knowing they will have a concerned, flexible, knowledgeable and certain response. This chapter assumes that the services do find it possible to appoint a key worker/care manager for life and examines the work and challenges at different life stages. Other chapters deal in more detail with the structure of the services. Whether for life or more sporadically and episodically, key-workers and care managers will recognize many of the issues raised in this chapter.

People with learning disabilities either living alone or with a family need an identified key-worker who will remain a consistent figure through their life. Ideally, this worker will be the person who supports the person experiencing difficulties through the process that decides whether the person receives a service. The key-worker then identifies need with the person and family in collaboration with other professions. He/she plans the care with the person and family, orchestrating necessary interventions of other professions and reviews and monitors the continuing care. The worker will carry responsibility for identifying whether a person is at risk and needs protection and will act as an advocate for the person and/or the family with other professions, agencies and local communities.

This key role has become known as the care manager role, but the term implies care always has to be managed by people other than the person receiving it, which can lead us to forget that work with people with learning difficulties and their families should be about an equal partnership in all the processes of giving and receiving care.

A person with severe learning difficulties requires help with many aspects of their daily life if they are to have a reasonable level of physical, social and emotional well-being. In many instances families meet the majority of the daily tasks that need to be done but families will rely on Health, Education and Social Services to support their activities or, on occasion, to take over the totality of such activities. The need to work in partnership with people and families should be an accepted principle underpinning all the activities of the team.

Care must be given in a sensitive and thoughtful way based on an appreciation of common human needs, and underpinned by an agreed value base. All professions concerned in caring for others have an obligation to their clients to spell out their values to clients and other professions and demonstrate how such values are carried through in practice. At all times practice must be viewed alongside these values and principles to ensure they are being upheld.

Interdisciplinary work demands a sharing of each profession's values and principles to ensure all are working to common goals. One of the first requirements for good team-working is to share the differing ethical base of each profession and to reach an understanding about the basis for the teamwork. The values that should underpin work with disabled people should be a commitment to social justice and social welfare; to enhancing the quality of life of individuals, families and groups within the community; and a repudiation of all forms of negative justice. This implies each worker should have a commitment to:

- the value and dignity of individuals;
- the rights to respect, privacy and confidentiality;
- the rights of individuals and families to choose;
- the strength and skills embodied in local communities;
- the right to protection of those at risk of abuse and exploitation and violence to themselves and others.

Tasks of the Key-worker/Care Managers

Assessment for provision of service

The first task of the worker is to support the person and their family through the process that decides the eligibility for service. Health and Social Service agencies must agree and publicize eligibility for services outlining, for example, whether people with mild learning difficulties will be excluded. The target groups will be identified in community care plans.

Those working with people who have severe learning difficulties must have strategies for reaching out to people eligible for service ensuring that other professions and agencies make relevant referrals and that families know of access points to service. An initial assessment will then be undertaken of the person's functioning to agree whether the service for people with severe learning difficulties is the appropriate place to locate future work. Such assessment will often require the involvement of a range of professions and be a lengthy process. It is a very stressful time for families, particularly the initial assessments involving the first diagnosis or suggestion that someone is experiencing learning disability. This period of 'not knowing' whether a child or adult is going to suffer from severe intellectual impairment can be more stressful than having to face a known and understandable condition.

The involvement of a series of professions each trying to add their knowledge into the process of diagnosis adds extra stress. The person and family may be expected to make many attendances at hospital or day centres or undergo long series of tests. Families may feel threatened by constant questions and be fearful of the results of this assessment. Usually, screening is done by a health service team, where the assumption is that the doctors lead the team. However, doctors will lead the professional team in decisions about medical interventions and investigations but they rarely accept responsibility for enabling the team to modify its activities to more ably incorporate family needs.

A worker should be appointed to work with the person and family until it is agreed they should or should not receive a service. The worker must be recognized as responsible for ensuring the assessment process is as comfortable as possible for that family. The worker must take responsibility for ensuring that the family have access to the results of all the tests, that information is not kept secret. Professions are often fearful of sharing their thinking, preferring to wait until they are sure of their assessment;

families usually prefer to be involved in the thinking and have to wait, uncertain and distressed by professional silence, which is usually interpreted as bad news!

The worker may have to interpret the language of professionals for families and constantly remind colleagues to speak in plain understandable language not peppered by professional jargon or terminology. The worker must ensure that the language requirements of ethnic minorities are met. The worker must ensure the families' right to attend and share in all discussions and help the family and person understand why the various processes are taking place; make sure all questions are answered freely; time appointments to fit more appropriately into other family matters; make sure that families can afford the high costs of travelling, meals and so on which occur; help with childminding; and deal with all the other matters which significantly affect the family.

The worker must ensure the family understands the final decisions and if a service is not to be offered outline alternatives and make appropriate referral. The results of the screening and decisions made should be given in writing. Families should have access to second opinions or to appeals or complaints procedures and the worker has responsibility to see the family is aware of its rights in these respects.

Identifying need

Having agreed that the person can be offered a service, the process of identifying need begins – a process again referred to as assessment, a word implying a dispassionate observation of the person with disability by a professional. Identifying need is, however, a joint process undertaken by the family, the person and worker in partnership, all sharing knowledge and experience and working to find agreed objectives.

The desired outcome is to help the person experiencing difficulties to, as far as possible, take responsibility for their own life. The process will require that the family and person have all the knowledge required to understand the disability and its causes, the prognosis as far as it can be given, an appreciation of the range of services available, an understanding of service deficiency, access to user groups and advocacy services as of right. They will have to reach an acceptance of the differing needs of the family and the person and be able to manage the tensions that result from these differences.

Identifying need demands from the worker complete openness, not withholding any information, and ensuring information is given clearly and as often as is necessary for people to be able to absorb it. For example, families who have just been told their child will experience severe disabilities will need to work through their distress, fear and anxiety; new knowledge will only be acquired when the family is ready for it. However, the worker will not know when is the right time, so new knowledge has to be repeated in varying ways until it can be seen to be clearly absorbed.

The worker must have an understanding of the disability, and of the knowledge and skills owned by other professions in the team and take responsibility for bringing these professions into the family at appropriate times in the process of identifying and meeting need. The family must be enabled to understand why different professions have to be involved and what knowledge and skills they will be bringing. The family should, if possible, agree to the involvement of different professions but their right to choose and agree cannot be paramount. The worker will be knowledgeable about the skills and knowledge that can help the service user reach his or her potential and at times it will be necessary to insist on another profession's involvement.

What needs and whose needs?

People have common needs: to be well fed, to be able to carry out bodily functions in order to remain clean and comfortable; to be appropriately clothed for their age and the weather; to have sufficient money to meet social needs beyond basic daily living needs, for example for entertainment or travel; to have social interactions which are interesting to the individual; to have close and loving relationships which add to the person's self-esteem; to have sexual relationships; and to be valued by the wider community.

These are the needs which have to be addressed but usually the person will be part of a family network and other needs have to be considered. Legislation lays a duty upon Local Authorities when identifying need to pay consideration to abilities of carers and therefore whatever the profession of the appointed worker, he or she will have to ensure that carers' needs are considered separately and are taken into account when planning care.

The needs of the disabled person may be different from the individual family member's needs and/or their wishes for the person. The needs of the family may be in conflict with the best interests of the person and vice versa. The worker must give respect to the needs of every individual involved, identifying for themselves, the family members and the person, the points at which needs are in opposition, or are causing tension or distress.

It is easy to identify the needs of each individual in isolation, the difficult process is defining which needs are paramount and negotiating between people with differing needs to reach agreements that to some extent satisfy all. Although the disabled person is the worker's primary client, it cannot be assumed that their needs will always be paramount.

A common fault in work with people with severe learning difficulties is assuming that the person is not able to appreciate the needs of their families. He or she is often allowed to continue with selfish demanding behaviour by the family and by others involved. The worker can over-identify with the person with difficulties and in trying to help him/her fulfil his or her own full potential can fail to acknowledge the importance of the family to that person and fail to accept that being part of a family can sometimes mean full potential cannot be reached. To belong to others we all have to give up part of ourselves.

The worker cannot judge or place values on family behaviour which is loving and caring but inhibits the development. The worker cannot determine which matters most to the person with disabilities, the wish for personal fulfilment or the wish to be secure in a loving but smothering family. In such families, the worker's responsibility is to enable the person with a disability to acknowledge the needs of family members or to teach him or her new behaviours which are more caring of others, whilst family members have to be helped to rethink their expectations of the person and enable them to appreciate the person's right to reach fuller potential. Family members will have to be helped to accept the importance and right to have other interests and concerns in life, to allow the person separation from the family or to allow their own separation from the person.

There will be families where these tensions between rights and responsibilities of each individual will be irreconcilable and the worker then has to make decisions about whether the impact of these behaviours is detrimental to the person with disabilities well-being to the extent that he or she needs protection. The worker's responsibilities in all the work with people and their families will be to identify the person's needs; ensure they are properly met; act as an advocate for the person in relation to his family; and identify whether the person is at risk either by their own or other's actions and take appropriate action to protect them.

Making choices

When identifying need the worker has to clarify what choices the person makes; what things are imposed on him or her by others; what opportunities can be given to allow him or her more choice; and what skills and knowledge are required so choices can be made. Being able to make choices is part of normal living, often denied to people with learning disabilities who are surrounded by people who 'know best'. To develop ability to manage his or her own life, opportunities to make choices, to take risks and learn from the results of choice are essential.

However, to make a choice people have to have experience and understand the options available to them. They have to have had the opportunity to learn how choices are circumscribed by social manners, for example how we eat and dress, and by the needs and expectations of other people who are part of their lives.

For a person with a severe learning difficulty the process of learning to make appropriate choices will be more lengthy than for most. The person will need to be given access to a range of options and to experiment with choices. For many aspects of their lives, choices will have to be made for them by their carers.

The worker has to therefore ensure the opportunity to experiment is given, that the choices made on their behalf do not further disadvantage them (e.g. it is not unusual to see disabled people in care who are badly dressed or have poor haircuts). The worker will have to act as an advocate for the person with carers as well as helping carers to work with the person to allow them to be party to choices made.

Identifying need through life

Childhood
A worker should be appointed immediately a child is diagnosed as potentially having a severe learning difficulty. If this is at birth, this worker should preferably be with the paediatrician when the parents are involved and will take responsibility for helping the family from that point.

The work for the next few years will be with the parents to ensure that the child is given the best start in life. Parents have to face an uncharted future for their child; all their wishes for the child's life will be broken. Parents will want to know what a learning difficulty means, what sort of school will she/he go to, will she/he ever work, will she/he ever leave home; what is day care? Things familiar to the worker will mostly be unknown to the parents. Extended family and families, even at early parts in a child's life, will often want to go and see a school or day centre to give them a concrete view of the future. The worker must help them to explore this new world by informing them about it and ensuring the family can meet other staff in the service and visit facilities as and when they want. The parents may wish to meet other parents; the key-worker should keep them informed of parents' groups and introduce them at a point the family feels is appropriate.

Learning of the child's disability can lead to severe marital tensions. The incidence of marriage breakdown is high and parents may need help with personal problems. The key-worker will be concerned primarily for the child, but the well-being of the parents is crucial for the child. They should be offered all counselling and other help needed so that the child is given consistent loving care which allows him or her appropriate stimulations and exposure to new experiences, not to be over-protected and cocooned; to be, in fact, treated like a child without disability.

Grandparents have a significant part to play and their fears, lack of knowledge and wishes must be given credence. They must be involved in the work, the timing of such interventions being in line with parents' wishes.

Brothers' and sisters' needs often get lost as the parents concentrate on the disabled child. The key-worker must remember their needs and help parents to continue to meet these appropriately and/or provide opportunities for brothers and sisters to have interests outside the home away from their disabled brother or sister.

The rejected child
Sometimes parents reject the disabled child and work with such parents should be done by a social worker who will carry the responsibilities of Local Authority for the care of children. The social worker has to help the parents explore their rejection and, if possible, work through it; but also has to be aware of the child's need for a stable family home and therefore for rapid decisions to be arrived at with regard to alternative family placements. The worker undertaking such activities must be experienced in and given the support of other experts in the field of adoption and fostering.

Practical needs of parents with young children
The trauma of diagnosis can lead to the worker's neglect of practical issues which are as important as the emotional impact on the family.

If the child has a physical handicap the parents may find extra difficulties in handling the child and carrying out basic nursing tasks. They must be given advice and practical demonstration by appropriate professionals. The importance of parents playing with children cannot be over-emphasized but they are often anxious about play with disabled children, involvement in play groups or day nurseries; help from the occupational therapist with play is important. The child should attend a play group or day nursery that caters for all children, he or she should not be identified as separate and different at an early age. Preferably, play groups and nurseries should be in the family's local area, as this helps families to know other parents and build supportive relationships with peers. The disabled child will become known and accepted in the area. If local facilities do not cater for disabled children, the key-worker should, with groups of parents, use all means to change attitudes of service providers in their area.

The key-worker must ensure families receive benefit entitlements, remembering that the extra costs of disability arise at an early age.

The occupational therapist should be considering with the family future housing needs: will adaptations or rehousing be required or what could be done to help parents within present housing? Housing matters can take a long time to resolve. It is important to act before major problems arise preventing future stress.

The school years

The attendance and involvement of the child and family with the school will be the foundation on which the child's future capacities will be built. The full involvement of parents with the school is essential. Most schools are now skilled at reaching out to families but there remain some parents who find difficulties in relationships with school and some schools are reluctant to involve parents in their activities. The worker in such instances needs to be an advocate for the family, negotiating with the school to ease tensions and develop an effective partnership. The worker will be involved in the assessments mandatory under the various Education Acts (see Chapter 5). The family should be involved in all procedures and discussions; they should have copies of all written material. The worker has to ensure that the family is fully involved and understands the procedures, discussions and outcomes.

Other needs during school years

The worker will see the family at regular intervals not only to check that schooling and school relationships are fruitful but to consider any other issues of concern. The child is growing and physical caring may be becoming more wearying; schooling entails extra costs and benefits need to be checked. The family may require relief from caring either over-night, for brief holidays, or after school. Access to relief-care should be as of right, with parents able to make their own arrangements. However, the workers should be aware of how much relief-care families are using. Its overuse can mask problems, which raises questions as to whether the child's interests are best met by staying in the family.

Protection of children and adults at risk

As community care becomes more of a reality then more people with disabilities will be at risk of abuse by others. Abuse can be by other family members, other carers including residential staff and home carers, and other people who are part of the disabled person's life.

Physical abuse results from acts of omission or commission and includes bodily assaults, burns, bruises, fractures, etc.; inadequate feeding – malnutrition or dehydration; poor hygiene; and improper use of medication (too much or too little). Emotional abuse is seen as constant humiliation and ridiculing of the disabled person; harassment and intimidation; and deprivation of other social contacts. Sexual abuse is using the disabled person for the other person's satisfaction or perverse needs without the willingness and proper understanding and a wish to be involved. Other abuse involves the misuse of the person's money, property or possessions by another, or not allowing the person access to such monies.

When such abuse is recognized the worker has an absolute duty to take action, however uncomfortable this may be. The employing agencies should have an agreed policy on how to manage such situations. For children, the guidelines that apply in each local area must be followed and childrens' future care planned through the use of these procedures.

For adults, the legal frameworks are less clear and the lack of appropriate legislation has led to teams not taking action or being unable properly to protect adults at risk. Guidelines similar to those used for children should be agreed between local agencies. Case conferences should be held immediately abuse is suspected, and clear plans made and agreed about future care. If abuse is by a family member that person must be clearly informed of the concern and the actions to be taken. If the abuse is by paid caretakers, the employing body must use its disciplinary codes to agree action against the caretaker. The involvement of the police can help considerably in changing behaviours.

An abusing family must be fully informed of suspicions from the moment they occur and be involved in all stages of investigation and treatment planning. In all cases of abuse a social worker must be involved.

Leaving school

Most Local Authorities are providing extended educational opportunities so that people with disabilities can attend classes into their early twenties. Good models can be found where day centres and further education colleges work together to provide programmes which allow a flexible interchange between the two, enabling the person to move, without disruption, from school to day centre attendance.

Work opportunities should be available. The worker should, through relationships with Job Centres and local industries, encourage the development of these opportunities.

Many children will become involved in some way with adult day services and day centres. There is a debate amongst professions working with people with severe learning difficulties as to whether day centres meet requirements for disabled people to have a normal life. Some professions suggest that all post-school activities should be in normal employment, with professional energies going solely towards developing and supporting such opportunities. The debate is long and involved but for families the arguments as to whether work opportunities are more normal than day centre attendance are of academic importance only. The worker must ensure debate does not get in the way of meeting immediate needs. Family needs can be ignored by professions concerned to provide a normal life for the disabled person. For many families, day centre attendance not only provides a respite from caring but gives the disabled person a life with some semblance of normality in that they leave home each day. The worker, however, must be part of the development of day centres and enable families to understand and work with changes in the way care is given but always carry the role of acting as advocate for the concerns of the family as well as promoting new approaches (see Joan Vagg's comments on day centres, Chapter 17).

Sexuality

The most sensitive area for the worker's consideration during the early teens and adulthood is sexuality – an issue which is sufficiently fraught in children without disabilities! Disabled people live in a malign social system that labels, scapegoats, disempowers, intimidates, stigmatizes and objectifies them. The beginnings of sexuality in people with learning difficulties brings all such attitudes to the fore, sexuality says to the outside world 'I am a person in my own right, I can no longer be ignored'.

The person with disabilities, like all other people, has to learn how to manage their sexual drive without selfishly imposing their needs and wishes on others. Family attitudes and relationships will have taught most children how to manage themselves but for others special learning programmes will have to be developed. The worker should instigate discussions with the family about sexuality, sexual relationships and marriage. For many families the exploration of such matters may be most comfortable in a group with other families; the family will feel their attitudes may be better understood by their peers. The worker with responsibility for considering and being an advocate for the person may be seen as 'biased' and not understanding the legitimate concerns of the family.

The timing of such interventions is important but for families involved in parents' groups the subject arises naturally before the person is reaching sexual maturity. The worker may need to help some families face these issues which for them are of particular difficulty.

There are many questions which need to be asked, for example if there is a likelihood of children being born from such relationships, is the person able to comprehend fully the needs of a child; should the pregnancy be allowed to continue? The concerns and fears of families, and the wish of the professions to do what they perceive as best, are very understandable.

The worker will have to ensure in any developing relationship that the person is not being sexually exploited, will provide access to family planning, and if a relationship is developing between two people in a hostel or a residential service, ensure they are given proper respect and privacy. The staff will be responsible for ensuring such a relationship does not intrude on the rights of other residents for privacy and respect.

The moral, ethical and other issues of sexuality in people with severe learning difficulties cannot be covered in depth here. The major responsiblity of the worker in this issue is to consider properly their own attitudes to sexuality and to the ethical issues about sexuality in people with severe learning difficulties, ensuring that in their assessment of situations and the action they take, objectivity is maintained.

Adult life

The major needs to be considered in adult life are a continuation of the concerns – where to live; who to live with; who gives care; work opportunities; monies; social and leisure opportunities; and continuing learning.

It is suggested that it is 'normal' for adults to leave their parental home and live elsewhere and such opportunities should be given to people with learning disabilities. The worker should be opening up discussion around this issue with parents and in parents' groups at early points in a child's life. The parents must be given permission not to need to continue to care for all their child's life and also have the opportunity to consider what would happen if they were no longer there to care. The person must be given opportunities to express their wishes about remaining in the parental home without professional people involved forcing their views on either party.

The worker must identify situations where a person's development is being inappropriately delayed by remaining in the parental home and bring such issues to the attention of the parents. However, the present legislation on protection of adults makes it very difficult to take action other than through persuasion unless the person is actually the victim of a crime against them.

Planning care to meet identified needs

Through the person's life the worker will be considering their daily living needs, identifying needs not met, providing services to meet priority needs and seeking to enhance independence. The worker will not be responsible for all the work but will be responsible for co-ordinating the activities of people responsible for various aspects of the plan. The worker will have to ensure that needs are met, and that interventions are carried out in such a way that the disabled person is allowed personal space and privacy and is not unduly stressed.

Issues to be addressed and some actions that could be taken

Issues to be addressed and some actions that could be taken are outlined in Box 1. The actions are the responsibilities of a wide range of disciplines: the worker's overall responsibility is to co-ordinate them.

Managing care

The person who gives daily care and the people with disabilities themselves have responsiblity for managing the care day-to-day. The carer, whether parent, family member or paid staff, is the only person able to review the appropriateness of all the arrangements made by the worker.

The prime carer must be fully involved in the treatment plans, understand and take part in skills training programmes and be given appropriate training for tasks they undertake, for example, lifting, bathing, toileting, etc. They must have an appreciation of the problems that may arise so that rapid changes can be made to plans and actions. The prime carer should have direct access to the worker, have a right to a rapid response to queries and problems, have the right to change the worker through an agreed system which would involve an independent arbitrator (i.e. not the worker's line manager), have access to all appropriate records and to a complaints system.

Reviewing and monitoring care

The monitoring of day-to-day care will be done through the prime carer but regular reviews of plans should be held to ensure they remain appropriate. In adult life, formal reviewing should probably be at yearly intervals unless issues have been identified which demand more frequent consideration.

The worker should be responsible for gathering all information in writing as well as through discussion with the people involved, such as day-care staff, residential staff and prime carer. From this information, the worker should decide if a meeting should be held and, if so, who should be invited. As few people as possible should attend with the person with disability. People such as concerned family members and the prime carer if this person is not a family member. All people involved in the care should have a written record of the review and its decisions.

The adult in care

If the adult person is being cared for by a paid carer either in a hostel or their own house, the worker's relationship with that

The needs of the person with a learning disability

Issues

1. Food

- What food is being eaten; is it appropriate?
- Who buys the food?
- Who cooks the food?
- Does the person have choice about what to eat?
- Who feeds the person?
- Who washes up and cleans the kitchen?

2. Personal hygiene

- How is toiletting achieved?
- Is there any incontinence?
- Who washes, baths, shaves the person?
- Does the person have any choice about when to shave, wash, etc.?

3. Clothing

- Who buys clothes?
- Is clothing appropriate for age, environment?
- Is the person allowed choices and are the choices appropriate?
- Who does the laundry?
- Who decides what will be worn, what needs washing and when?

4. Finance

- Is the person receiving appropriate benefit?
- Who decides how to spend the money, manages bank accounts, and pays bills?

Action

- Make changes to diet, teach about dietary needs, teach to make appropriate choices.
- Teach person to do shopping, provide special equipment, solve mobility problems in and out of the home.
- Promote independence by teaching new skills.

- Ensure there is no medical reason for incontinence.
- Plan behavioural programmes, determine who will carry them out.
- Teach new skills, provide special equipment and adaptations.

- Ensure the person experiences a range of options available.
- Teach new skills to enable the person to make choices.
- Provide special equipment.
- Solve mobility problems.
- Know the shops which can provide access and support learning.

- Develop a relationship with a bank that will help with specific problems.
- Ensure the person has their own bank account.
- Protect client's financial interests, if necessary through legal means.
- Plan programmes to teach about money, its use and management.

continued overleaf

continued

5. Housing

- Is the house appropriate for the needs of all who live in it (including carers)?
- Is it warm and dry?
- What type of area is it in?
- Does the person suffer from poor community attitudes to disability?

- Identify housing problems and determine actions to be taken.
- Provide adaptations and equipment.
- Work with local communities to be more accepting of and helpful to people with learning disabilities.

6. Social interactions

- Does the person have friends/acquaintances other than family?
- What opportunities are there for meeting and making friends?
- Is the person given freedom to choose own friends?
- Is the person concerned and caring of others?
- Are there maladaptive behaviours which need to be altered to develop better relationships?

- Make opportunities using local groups, etc. to meet people and develop friendships.
- Address the mobility problems which prevent friends meeting.
- Help the person with social skills through training programmes.

7. Personal interests

- Does the person have special interests — music, dance, cards, etc?
- Do they have opportunity to experiment and find special interests?
- Are they encouraged by family, etc. to pursue special interests?

- Find local groups, colleges, etc. where the client can join activities and test out interests.
- Give the person opportunity to use their skills.

8. Employment

- Is the person able to work in open or sheltered employment?
- Have they been given appropriate opportunities to test out skills?

- Ensure employment training schemes are used.
- Work with local employers to ensure the needs of disabled people are understood.
- Solve mobility problems that prevent use of work opportunities.

continued opposite

The carer's needs

Issues

1. Help with physical tasks

- Which tasks do family members find difficult – shopping, cleaning, washing, toiletting, bathing, feeding?
- Has the carer health problems?
- Does the carer dislike having to carry out some personal tasks for the person, e.g. toiletting?

2. Relief from caring

- When does the main carer want time out – hours, days, weeks?

3. Alternative interests/relationships

- Does the carer have other adult relationships?
- Does the carer have interests separate from the disabled person?
- Does the carer want paid employment?

4. Money

- Is the carer receiving all benefits?
- Does the carer spend money on themselves – clothing, entertainment, etc?
- Is the carer managing the person's money – is this appropriate?

5. Housing

- Does the house allow the carer some personal space?
- Is it cluttered with the disabled person's equipment?
- Is it warm, dry, clean?
- Does the carer have friends in the local community?
- Does the carer want action on housing matters?

Action

- Teach appropriate skills.
- Provide equipment.
- Ensure person is as independent as possible, help family to allow independence.
- Put in paid staff to do tasks which the family want met.
- Meet carer's health needs.

- Provide a service which will give care in arrangement with the carer, e.g. foster parents, small hostel/day centre.

- Work with carer to encourage the right to live separately from the person with disability.
- Support moves to independence, identify opportunities to meet others out of the disability world.

- Help the carer apply for benefits.
- Discuss money matters, encourage and support the carer in using money for their own needs.
- Consider and arrange alternatives for the management of the disabled person's money if appropriate.

- Work with the carer to solve issues seen as important.
- Ensure the carer has full understanding of alternatives.
- Provide equipment and adaptations.

continued overleaf

continued

6. Does the carer want to care?
Over the years the worker must constantly review with the family carer the satisfactions and dissatisfactions of giving care, acknowledging with the carer their own needs and their right to cease giving practical care. However, it must be remembered that a parent has specific responsibilities for their child; to the age of 18 years the legislation for children applies to any situation where parents wish to stop providing care and parents will have to undergo the legal processes that arise making them face uncomfortable questions about parental duties. Parents are parents, not carers! After the age of 18 years, parents have no obligation to continue caring, nor are they any longer the guardians of the person with disabilities. It is important that parents understand this, as the worker acting as advocate for the adult person may come into conflict with parents who continue to treat their child as a legal dependant. The worker must work with parents so they know of alternative living options for the disabled person and have opportunity to see such alternatives, talk to staff and explore fully the living environment their child could move to.

Box 1 Issues and action

paid carer will have similarities to the relationship the worker has with parents. The paid carer will take responsibilities for managing monies, ensuring daily needs are met, developing social and leisure opportunities, working closely with staff in day care to develop and effect learning programmes. In all work with adults, wherever they live and whoever gives daily care, the worker's responsibilities will be to act as an advocate for the disabled person, to identify that their priority needs are being met, that they have opportunities to continue to develop and explore other social and leisure activities, that they can have relationships with people other than the prime carer, that plans are relevant and are reviewed appropriately. The worker will have responsibility for ensuring the overall safety and well-being of the person and for taking protective action if required.

Interdisciplinary work and the role of key-worker
The actions needed to meet issues which need resolving will be the responsibility of different professions, for example the planning of skills learning programmes will be done by psychologists, educationalists, day centre or residential staff. The carrying through of programmes will be by families or paid carers in the person's home or a centre. The occupational therapist will be involved in assessment and provision of aids adaptations and the teaching of daily living tasks.

The worker will at times be the person to carry through specific programmes but usually they will have the task of helping the person with disability to take an active part in programmes; ensuring the family supports the activity; ensuring financial and mobility issues are not prohibiting involvement in programmes; ensuring that programmes are monitored so they are not putting the person under stress; and undertaking formal reviews of work.

Key-worker skills
To carry out the identification of need, the planning and the monitoring of care, the worker needs to be skilled in the following activities.

Gathering information

Carrying out purposeful interviews which enable the person with disabilities and family to trust the worker and explore matters pertinent to the person's well-being. The worker must have ability to use open-ended questions, be sensitive to non-verbal cues, to use language appropriate to the people being interviewed, to appreciate feelings and thoughts which may be foreign to the worker, but not to patronize by pretended understanding. The worker must give new knowledge freely, and offer new skills appropriately. The worker must not identify issues in terms of 'problems'.

Hypothesizing

The worker must be able to consider the information gained within the context of the worker's knowledge of human growth and behaviour, social, emotional and other needs and be able to use the knowledge and skills of other professions to develop thinking. The worker must be able to identify areas which are causing maladaptive behaviour, identify needs which must be met by others (e.g. medical needs, hearing problems, special aids, etc.) and identify carers' needs.

Testing out

The worker must be able to explore whether the person and/or their carers see these behaviours and needs as requiring intervention, to share thinking with all involved and reach compromises on issues to be tackled.

Planning

The worker must be able to identify how areas of difficulty can be tackled, identifying and agreeing who should carry out specific tasks – and who on a daily basis manages the care.

Reviewing and monitoring

The worker must be available to the prime carer and person to solve new problems, support on-going work and formally review at appropriate intervals that planned care continues to be meeting needs.

Networking

The worker must have a knowledge of community networks that would offer help – individuals, groups, clubs, helpful shopkeepers, etc.

Working with other disciplines

The worker must be able to identify the specific skills they bring to the task and know of the specific skills of others that will be of benefit in meeting need. The worker must know how to ensure these others are used appropriately in the care and to co-ordinate activities.

Knowledge of statutory services and their resources

The worker must be able to maximize financial benefits, know when to call upon leisure services, housing; know the responsibilities of social services/social work departments for child protection, mental health inputs or other statutory provisions; know how to get access to day care, paid carers, residential care, etc.

Service planning

The worker must be able to identify how services should be developed and how to make this information available to service planners. The worker must be able to involve people with disabilities, their families and service planners in formal and informal processes to ensure services are meeting the needs identified by users.

Managing and allocating resources

The worker must be able to set priorities and manage resources, and work with resource holders, such as officers-in-charge of day centres, to ensure priority needs are met. If the worker has a budget they should be able to manage it appropriately.

Be imaginative

The worker should be able to look for new solutions, and be prepared to take risks in trying new approaches.

Advocacy

The worker must be able to inform others of the client's thoughts and wishes if the client is unable to do this or wishes the worker to do it on their behalf. With the client, the worker must be able to represent the client's needs to resource holders so these needs are properly met.

Discussion Questions

'It is easy to identify the needs of each individual in isolation, the difficult process is defining what needs are paramount and negotiating between people with differing needs to reach agreement that to some extent satisfy all.'

- Do you agree? In what sort of ways might needs conflict? How could this be overcome?
- What are the key skills and knowledge required in assessment and care management?
- Do you have them?

Chapter 10

Balancing Risks and Needs

Ruth Prime

Key Issues

- Defining risk
- Identifying elements of risk
- Multidisciplinary assessments
- Consultation with black and minority ethnic communities
- Risk to self
- Risk to carers
- Risk from carers
- Risk from community/neighbourhood
- Issues of culture
- Issues of race
- Legislation
- Policy
- Staffing
- Training

Introduction

Perhaps one of the most fundamental and helpful principles to be learned and accepted by those preparing for practice is that policies and practice in social work must be viewed within the context of a multiracial, multicultural society. Although, on the face of it, this seems a very simple concept, in reality it is most difficult to communicate. The difficulty stems from the persistent tendency to treat issues of culture, and of race in particular, as though they are separate from the people concerned. Furthermore, there is a strong misconception that culture is the same as race. Moreover, when issues of culture are addressed, negative conclusions are often drawn.

Issues of race are concerned with the combined use of prejudice and power against people from black and minority ethnic communities to create differential access to housing, employment, education and social services, and resulting also in racial harassment and hostility. The impact on the lives of the recipients could sometimes be devastating. Issues of culture are concerned with the specific mores that characterize a group of people and which are passed on from one generation to another by learning. Account must be taken of:

- attitudes
- beliefs
- kinship systems
- child-rearing patterns

- music
- food
- religion
- political systems
- class systems.

Although our primary concern is with those who suffer from a learning disability, many of the basic principles which are discussed apply to all client groups. It is of extreme importance to keep in mind that people who experience learning disability are first and foremost people who have the same basic needs and are entitled to be treated with the same dignity and respect as the rest of the population. At the same time they have particular needs. In addition, societal attitudes create problems for people with disabilities and for black and minority ethnic communities; racism within society produces a range of further problems.

It is within the context of a multicultural, multiracial society that some analysis of 'risk-taking' in working with people with learning disabilities and their carers will be attempted.

Defining Risk

In social work, phrases such as 'at risk' and 'taking risks' are frequently used, but what exactly do they mean and what are the implications?

Longman's dictionary defines 'at risk' as a situation or circumstances where loss, injury, etc. are possible. 'Taking risks' is defined as placing in a dangerous situation; liable to mischance. Both definitions are pertinent in social work where the mischance can lead to physical, emotional, psychological abuse, neglect, injury and even loss of life.

Climate

Risk is an inherent element in the process of social work and related professions. The nature of the work makes risk inevitable and it increases when dealing with vulnerable clients. Although we would all agree with the inevitability of risk, it does not follow that clients must be placed in dangerous situations liable to mischance, loss or injury. Risks can be estimated, that is to say, taken in the light of a wide range of knowledge – a well-informed stance which contributes to the decision-making process of balancing risks and needs. In calculating risk, some assessment must be made of the possibility of failure, the degree of which must be estimated and taken into account before a venture is undertaken.

In social work, situations which lend themselves to risk vary, but in principle there are many elements common to all situations and which can be identified.

Identification of Elements of Risk through Assessment

Elements of risk are identified through the assessment process. The value of good assessment procedures cannot therefore be sufficiently stressed. An assessment is carried out to determine whether there are factors, the absence or presence of which may cause problems or have adverse effect on the quality of life. Having identified these factors, an evaluation is made, conclusions are drawn and decisions arrived at.

The assessment process covers six stages. The first stage of information gathering is crucial. The purpose of the information should be to get a comprehensive picture of the person within his or her total environment, how she or he functions within the environment and the impact of the environment on the functioning. A number of pertinent factors need to be considered including:

- physical environment of the home and neighbourhood
- health factors
- financial factors
- the client's abilities
- formal networks
- informal networks
- friends
- neighbours
- main carers
- abilities and wishes
- emotional and physical needs of client and carer(s)
- attitudes of carers towards handicap
- attitudes of the neighbourhood to and relationship with the person and family
- strengths and weaknesses of the handicapped person and family
- issues of race and culture.

- Gather information
- Evaluate information
- Draw conclusions
- Decide action
- Implement decision
- Monitor and review

Box I Assessment process

Evaluating the information needs skills and objectivity. Each facet of the information gathered interlocks to form a comprehensive picture to enable conclusions to be drawn about the way in which the needs of the individual and carer can be best met. Based on the conclusions drawn, decisions

are made on action to be taken. The range of actions include:

- assurance
- information giving
- advice
- advocacy
- provision of a single service or services
- a care planning meeting where all relevant people involved or likely to be involved come together to:
  - share information
  - discuss needs
  - decide on the most appropriate way of   meeting those needs.

A 'package of care' or care plan should then be drawn up, outlining the implementation of the plan in a clear and detailed manner so that everyone is clear about:

- responsibilities
- tasks
- time limits
- achievements of goals
- back-up systems
- lines of reporting
- support for workers
- key-worker.

Finally, a review date is set. An appropriate plan of care would be designed to ensure that the needs of the individual and carer are met effectively with the minimum amount of confusion and intrusion.

Close monitoring and reviewing are essential so that plans can be adapted to meet changing situations. It follows then that if assessments are to be comprehensive they must be multidisciplinary, consultation with representatives from the black and minority ethnic communities who are aware of the needs of people with learning disabilities must take place, and the needs and abilities of carers must be determined.

Multidisciplinary Assessments

Multidisciplinary assessments are essential because the needs of the person with a learning disability are highly likely to cover a wide span requiring specialist knowledge and expertise. Furthermore, people come from all age groups, therefore some of the specialist knowledge will be related to the needs of the particular age group. Children, for example, may need the expertise of a paediatrician and a child psychologist, while an elderly person may need the expertise of a geriatrician or psychogeriatrician. The White Paper *Caring for People* (DOH, 1990) made the following statement:

All agencies and professions involved with the individual and his or her problems should be brought into the assessment procedure when necessary. These may include:

- social workers;
- general practitioners;
- community nurses;
- consultants in geriatric medicine, psychiatry, rehabilitation and other hospital specialities;
- nurses;
- physiotherapists;
- occupational therapists;
- speech therapists;
- continence advisers;
- community psychiatric nurses;
- staff involved in vision and hearing;
- housing officers;
- the Employment Department's Resettlement and Employment Rehabilitation Service;
- home helps;
- home-care assistants;
- voluntary workers.

This is indeed an impressive list to which others may still be added such as educationalists in the case of a child. It is not, however, a prescription for involving all these people in every case. The statement makes the point 'when necessary', therefore people should be involved where their expertise is deemed appropriate or of value.

Assessment of Carers

The needs of carers were given a very high profile in the White Paper *Caring for People*. One of the six key objectives of service delivery is to ensure that service providers make practical support for carers a high priority. Assessment of care needs should always take account of needs of the caring family, friends and neighbours. One of the stated principles of assessment is that 'assessments should take account of the wishes of the individual and his or her carer and of the carer's ability to continue to provide care and where possible include their active participation. Effort should be made to offer flexible services which enable individuals and carers to make choices'. Considering the strengths, weaknesses and wishes of the carers cannot be sufficiently stressed. If these elements remain unknown, then vital pieces of the puzzle will be missing and decisions will be based on partial knowledge – a dangerous practice. Equally, as far as it is possible to do so, the client must be consulted and his/her wishes taken into consideration.

The Wagner Report (1988) though addressing the needs of the elderly, makes the following statement which is pertinent to all carers.

We believe that community care services should use every means available to contact as many of the informal carers in their area so as to find out what support of all kinds they may need. Even where it appears that they require no regular support, it will still be important to ensure whether the carers ever had a holiday since if they do not, the whole caring arrangement should be regarded as potentially 'at risk' or under stress of a sudden breakdown of damage to the mental and physical health of the carer, and consequent danger to the person cared for.

Consultation with Representatives from Black and Minority Ethnic Communities

The White Paper gave recognition to the fact that 'people from different cultural backgrounds may have particular care needs and problems. Minority communities may have different concepts of community care and it is important that service providers are sensitive to these variations. Good community care will take account of the circumstances of minority communities and will be planned in consultation with them'.

A recurrent error is the belief that in the consultation process any black representative would do. This error must be avoided. Representatives must have an understanding of the general needs of people who experience a learning disability and the particular needs of those from black and minority ethnic communities. Knowledge of the beliefs, attitudes and reaction of different groups to learning disability is an important feature.

Elements of Risk

A comprehensive assessment should identify whether the following elements of risk are present or not:

- risk from self
- risk from carers
- risk to carers
- risk from the community/neighbourhood.

It is not sufficient however to identify these elements of risks. Positive steps need to be taken to eliminate or minimize them.

Risk from self

Risk is inherent in social work because among the primary objectives of good-quality care are independence, choice, fulfilment and dignity. In *Homes are for Living In* (DOH Social Services Inspectorate, 1989) independence is defined as 'opportunities to think and act without reference to another including a willingness to incur a degree of calculated risk'. The extent to which each individual can be independent will obviously vary but opportunities must be provided for the testing out and development of independence. Choice is 'an opportunity to choose independently from a range of options'. If independence is to be encouraged, then choice must also be given. If, for example, an individual chooses to live independently after being given a range of options, independence could be made possible but risk will be involved.

In the course of day-to-day living there are a number of activities which must be carried out, ranging from the simple to the complex. Decision-making is also a part of day-to-day living, and in both areas regard must be given to physical, emotional and mental development of the individual. Some of the areas which can be examined are ability to perform tasks which are related to:

- personal care
- home care
- shopping
- use of public transport
- attending school
- going out to work
- participating in social activities.

This is not an exhaustive list but it does give a good indication of what needs to be considered. Any of the items listed can be used to illustrate how elements of 'risk from self' can be identified. *Personal care* will be used for this purpose.

Personal care involves numerous activities which the vast majority of the population take for granted but which, for those who experience learning disability, can present an incredible number of problems. Assessment should focus on the extent to which the individual is able to perform tasks, the element of risk, if any, in performing the tasks, and steps which could be taken to simplify the tasks as well as remove or minimize the element of risk. The skills and expertise of an occupational therapist or equivalent practitioners are essential. Personal care includes:

- bathing/washing
- toiletry
- dressing
- brushing teeth
- combing hair
- putting on make-up
- shaving.

All these tasks call for a measure of co-ordination, balance and judgement. For the handicapped person, some of the risks are injury from falling, and accidents in using implements such as make-up, brushes and razors.

There is another area of risk from self which stems from limitation of the individual's ability to conceptualize or assess danger. The extent of the limitation will determine what degree of risk is permissible.

Risk from carers

The term 'carers' is generally used to describe relatives, friends or neighbours who care for dependent people without payment. They are often referred to as informal carers. Relatives include parents, grandparents, spouses, children and others.

There is, however, another group of carers, often referred to as formal carers who are paid to provide care. The risk to clients from this group is mainly associated with staff in institutions or residential care, but there are paid carers in the community. Employers must be alert to the fact that those for whom they care can be equally exposed to physical, financial, emotional and psychological risks of abuse and neglect. In this chapter, informal carers are the focus of concern.

Reference has already been made to the high profile given to the needs and abilities of carers in the Government White Paper *Caring for People* and the recommendations of the Wagner Report.

Although high priority is given to independence of the individual, it is common knowledge that in many instances total independence cannot be achieved and dependence for care, which is often provided by carers, can be minimal or extreme both physically and emotionally.

Assessing the needs and abilities of the carer is therefore as important as assessing the needs of the individual. It would be true to say that no assessment is complete without exploring the needs and abilities of carers.

Many people take on the caring role out of love, humanity and duty to those they love. The problem for them is societal attitudes. Society places responsibility for care firmly on the shoulders of the carers, usually women, and this attitude is reflected in social services. Thankfully, attitudes are beginning to change and realization is dawning that love and willingness to care are not enough to sustain carers. The harsh reality of stress is inescapable.

Stress is a word which very aptly describes the problems endured by carers. Various factors combine to produce stress. Broadly speaking, stress is classified as physical and emotional and while in some instances they are clearly independent and identifiable, often one can lead to the other. Physical stress stems partly from the practical tasks involved in caring, some of which can be very strenuous (e.g. lifting) and some frequent and repetitive. Physical stress can lead to emotional stress. Emotional stress comes in many guises. The emotional demands made by the client, the carer's inability to lead a social life and the ensuing isolation, sometimes the inability to go out to work or having to give up a career, all of which can produce resentment and the guilt which resentment often brings. The wearing effect of it all when faced at times with the relentlessness of the situation can eventually lead to depression. In addition, carers may be faced with their own personal problems.

Although workers can be aware, in any given situation, of factors that produce stress and can identify clusters of factors which have the potential to produce high-level stress, they must be mindful of the fact that individuals vary and their tolerance levels will fluctuate in relation to variables such as health and emotional needs. Assumptions therefore must be made with caution and help must be tailored to meet individual need.

Within this context, due account must be taken of the abilities of carers. There are those who are in the role of carers but who are incapable of caring for themselves and need to be cared for in their own right. Failure to assess their needs puts both client and carer at risk. Some workers argue that the carer is not the 'client' and that it is the needs of the client with which they are concerned. Certainly assessing the needs of the carer is not an implication that he or she is a client, nor does it imply putting the needs of the carer above those of the client. The value of the assessment is that it can identify the strengths and weaknesses of the carer and conflict between the needs of the carer and cared for. It can provide information which assists in the balancing of the needs of the one against the other, and ultimately contribute to judgements about the risks involved. In the process it might well be discovered that the carer is a 'client'. Conflict between the needs of the carer and cared for heightens the risk and yet it is an element which is often unidentified or unaddressed when identified.

So far the emphasis has been on those who are in the caring role and may wish to continue to do so with appropriate help or those who sadly will continue to do so even without help. There are, however, those in the caring role who either do not accept the role of carers or do not have the necessary patience and understanding to perform the required tasks. The potential risk of physical and emotional abuse to those being cared for by such individuals is extremely high. It is essential therefore that in assessing the abilities of carers we try to elicit their attitudes to being in the caring role

Risks to carers

All the determinants of risk to the individual from carers indirectly put carers at risk. Firstly, if carers subject those for whom they are caring to physical abuse, they may put themselves at risk legally. Secondly, when due to stress they subject the client to emotional or psychological abuse, they may suffer from guilt, remorse and depression. Carers are therefore at risk of physical and emotional ill-health. Moreover, there is the risk of physical and emotional abuse to the carers from those being cared for – risks that should not be under-estimated.

Risk from the community/ neighbourhood

In general, the community does not respond positively to people with learning disabilities. It is quite likely, therefore, that those who suffer from such disabilities may suffer from ridicule, be the subject of jokes and even be easy targets for physical attacks in their neighbourhood. In some instances, families can become very isolated and frightened and for black and minority ethnic people this can be compounded by racial harassment.

Issues of Culture

Dearnley and Prime (1989) draw attention to the fact that workers in many professions when working with people from black and minority ethnic communities use cultural factors negatively. The most commonly held view often referred to as a myth is 'they look after their own'. On the face of it, this can be a positive view implying that people from black and minority ethnic communities are caring and accept the responsibility for looking after their relatives. In reality it is an obstacle to their getting needed help, for as much as they might love to 'look after their own' there are factors such as housing and low income which work against them. Further, willingness to care is not an antidote to stress.

Another tendency is to use cultural norms to explain other types of behaviour. In so doing, unacceptable behaviour is ignored. The cause is not investigated and risk factors remain unidentified. In a case cited by Dearnley and Prime the psychiatric problems of the mother were not identified because her behaviour was attributed to cultural norms and the children were left in a situation of risk for a long time.

Issues of Race

Racism has an impact on the lives of recipients in various ways, such as poor housing, low income and low self-esteem. These factors are problematic wherever present but for those who suffer from a learning disability and their carers they can be greater. Personal and institutionalized racism can also affect the way services are designed and delivered and workers need to be aware of this. Good practice would demand that instead of drawing conclusions on erroneous assumptions, workers with relevant knowledge and understanding of issues of culture and of race should be involved in the assessment process either at fieldwork or consultant level or both.

Service Delivery

Good assessment though absolutely necessary is not enough to ensure appropriate service delivery. A knowledge of resources in the statutory private and voluntary sectors, is fundamental. Resources in the broadest sense covers:

- information about benefits
- funds
- medical and social aspects of disability
- supportive networks
- day-care services
- respite-care
- employment
- education.

If people are to be given choice they must be informed about what is available so that they can make informed choices. Services should be tailored to individual need; therefore, a flexible and imaginative and sensitive approach is necessary. Respite care in a residential establishment may be acceptable to some and not to others. If the service delivered is not appropriate, the element of risk remains or may even be heightened, and while this is true in all situations the likelihood of inappropriate service delivery is greater for people from black and minority ethnic communities.

Managerial Responsibility

Issues of practice have been the main thrust of this chapter but managers have a responsibility to provide the framework within which fieldworkers can carry out their duties. The following key issues must therefore be addressed:

- legislation
- policy
- staffing
- training.

Each issue provides scope for wide-ranging discussion (see other chapters in this volume), and the main aspects are summarized here.

Legislation

Legislation has changed rapidly in the 1990s and that applying to particular services is described in other chapters. However, it is worth reflecting for a moment on the Race Relations Act, 1976, which states:

Section 71: It shall be the duty of every local authority to make appropriate arrangements with a view to securing that their various functions are carried out with due regard to the need:

(a) to eliminate unlawful discrimination,
(b) to promote equality of opportunity and good relations between persons of different racial groups.

This legislation provides foundation on which Local Authorities can build, the end-product being their service delivery to a multiracial, multicultural society. The extent to which they take it on board will be reflected in their policy statement, training programmes and staffing levels.

Policy

Every agency concerned with work with people with learning disabilities should have a statement of policy (intent) and a strategy for implementing that policy. Further, there must be a system for monitoring and reviewing in order to give the strategy viability and credibility. The identification of sustainable targets for performance and an indication of time scales for their achievement is also an important aspect of this process. Policy statements should include the needs of black and minority ethnic communities and policy-makers and planners should consult with well-informed members of these committees.

Allied to policy for the person will be the implementation of an equal opportunity policy which should include guidelines for recruitment, interviewing, selection, ethnic recording, staff opportunities and the composition of interviewing panels. Very often an equal opportunity policy amounts to little more than a statement which is included in advertisements and is no more than a paper exercise.

Staffing

If an effective equal opportunity policy is in place, the probability of a work force which reflects a multicultural community will increase. A representative work force is likely to enhance the quality of service delivery and its sensitivity to the range of community expectations. However, the creation of a multicultural work force does not in itself guarantee that all sections of the community will receive a service or that the service will be delivered with cultural sensitivity or free from racism. The organization's strategy and the effective and appropriate use of staff will be the determining factors.

Training

Training of staff is fundamental to the implementation of an equal opportunity policy and of anti-racist strategies. Anti-racist training should assist workers in the understanding of personal and institutionalized racism and in recognizing how racist conditioning may affect their feelings and attitudes. If staff lack this understanding, they are unlikely to respond to the anti-racist strategies which are designed for effective service delivery and for dealing with racism in the workplace.

It must be stressed that training for work in a multiracial, multicultural society should be an underlying theme of all social work training. If preparation for work in such a society is to be treated seriously, it cannot be achieved by devoting a few days to the issue of race; it should be an integral unit of all aspects of training courses for social services and health and voluntary organizations and should be revised and refined as appropriate. On-going training for working with those who experience learing disability must also be addressed by managers.

With the key issues addressed, the foundation will be laid for the fieldworkers to undertake the tasks of identification of need, assessment and service delivery.

Conclusion

In summary it would seem fair to say that risk, though an inherent element in the process of social work, can be identified, estimated and ultimately prevented or minimized.

Assessment is not only the key determinant of need; it is also the process through which risk factors and the potential danger to the individual and carer can be identified,

after which careful balancing of risk and need can ensue. During the assessment process, distinction must be made between the needs and abilities of the individual and those of the carer, and areas of conflict can be recognized.

A good assessment is one that takes account of the individual as a whole within his or her total environment. Because the needs of those people experiencing learning disability are likely to cover a wide span requiring specialist knowledge and expertise, multidisciplinary assessments are essential. Furthermore, where people from black and minority ethnic communities are being assessed, issues of race and culture must be addressed. The end-product of the assessment – the effective delivery of service – must be well planned, co-ordinated and tailored to meet individual need if risk is to be minimized or prevented. If the outlined process is adhered to, risk will be taken in the light of a wide range of knowledge – a well-informed stance which would contribute to the decision-making process of balancing risk and need, and the likelihood of disaster will be greatly reduced.

Finally, it is incumbent on managers within the legislative context to provide the framework within which fieldworkers can operate effectively, through policies, procedures, training and staffing.

Discussion Questions

- Identify the elements of risk in your particular area of work.
- Who are affected by these elements of risk.
- What in your view are the specific issues to be addressed where working with black and minority ethnic communities.

- If your department has no policy/procedure for dealing with risk, how would you go about developing one with the help of other relevant people.

References

Dearnley, J. and Prime, R. (1989). *Inspection of Social Work with Afro-Caribbean and Asian Families in Avon*. Department of Health, Social Services Inspectorate. HMSO, London.

DOH (1988). *A Positive Choice: Residential Care – Report of Independent Review* (Wagner Report). HMSO, London.

DOH Social Services Inspectorate (1989). *Homes are for Living In*. HMSO, London.

DOH (1990). *Caring for People: Community Care in the Next Decade and Beyond*. Cmnd 849. HMSO, London.

Prime, R. (1984). No longer a second class service. *Community Care*, **536**, 25–9.

The Wagner Report (1988). *Residential Care: A Positive Choice*. The National Institute of Social Work.

Chapter 11

Implementing the Care Programme Approach

Mike Musker

Key Issues

- Origins of the care programme approach
- The process
- Implementation
    views of team members
    a care programme plan
- Implications

Introduction

This chapter considers the practical implications of introducing an avowedly interprofessional care programme approach (CPA) into a high-security setting, illustrating its potential by describing its use on behalf of someone experiencing learning disability and behavioural disorder.

The CPA was introduced in April 1991 (DOH, 1990) as part of the response to tragedies that had occurred in the community, carried out by patients who had not been appropriately monitored. These cases included Christopher Clunis, who because of his severe mental illness murdered an innocent bystander, Jonathan Zito (Ritchie and Lingham, 1994); and the murder of the occupational therapist Georgina Robinson, who was brutally stabbed to death by a patient who had previously committed the serious offence of attempting to shoot his girlfriend (Blom-Cooper *et al.*, 1995). These cases demonstrated how poor networking and breakdowns of interdisciplinary communication can result in traumatic situations in the community for innocent people, their families, and for the individual themselves.

If we consider the complexities and difficulty of accessing services within the community, we can begin to imagine how someone who has a learning disability and mental health difficulties might manage under such circumstances. Whilst in hospital, an individual has relatively co-ordinated access to professionals and other resources. It is when they return to the community, which may consist of a large catchment area of around 180 000 people or more and where a Health Authority often has to deal with up to 900 acute admissions a year, that they may find their access to care begins to fragment (Hamilton and Roy, 1995).

An information system that spans all levels of care, so that it follows the service user wherever he or she goes, should bring about resource savings, and prevent the user having to go through the same burdensome assessments repeatedly. CPA is a systematic process of care that has been developed to reduce the failings of the caring services, and can be applied to all service users who come into contact with the specialist psychiatric services and all patients considered for discharge (DOH, 1994a). It is not necessary for all service users to be covered by the CPA system, but a consistent approach across all services and for all individuals makes sense and would be good practice. The main emphasis is to prevent people being discharged inappropriately to services or situations that are unsuitable, and to ensure that care is available where it is needed.

CPA has been tiered into three categories to ensure that time and resources are used efficiently. These are:

- *minimum CPA* which may involve contact by just one carer;
- *more complex CPA* involving a few members of the team who will need to be in contact with each other;
- *full multidisciplinary CPA* which incorporates full multidisciplinary assessments, a care plan and reviews.

The *Building Bridges* guide to the care programme approach (DOH, 1996) sets out several tenets that care teams should consider when developing care programmes for their service users:

- There is a single *care plan* that is agreed by all the agencies involved in the delivery of care.

- A *key worker* will take responsibility for the implementation of the plan and can call for a review.
- A full *assessment of risk* should be part of the assessment process.
- The *service user* must be involved in all planning, reviews and implementation of the care programme.
- The *supervision register* (DOH, 1994b) is a subsection of the CPA.

The National Health Service (NHS) Executive has stated that the CPA is just what it says – 'an approach'; they have no intention of being prescriptive about how it is implemented, providing latitude for each hospital or care team to apply their own interpretation. There is now an audit pack (NHS Executive, 1996) which allows teams to assess the quality of interventions against a set of basic care standards. Participation of the service user is the key premise which has inspired the need to change the management of health care. The key-worker should attempt to gain consensus about the care programme from the service user, their family, and other people that may be involved. When this is not the case, attempts should be made to change the care plan to how the service user wants it designed (DOH, 1996). This pledge of commitment and involvement will ensure that the person will feel valued and is more likely to co-operate with their care.

The CPA seems very similar to the notions put forward by care management, and this is because they are essentially the same process. CPA is about how Health Authorities provide care, and care management is more about the provision of support by the Social Services. It is important that both these systems work in harmony and they should use the same assessment process to avoid duplication and inefficient use of resources. The reasons why services are still managed separately are set out in the

White Paper *Caring for People* (DOH, 1989), which describes the roles and responsibilities of the Social Service Authorities and the Health Authorities. Some patients may require exclusive Social or Health Services care but the CPA should pay particular attention to those service users who have learning disabilities who need to receive integrated services:

In some cases it may well be difficult to draw a clear distinction between the needs of an individual for health and for social care. In such cases it will be critically important for the responsible authorities to work together.

(DOH, 1989)

Emphasis is placed on the need for the development of healthy alliances, which will provide strategies to promote health through intersectoral collaboration and interagency working. This can be done by health service providers working closely with representatives of the people in the community, voluntary organizations and Local Government (Simnett, 1996).

The Process

Our care team has been developing the CPA over the past 3 years. The initiative was led by our hospital CPA liaison manager, Chris Maher, who researched and developed the main documentation layout and provided some workshops to cascade the ideals of the CPA to all staff. Initially, the team was unsure how to put the new ideas into practice. However, it was discussed at the care team meeting and the following agreements reached over a number of months:

- Each service user would have a case worker (i.e. key-worker) and up to three associates case workers of their choice. As this is a closed ward setting the people who were best suited to this role were nurses, as they had more contact time with the service user.
- A case manager who would chair the care team assessment and reviews, in conjunction with the case worker, would be designated to each service user. Any discipline could be the case manager for specific service users, supporting the nurses in the implementation of the care programme. This would provide a strong link for the case worker at care programme meetings, as the case managers attended almost every week.
- A case co-ordinator would oversee all the care programmes, reviews and resources. The clinical leader was best suited to this role, as they had access to budgets and management initiatives. They were also based on the ward Monday to Friday, and were present when any visitors or external personnel attended the ward. This would enable the case co-ordinator to maintain an overall view of care and thus ensure consistency within care programmes.
- Care programmes would be discussed on a 2-weekly basis, with full reviews set for between 4 and 6 months as required. An up-to-date report would then be supplied by each discipline against the service user's needs.
- Each discipline would ensure they provided time for service users on a one to one basis in between care programme meetings. This could be by appointment or during their visit to the ward on a specific day of the week, which we decided to call 'clinics'.
- Service users were welcome at all meetings. In practice only one or two service users would request to see the care team, because they had adequate liaison through their case worker or they would speak to the specific professional concerned during their regular ward clinics.

Advocates or family members were also welcomed. When necessary, specialists such as the pharmacist were also invited to provide specific advice.

Two major changes have occurred with the introduction of the CPA. First, the service user is involved at every stage of the programme. Second, the roles of the professionals have blended together, sharing the caring role without any hierarchical power struggles. The whole process has encouraged real interdisciplinary working, demonstrating respect for each profession's contribution to the care programme. This has enhanced the team work within our meetings. It has emphasized equity within the team, encouraging debate and conflict where necessary as part of a democratic process.

The introduction of an information system that would flow between the disciplines was one of the most important steps of the CPA. We have moved away from nursing notes and clinical notes, toward care programme notes, where all professionals record their contributions and any progress in relation to service-user needs. The key parts to the system are:

- *case discussion* – a brief synopsis of the meeting;
- *case review* – essential information of all the carers and team involved;
- *a risk assessment* – specialized information assessing dangerousness to self or others;
- *interdisciplinary reports* and a summary;
- *the care programme* – a list of needs, outcomes and interventions;
- *the post-communication review* – a list of contact information including family/future carers; home details; the Local Authority; and other agencies.

The Team's Comments on Care Programme Implementation

Each member of the team was asked to give their opinion on how they contribute to the CPA and what improvements they saw in the process. The team is currently working on a ward which provides specialized care for people who display severe challenging behaviours, who are likely to require long-term health and social care interventions due to their learning disabilities and the complications of brain damage. The ward is situated in a high-security setting. Here are the opinions and comments from one service user and the team that cares for him.

The service user

Billy (a pseudonym) cannot write but when asked about his care, he felt that the nurses helped him and he looked forward to being transferred to a new unit where he could live more independently. Billy has learning disabilities and he finds it difficult to understand the care process, but every effort has been made to consult him. Billy has a particularly good memory for names and he can explain each role of the care team members. He does have difficulty, however, interpreting what people are saying to him, requiring time, and re-interpretation of complicated phrases. Billy frequently states: 'What does that mean?', asking this so often that he really just needs some time to take in what has been said. His care programme was explained to him and he was asked to sign it to demonstrate that he had been fully involved. Billy was excited by the idea that someone had written something about him, and his case worker helped him to recognize some words in his programme. He is particularly good at reading names and this enabled him to recognize who was involved in his care (see case study below).

The consultant registered medical officer (RMO) (Psychiatrist – Dr D. Kumarajeewa)

The exact method of CPA to be used in clinical care was not specified, but the Government circulars stressed the importance of multidisciplinary working in the approach. The key-worker or case worker was defined as a named person appointed to keep in close touch with the service user and to monitor that the agreed health and social care was given. Although a consistent case worker or key-worker was already commonly used in mental health services, written multidisciplinary care plans and CPA were not. Initially, this important change was brought about by the introduction of the CPA for hospital patients who were going to be discharged into the community. The CPA is now commenced when the patient first enters hospital. The person's needs are identified and the responsibility of meeting these needs is taken by relevant professionals who make up the multidisciplinary team. Regular reviews are co-ordinated with the key- or case worker to assess to what extent the needs of the service user are met. Although CPA was seen as a valuable instrument to monitor and measure the type of care received by a particular category of patient, soon this became popular for other people who could benefit from a written care plan or CPA. This was viewed as good clinical practice by which care is provided according to the needs of the service user. Introduction of CPA in this high-security setting with people who require a highly structured care plan became a real asset over and above the institutional care they had been receiving. The remit of the care team is to establish CPA and carry out regular reviews. Service users may wish to express their views about their care programme. It is the responsibility of the RMO to ensure that discussions take place to establish a care plan to organize the management of the person's continuing health and social care needs.

The long-term objective for each person in this setting should be to prepare the individual to live an independent life in the community in the foreseeable future, wherever possible. Nursing staff and the care team are committed to achieve the initial steps of this long-term goal. Properly conducted CPA should allow patients and their relatives (with the patient's consent) to take an active role in their care plan. When the patient agrees with their individualized care programme, they should be asked to sign the CPA documentation to demonstrate their involvement. The patient should be told that they are entitled to have a copy of their care programme. It is also the responsibility of the care team to invite relatives to review meetings. Again, this should be done with the patient's consent.

The senior social worker (Doug Hicks)

There has been a clear achievement of objectives in the implementation of the CPA over the past 12 months. The multidisciplinary care team has become accustomed to the requirement of producing individual assessment reports that focus on a needs-led approach to health and social needs. These reports pinpoint individual needs rather than provide a general narrative. Care team members have been able to shift away from a problem-orientated report, which in the past had often emphasized individual pathology and a negative description of patients, to a more positive reformulation based on concept of need. The care team has demonstrated its ability to work in a collaborative way to produce individual care programmes which are multidisciplinary and do not overemphasize the contribution of any particular discipline. This has been part of a holistic approach to health and social care needs and has moved away from a more medically oriented model.

In line with the 'Empowerment Model' of care and treatment, patients have been closely involved in drawing up their care programme. They have been able to give their views on what they feel are their health and social care needs, prior to the care programme review meeting; thus, those views have been part of the input from which the care programme has been devised. Also, they have been encouraged to attend the meeting to give any additional views and to ask any questions that they may have. Patients appear to have appreciated their close involvement in the care programme process. In addition, patients' relatives and families have been encouraged to express their views and these have been used in the CPA process. The care team has taken steps to ensure that there is a review system for actions and interventions in the care programme. These are given a specific date for implementation and 'actioned' by a particular individual. In addition, there is a half-yearly review of the needs action plan, when it can be refined if necessary, as well as a full review at 12 months with the provision of new assessment reports by team members. Significant progress has indeed been made in implementing a needs-led approach to health and social care based on multidisciplinary collaboration.

Rehabilitation liaison (Jonathan Duff)

I have represented the Rehabilitation Services within the specialist services unit for approximately 12 months, previously playing a role as part of the ward liaison service. I perform a number of roles in relation to the CPA process. One important role is to form part of a multidisciplinary team to aid the decision-making with regard to care programmes. A second role is to act as a representative of the Rehabilitation Service at the care programme meetings. A third role is to provide a communications link between education and training, vocational and recreational therapies and the ward environment. A fourth role can be seen as representing specific patients such as those on the ward in relation to their rehabilitation needs or aspirations. The duties that I perform include: attendance at the care programme meeting on a weekly basis and taking an active part in discussions and decision-making; assessing patient need with regard to rehabilitation areas; advising patients and the care programme meeting on suitable placements within the rehabilitation departments; and making arrangements for these placements and any necessary changes as patients request them.

My main role is reporting regularly on patient progress within the Rehabilitation Service. I co-ordinate the preparation of these reports for case reviews, assessments, Mental Health Review Tribunals, or by specific request of the care team. I offer guidance and counselling to patients on their placements. I report on care programme decisions and discussions to colleagues involved in the treatment and rehabilitation, by ensuring I am familiar with specific individual treatment plans and discussing these with my colleagues. There is a monitoring of attendance by individuals at programmed rehabilitation activities. It is necessary to gather information and requests from key personnel to present at the next care programme meeting. I am continually communicating with case workers to ensure that individual needs and interests of their patients are addressed. I have found it beneficial to hold a clinic on the ward on a regular basis to discuss with patients their individual needs. One particular role I enjoy is participating with the patient and case worker in rehabilitation excursions, when resources allow.

Lead consultant clinical psychologist (Kate Hellin) and assistant psychologist (Helen Ley)

The CPA provides a framework for structuring clinical work and communication in the multiprofessional team working with a complex client group. The CPA underpins the process of clinical assessment, which is needs-focused. Needs are identified through detailed multidisciplinary assessment and formulation. It is the specialized assessment skills of clinical psychologists that are perhaps most utilized in the CPA process. All patients should receive a full clinical psychology assessment. Ideally, this would be before the patient is admitted but resources have dictated that this is seldom possible. Assessment consists of a wide range of skills and techniques which would be applicable in any psychological setting: cognitive, behavioural, psychodynamic, neuropsychological and psychometric. Here, there are also further aspects of assessment, such as risk assessment with respect to physical violence, sex offending, arson, suicide and self-harm.

A clinical psychological approach to understanding people, their feelings and behaviours, rests upon functional analysis and formulation rather than pure diagnosis.

Formulation draws upon a wide range of information including historical and current records from all disciplines, interviews with patients, case workers and other relevant staff, psychometric assessments and theoretical and research knowledge. The clinical psychologist's role will be in producing a formulation which, with other team members' contributions, comprises the basis for care programme discussion and the identification of clinical needs.

The clinical psychologist may then follow on after an assessment, to work with the patient, individually or in a group setting, where psychological needs have been identified. Psychologists will play a central role in the monitoring and evaluation of CPA goals through the use of specific applied methodology such as single case design measurement and the use of sophisticated psychometrics.

Recruitment difficulties in clinical psychology have meant that psychologists have not been fully involved in all stages of CPA as was intended.

The behaviour nurse co-ordinator (Pete Stoddart)

The role of the behaviour nurse co-ordinator in the CPA is multifaceted. They have the responsibility for advising the care team with regard to behavioural principles, definitions, and techniques, either on an informal basis or more formally through a series of tutorials and multidisciplinary workshops. When they have identified a client as displaying challenging behaviour of such an intensity, frequency or duration as to warrant a behavioural intervention, the care team formally requests that a behavioural assessment be carried out and recommendations be presented as to which would be the most effective method of intervention. When the team formally refers a client, the two options for the behaviour nurse co-ordinator are either acceptance or rejection of the referral. If a client is rejected for behavioural intervention, which is a rare occurrence as the care team has attained a sound grasp of the behavioural approach, then we may refer the client back to the team or on to a relevant professional. Upon acceptance of the referral, the behaviour nurse co-ordinator will conduct a baseline assessment of the challenging behaviour; interview all relevant people involved in the care of the client; carry out observational assessments and conduct formal assessments with the client who is displaying the challenging behaviour.

Only when all the relevant data are gathered can a functional analysis be completed and a hypothesis of the function of the challenging behaviour be considered. This is pivotal when attempting to formulate effective behavioural intervention programmes. When a behavioural programme is drawn up for a client, the behaviour nurse co-ordinator presents the proposed intervention to the care team for ratification. If they ratify the plan, the behaviour nurse co-ordinator will liaise with the key nursing staff who have responsibility for the implementation and continuation of the programme. They then work through the plan together with the client to explain what the programme consists of, and what is expected of the client and the case worker. After implementation of the behavioural intervention the case worker carries out an ongoing evaluation, measuring the effectiveness of the intervention and, if necessary, we can then make alterations to the care programme. Any modifications to a behavioural programme are always presented for ratification to the care team.

The behaviour nurse co-ordinator works with clients, care staff, allied professionals, specialists, as well as any other agencies, with the aim of reducing behavioural challenges through the use of positive programming and reactive strategies. It is considered by the behaviour nurse co-ordinators that the development and maintenance of positive therapeutic relationships with clients and professional relationships with case-workers are fundamental to the effective implementation of behavioural interventions. The promotion of effective, efficient and consistent practice as a preventative tool is essential to the success of the behavioural approach. The behaviour nurse co-ordinator provides additional expertise, support, guidance, training and evaluation where necessary. The primary role is to support the efforts of the case worker and associates rather than replace them. Thus, the behaviour nurse co-ordinator works in tandem with clients, staff, carers and the care team as part of the CPA.

The case co-ordinator (clinical leader – Matthew Byrne)

The case co-ordinator is responsible for maintaining high standards of care, and this means the effective implementation of the CPA. Part of my role is to liaise with other managers within the hospital; to gain resources to implement care programmes; to audit and measure quality initiatives; and to maintain a link with hospital policy-makers. The role of the clinical leader involves balancing two systems: a managerial system which includes the managing of a nursing team, with three team leaders as subordinates, and the responsibility of maintaining the momentum of actions stated within care programmes for all service users. The two systems are juxtaposed, one being the nursing discipline, and the other being a shared multidisciplinary approach. The philosophy of the care programme approach means that any discipline can be a case worker, case manager or case co-ordinator.

I have been elected by the team to perform this role, and other members of the team have agreed to take on equally time-consuming roles. Each meeting is a dynamic learning process, we share ideas, view new challenges and develop new skills to deal with severe challenging behaviours. The relationships within the team have now evolved to a point where people feel confident in expressing their opinions; this can lead to heated argument or a real enthusiasm for new ideas. The atmosphere within a team can move through a continuum of being very humorous, to tension about a real concern for a service user's welfare. I personally prefer to be honest and open about my opinions, and I feel comfortable in sharing these with the team. The care team has moved beyond the insecurity of interdisciplinary roles to a place where skills and knowledge are used for actual problem-solving and facilitation. The clinical leader is based on one ward only, whereas the other members of the team have to work on a variety of wards. As case co-ordinator I am able to maintain a consistent approach and provide an overall picture of care to the team.

Resettlement nurse (Brian Devine)

The CPA has proved a more than useful tool in my role as resettlement and community nurse. Often I am the identified contact person for external agencies or provider units, in relation to patient transfers and leave of absence. By developing links through interagency networking, I am able to bring the respective clinicians together and this is part of integrating the seams of the CPA. When meeting with fellow clinicians, the information I hand over has to be both accurate and appropriate; utilization of the CPA format has assisted in this. Regular CPA reviews mean that when a patient is identified for transfer their needs will be re-evaluated, and pretransfer care plans are developed. For example, if a patient was identified for transfer to a community placement, one identified need might be that he/she requires road safety skills. By this process we hope to equip our patients with the skills necessary to make the transfer successful in a planned and co-ordinated manner.

Information relating to patient transfer is passed on in a variety of ways. There is the formal assessment, often carried out by a psychiatrist who will spend time with the patient as well as perusing case notes and other information sources. However, perhaps more important is the pretransfer meeting, convened immediately prior to the commencement of trial leave. At the meeting clinicians from the relevant care teams have the opportunity to meet formally to discuss current clinical issues and hand over care plans and to share information. Additionally, at this meeting we clarify to the receiving agency all identified needs of the patient, how we have addressed them, and what needs ought to be addressed by them as the receiving agency. Up-to-date copies of care programmes are provided within the 'Leave of Absence Care Programme' package at the pretransfer meeting. Also included in this package are for example a discharge risk assessment, after-care checklist and supervised discharge information.

We are able to monitor the implementation (or failure of implementation) of the care programmes by arranging a formal post-transfer clinical review, usually at approximately 12 weeks following transfer, when all aspects of the patient's care will be discussed. This meeting will be attended by clinicians from the respective clinical teams.

We would expect evidence to be produced by this time which showed that identified needs were being addressed. The pretransfer meeting is generally the time when those who have direct contact with the patient can meet. In some instances we have offered receiving agencies the opportunity to spend time with the patient here prior to transfer, this offer has been taken up several times now, and this has some obvious benefits. For instance, the clinician (ideally the identified key-worker/case worker) has the opportunity to meet with the patient and see how he or she spends their time in their current environment and they can see the type of facilities the patient has been used to. Also the patient can benefit from having somebody to relate to when they are transferred – this can help to allay any fears and anxieties that are likely to ensue. This, in turn, has led to staff exchanges which has enhanced the networking process with shared practices ultimately leading to improved patient care and understanding. CPA is clearly playing an important role in our treatment process and has by these examples proved the vehicle by which other initiatives are being developed. By handing over live documents relating to patient care we are able to assist the receiving agency in the early stages following transfer, at a later stage they are likely to do their own in-depth assessment.

Security/clinical liaison (team leader – Gary Illston)

Risk assessment as described in the hospital CPA manual is a specialized assessment for each patient of the clinical issues related to risk. There have been many academic papers regarding the introduction of an appropriate risk assessment strategy, all of which have contained similar premises:

- Documentation should provide a clear comprehensive assessment of risk.
- It should follow an integrated and structured working document process, which provides for planning and meeting the needs of patient-related clinical risk.
- Risk assessment is to be differentiated from risk management.
- Risk assessment can be utilized for hospital patients as well as being a tool for discharge planning.
- Risk assessment is an inexact science; as such, it should be recognized that certain exclusive environments do not provide an overall perspective sufficient to consider risk across a variety of settings.
- Risk assessment specific to hospital care planning should identify risk issues and implications for patient management, care and treatment, in the least restrictive environment. However, account needs to be taken of the needs of security of other patients, staff, visitors and the general public.

Care programme documentation should be considered as the starting point for discharge planning. Particular attention should be paid to the adage 'the best predictor of future behaviour is past behaviour'. Within this context it is incumbent on professionals to assess suitable future placements, and set in place safeguards that will minimize identified risks. It should also be overtly stated which professional is or will be responsible for ensuring that safeguards are not only in place, but that ongoing follow-up assessments are maintained. Finally, risk assessment cannot be about whether or not we can accurately predict risk. What it should be about is whether or not we have made informed, defensible decisions regarding a person's level of risk, in terms of 'social realities' and current 'scientific knowledge'. This must be a fundamental part of a care programme.

The case manager (team leader – Mike Musker)

I see the case manager's role as a facilitator within the team (a reticulist and change agent), they are at the hub of the CPA. The case manager is responsible for effective communication between all levels of the care process and should advocate on behalf of the service user at the care team. Any difficulties met by the case worker in accessing resources or prompting others to provide an efficient service should be taken up by the case manager. I take time to discuss the care programme developments with the case worker during the assessment; between major reviews; and at each step of the service user's development. The case manager should be up to date on what is happening in interdisciplinary areas, giving feedback to the case worker. The case worker can then concentrate on their relationship with and day-to-day care of the service user. Although the case worker takes on responsibility and accountability for care, the case manager in turn must reinforce the level of accountability and promote the highest quality of care. The case co-ordinator then supervises the whole process.

The case worker (senior enrolled nurse – Mick Flynn)

As Billy's case worker, I spend time with him throughout my shift, as well as working with other service users within the ward community. As part of his care programme, Billy and I have agreed that a minimun of 1 hour a week will be spent together specifically discussing needs, although this is invariably much higher as he likes to spend time in the company of the people he knows well, particularly nursing staff. He will often just sit in my vicinity and spend time with me, request to go for walks in the grounds, or visit other wards, both situations requiring supervision by a nurse. I do a weekly update (*weekly review*) of how Billy is doing with his identified needs as part of his care programme, as well as recording any unforeseen happenings. Billy's care programme is discussed with him and a formal review is done once a month (*monthly review*) to check whether services have been provided, and to ensure that each need is being addressed by all concerned. I have taken Billy to visit his proposed new service provider, and I have invited his future carers to spend a number of shifts with me, to develop consistency of care. I have regular meetings with Billy's case manager to discuss the implementation of the care programme, and any difficulties I might be having in accessing services or resources. I recently attended and prepared reports for a predischarge meeting. Attempts were made to involve as many people as possible who would be part of Billy's future care, including the purchasers (Local Authority), the new units care team and our current care team.

A Case Study Using the CPA

Billy: a brief outline

Nominated members of the team went to assess Billy on his previous ward. Billy, aged 25 years, has congenital achondroplasia (commonly referred to as dwarfism), which results in the person being born with short limbs and a normal-size body. He has had many developmental difficulties and has been in institutions since the age of 5 years. Billy is in a special hospital due to his attempts at sticking pens into carers' eyes and attacking them violently. He is also considered a danger to female carers, but when angry will attack anybody within range, initiating this with rapidity and ferocity. Once he initiates an assault, he enters a cycle of aggression which can last up to 3 days – requiring intensive management. Alternatively, when he is well, Billy is extremely co-operative. Owing to his previous ward's philosophy of minimal interference in the patient's day, Billy had developed a routine of staying in his room for most of the day, hiding there, away from social interaction. His room would quickly fill with rubbish, newspapers and foodstuffs, and unwashed clothing. He did not attend to his personal hygiene and would refuse to participate in any care programme. Billy would not eat with other patients, and at times would only accept food in his bare hands. He also refused to sleep in a bed. Any attempts at encouraging Billy to change his behaviour would lead to him smashing his room, breaking his bed up, attacking the nurses, throwing things and pressing fire alarms. This would happen over a number of days until he was allowed to live the way he wanted to live, which resulted in self-initiated social isolation in his own room.

A report was produced by members of our team to provide feedback to the care programme meeting, who decided to accept Billy as it was felt our ward could provide a structured day for him and the specialized interventions required. The increased staffing levels, and the behavioural training of the staff in dealing with severe challenging behaviours, meant that Billy would be provided with the motivation to change his target behaviours and to prepare him to live back in the community. The team requested the behaviour nurse therapist to assess Billy prior to his arrival on the ward, and after discussion with an identified case worker a behavioural contingency management plan was developed to deal with any immediate challenges that would arise.

The general idea was that Billy would assume what was considered to be a 'normal' day from the moment he arrived on the ward. This included eating with other patients at a table with crockery, sleeping in a normal bed and associating with others for a large part of his day. Initially, he had no problems accepting the new structure, but after around 2 days he decided to start testing the boundaries by refusing to eat with others and by refusing to leave his room. With persistence from the nursing staff and a contingency plan that had investigated all foreseeable behavioural relapses, each challenging behaviour could be addressed, consistently and with clear strategies. One example is the supply of a reinforced bed. Initially, Billy reverted to attacking staff, smashing things, throwing items, kicking, punching, screaming and pressing disturbance alarms. His objective was that he would be secluded away from other people, and be allowed to continue his anti-social behaviours. The main intervention was to take Billy to a quiet area of the ward until his violent attacks subsided, and move him back to the main social area at the earliest opportunity. This strategy was very effective, the outcome being that Billy learnt that his violent behaviours would not change the activities in his day. Billy now willingly eats with other patients, socializes with others for the majority of the day, attends every possible off-ward activity at his own request, and goes for walks in the grounds with the nurses. He now yearns social interactions so often that we can use such activities as rewards within his care programme.

Billy's improvements have resulted in the purchasers (Local Health Authority) pursuing a place for him within a less secure facility, with the long-term aim of providing him with a sheltered flat where he can live independently. However, Billy continues to be unpredictable. He has spontaneously attacked female staff three times, punched and bitten his case worker without provocation, and can become truculent at times unless carefully managed. This behaviour is now being explored through a functional analysis, and the psychologist from his new unit has been involved in this intervention.

Apart from these sporadic violent episodes, Billy now leads a healthy life. The relationship he has with his case worker has become pivotal in his care, and it would also appear he is currently the key person in Billy's life. He frequently asks other carers, 'What will Mick Flynn say?'. This may happen after he has cleaned his room, or carried out an activity that he wants to boast about. Billy's mother has now visited him twice, and she has expressed awe at the improvements in her son's quality of life. She kept stating with astonishment that she could not believe the difference in him. This was reinforced by the fact that Billy made a tray of tea for his mother, showed her around the ward introducing people, and spent an hour together with her in an interview room.

Carers from the next place of care have been involved in Billy's current management plan to provide a borderless connection of care. Ths collaboration prevents service users having to return to secure facilities and provides an opportunity for future carers to decide if their service has the facilities and staffing to manage the severe challenging behaviours when they arise.

The care programme

At the meeting a case discussion occurs which looks at Billy's needs, assessed and identified by all disciplines. This involves each discipline reporting on the person from their professional perspective. Once these reports have been read out at the meeting, an important discussion takes place which attempts to prioritize the identified needs. The following needs are those

that were identified and prioritized for Billy:

- request for a psychological assessment to support the behaviour management plan;
- sex education;
- sexual awareness;
- problem-solving skills;
- *Health of the Nation* targets for health (using Health of the Nation Outcome Scales);
- anxiety in respect to above;
- family contact;
- educational needs assessment;
- speech therapy.

Sometimes the total needs are too great to focus on at one time, so the team and the service user decide on which needs they want to target before the next review date. A manageable amount is around six needs, although this will vary between service users. Any unmet needs must also be identified – these may be due to the lack of services available or because the service user refuses to deal with this need at this moment in time. Where there is no service provided to meet the need the case manager, with support from the case co-ordinator, can make efforts to resolve this deficit, or seek to purchase the service from other outside agencies. Where there is a persistent service deficit, the care team use their group power to obtain such services. Alternatively, the hospital-based independent advocacy service or complaints procedure can be utilized by the service user. The Health Advisory Service and Mental Health Act Commissioners are constantly visiting to monitor the quality of interventions. Table 11.1 is an abbreviated view of the actual care programme in action, referring to the identified needs in the case study above.

The interventions in Table 11.1 have been 'actioned' successfully. Billy's behaviour has changed dramatically, and those unaware of his history would find it difficult to believe

Table 11.1 Billy's care programme (multidisciplinary)

Needs	Expected outcomes/aims	Interventions agreed	Action by and review date
Need No. 1 To investigate Billy's 'arrested hydroencephalitis', epilepsy, speech defect, hearing defect and squint	To investigate and provide up-to-date information on these disabilities	Review records of early childhood through family and GP. Make further investigations	Dr D. Kumarajeewa 12/1/97
Needs No. 2 To continue and develop current behavioural programme	To stabilize Billy's behaviours that are discussed in his behavioural schedule	For nursing staff to implement current management plan. To be monitored by behavioural nurse and case worker	Mick Flynn and Pete Stoddart 12/3/97
Needs No. 3 Functional analysis	To develop a full behavioural assessment of Billy's behaviours and abilities	To be assessed by Pete Stoddart and external psychologist (North Mersey Health Trust)	Pete Stoddart and external psychologist 12/3/97
Needs No. 4 Liaison with external agency regarding transfer Use community excursions to reduce institutionalization, getting Billy used to entering the community, which can also be used as part of a risk assessment	To reduce institutionalization To get Billy used to going out into the community To prepare Billy for external agency transfer To be more aware of Billy's risk behaviours	For case worker to plan regular trips for Billy into the community To plan a trip to external agency unit for Billy to have a look at his possible future, and to gain feedback from this for the team Case worker Mick Flynn to liaise with resettlement nurse Brian Devine regarding external agency and Liverpool Health Authority	Mick Flynn 12/3/97 Brian Devine 12/3/97

Billy's part. The chance of living in the community has become a rewarding idea rather than something to fear.

Billy's dependence upon institutions and his learning difficulties have left him with the outlook on life that might be expected from a teenager; he is excited at the idea of moving on and relishes the idea of a new challenge. The vigour and vitality he now shows is a total contrast to his circumstances on his previous ward. Through appropriate planning and team work, the care team has provided Billy with support and new opportunities to develop. The CPA has enabled the care team to provide a package of care that is holistic. The objectives have been determined from a shared vision from a team of carers and the service user, which is implemented as a systematic plan with a clear review system. This differs from the old multidisciplinary approach which relied on self-promoting disciplines vying for a share in hierarchical power (Simnett, 1996). Once Billy is transferred to his new unit, he will continue to have the support from the hospital through the newly developed liaison system which maintains the continuance of care. Where necessary, it can be arranged for his current case worker to spend time with Billy at his new placement. This may require overnight placements at distant hospitals and providers need to think about incorporating such facilities into their care systems.

The ideal of the care programme documentation is that other services will be able to adapt the process easily to their own system, but it would be preferable that we all share the same system. A copy of the care programme has been sent to his new unit so they can plan services, and so they do not have to repeat the information-gathering process.

Summary

Although the CPA was supposedly introduced in April 1991, it has not gained universality in community- and hospital-based services. In the new purchaser–provider market, care teams and service providers must be able to demonstrate their quality of care (Audit Commission, 1992). If we begin to use a consistent approach as put forward by the Department of Health's advisory document *Building Bridges* (DOH, 1996), which is supported by a specific auditing system produced by the NHS Executive (1996), a comprehensive service that is safe and effective should be developed. This will help to prevent the tragedies like those discussed in the opening paragraph, by providing a consistent approach toward supervised discharge and smooth links between agencies. Billy's case study is just one example of how service users must become the fulcrum of the care process. The number of people with learning disabilities living in institutions in 1979 was 45 400; by 1993 this has been reduced to 16 000 people (DOH, 1995). The CPA can assist in a further reduction by supporting people with effective after-care in the community. It is believed that this will reduce the amount of admissions and re-admissions. Interdisciplinary in-service training and development, team building exercises and shared workshops can help to achieve this objective.

Discussion Questions

- What is the care programme approach (CPA) and how does it differ from care management?
- How is the CPA implemented in practice?

- How does the multidisciplinary care team work together to develop an integrated care programme?
- What method can the care team use to prioritize needs and audit their implementation?

References

Audit Commission (1992). *Community Care: Managing the Cascade of Change*. HMSO, London.

Blom-Cooper, L., Hally, H. and Murphy, E. (1995). *The Falling Shadow: One Patient's Mental Health Care 1978–1993*, Duckworth, London.

Department of Health (1989). *Caring for People: Community Care in the Next Decade and Beyond*. HMSO, London.

Department of Health (1990). *The Care Programme Approach for People with a Mental Illness Referred to the Specialist Psychiatric Services*. HMSO, London.

Department of Health (1994a). *Key Area Handbook: Mental Illness*, 2nd edn. HMSO, London.

Department of Health (1994b). *Guidance on the Discharge of Mentally Disordered People and Their Continuing Care in the Community*. HMSO, London.

Department of Health (1995). *The Health of the Nation: A Strategy for People with Learning Disabilities*. HMSO, London.

Department of Health (1996). *The Health of the Nation: Building Bridges*. HMSO, London.

Hamilton, I. and Roy, D. (1995). The care programme approach at work in mental health care. *Nursing Times*, **91**(51), 35–7.

NHS Executive (1996). *An Audit Pack for Monitoring the Care Programme Approach: Monitoring Tool*. HMSO, London.

Ritchie, D. and Lingham, R. (1994). *The Report of Inquiry into the Care and Treatment of Christopher Clunis*. HMSO, London.

Simnett, I. (1996). *Managing Health Promotion: Developing Healthy Organisations and Communities*. Wiley, Chichester.

feel valued as people, as professionals and as colleagues. Feeling valued has two related aspects:

- it involves nurses believing that what they are doing professionally is valuable, credible and worthwhile;
- it involves feeling that what they are doing is valued by others whose views are respected and needed (employers, colleagues, clients and their significant others).

Within a broad framework of staff development the particular professional relationship within which the above can be systematically explored is *clinical supervision*.

Why do Professionals Working with People who have a Learning Disability need Clinical Supervision?

For the majority of nurses working in the field of learning disability, the type of formal training they received was premised on hospital-based care. Policy, legislation and attitudes in the past two decades has led to large numbers of people with learning disability living in the community. For nurses, this has meant substantial changes to the care they can provide.

The form in which they can receive and provide support for one another has also changed. Within a hospital environment nurses could and usually did, find that the level of supervision they received could be high, even if this only took the form of making sure that the daily routine was continued. The hierarchy of senior nurses (e.g. ward sisters) overseeing their members of staffs' work, at least provided nurses with the feeling that there was somebody who could help (or take over) if they got into professional difficulties.

The development of community services and the role of the practitioner in the provision of care to people with learning disabilities has required the nurse to be a far more autonomous practitioner. It has also led in many instances to the nurse finding support and help from other professionals from different disciplines. Cooke (1994) raises a pertinent point, felt by many nurses working in the field of learning disability. She highlights that nurses working in the field of learning disability are required (and have been for many years) to liaise with many professionals, and utilize a multidisciplinary approach to care provision. For many nurses working in this field, it has necessitated working in departments/offices other than nursing and, for some, having line managers other than nurses. Geographical isolation from other nursing colleagues is yet another example of how nurses working in the community with people who have learning disabilities have moved away from the traditional hierarchical structure of nursing management.

There does not appear to be a uniform, standard model for the provision of care for people with learning disabilities. Recommendations by the National Development Team (1982) have been widely interpreted. Reasons for the differences in care provision with this particular client group include:

- varying needs of the 'community' identified;
- service provision identified as being 'priority' in terms of no existing service;
- service provision being defined by groups of people, for example resettlement teams, challenging behaviour teams, children's teams;
- varying availability of range of professionals;
- financial constraints.

However, for many nurses working in this field they will be in contact with a number of professionals involved in the care delivery to an individual. All these factors therefore require the provision of some mechanism by which the nurses working in this field can gain the support, education and facilitation that they need, in order to provide effective, competent, quality care.

Clinical supervision can also ensure that the person receiving the care provided by the nurse is the best possible care. Nurses are encouraged to be 'empowerers', facilitating appropriate and optimal levels of independence for their clients. For many clients and their families, the nurse is a new experience. Often such care provision has been absent. It is therefore sometimes difficult for the client or their carer to fully 'know' whether the 'advice' and 'support' they are receiving is the best for them. To offer advice and support is a powerful element of the nurses' work, so the provision of an external person to that client/nurse relationship, in the role of supervisor, can provide the necessary balance.

Interdisciplinary Clinical Supervision

Community nurses may argue that, for them, regular meetings with colleagues to discuss referrals provides the support they need. Where there is the provision of a truly multidisciplinary team, and there is the time available to discuss the clients' needs fully, this may be so. However, this is dependent on trusting relationships between the professionals represented in the team, and again adequate time. It may also be a very informal way of support, and lacking the structure that more 'formal' methods of supervision could provide. Very often the time when such discussions can occur is during case management, or individual programme planning meetings. For support to be given fully to the nurse, however, time between a designated person and themselves to discuss particular aspects of their professional life is essential.

Learning disability nurses can and do play a pivotal role in the provision of care to people with learning disabilities, yet they are still relatively small in number. For some this may mean that their supervisor is from a different professional background to their own. Whether this is successful or problematic may be due to several factors, including:

- trust between the supervisor and supervisee;
- professional relationships within the team;
- potential (and actual) interprofessional tensions;
- perceived role and purpose of clinical supervision.

It is now accepted, however, that multidisciplinary teamwork and interagency collaboration are essential prerequisites for effective, high quality service provision to people who have learning disabilities and their carers. Changes in service delivery and service organization have meant that professionals working in this area have a responsibility to develop and maintain good working relationships with all their multidisciplinary colleagues. The advent of care management means that interagency and multidisciplinary practice are even more bound together. It would make sense therefore that if a practitioner is used to working alongside another professional on a regular basis, that clinical supervision across disciplines can be beneficial both for the practitioners, where there may well be an exchange of knowledge and information, and for the client whose care package may well be organized, developed and maintained by several members of a multidisciplinary team.

However, Thomas and Reid (1995) highlight the causes of problems that can occur between the professionals working within a multidisciplinary team. These include stereotyped views about each professional's role and function, lack of understanding about each team member's role, working from different theoretical and knowledge bases, functional isolation and hierarchies. One of the ways to combat all of these problems, which could begin with the understanding of each team member's role, leading to less professional jealousy and protectivism, is through interdisciplinary clinical supervision.

Many practitioners working in the field of learning disability have faced recent changes in their role with the implementation of market strategies and the purchaser/provider split. For some nurses the introduction of case management has changed their relationships with their clients. They are now in the business of purchasing, contracting and arranging care, sometimes with the added responsibility of costing out that care. For the majority of nurses working in the direct provision of care to people with learning disabilities this represents a fundamental shift in their working relationships with their clients. Changing existing working practices is often fraught with anxiety. Nurses working in a field of care that has had many changes imposed upon it in the last two decades need support and supervision. According to a study by Jukes (1994a,b), nurses working in the field of learning disability consider that clinical supervision should be an integral part of their professional life, and appear to fully comprehend the valuable role it has to be in the delivery of effective, competent and high quality care.

The Purpose of Clinical Supervision

Supervision has many purposes, including the promotion of competent and accountable work which concerns both the client and the supervisee. Another purpose is the facilitation of professional and personal development.

Chris is a community nurse working with people who have learning disabilities. A family has recently been referred to Chris, in which the mother is due to give birth to a child who has been diagnosed as having Down's syndrome. Chris is concerned that she will not be able to support this family as well as she would like, because she has not experienced this type of referral before.

In clinical supervision, Chris raised this concern. The supervisor was able to provide practical advice in terms of giving Chris information about:

- support groups who might be able to help;
- the name of another nurse in a nearby town who was experienced in providing this type of support.

The supervisor also emphasized that Chris was not to feel 'alone' in this, and that this issue should be raised whenever it was necessary, in supervision sessions.

Box I Case study

The process of supervision closely parallels that of the practitioner–client relationship. Both should be a learning process, a process that takes place within the context of a relationship that facilitates positive change, both at a professional and personal level. Respect must be the foundation stone for any supervisory relationship, not only for the process of supervision, but also for the supervisor, the supervisee, the client and the organization in which supervision occurs.

Butterworth (1994) identifies that for nurses the development of their role as accountable, autonomous practitioners has evolved from the movement away from the medical model of health care by nurses. This development has left nurses with the need to develop strong 'protective' mechanisms, and to identify that with autonomous practice comes accountability. For nurses working in the learning disability field, the power and protection by medics was never as strong as for other nursing professions, yet by developing new roles, the need for support and supervision has never been more important.

For Booth (1994) the purpose of supervision is the provision of support to nurses but it may also provide a vehicle for stress reduction (Box 2).

Learning disability nurses are familiar with the designing of care plans and individual programme plans for their clients, yet this can provide a useful tool for the nurse to identify their own strengths and weaknesses, and priorities for care. The inclusion of a supervisor in this process can facilitate an objective viewpoint, provided the relationship between the supervisor and supervisee is based on trust, non-judgemental attitudes and facilitation.

Clinical supervision should be addressing the clinical and practical aspect of nursing. Training and research needs can be identified through effective clinical supervision, and can provide a link between research and practice. It should help nurses appreciate clients as individuals, and should also examine the contribution of the nurse to the multidisciplinary team. Effective clinical supervision should identify and develop innovative practice. Cooke (1994) identifies how, within traditional institutional settings, good practice could be seen even if it was not rewarded. Nurses working in the community are often isolated from colleagues and therefore examples of good practice may not be so readily identified. Finally, clinical supervision should support nurses with their feelings, thus leading to foster staff retention and morale.

There are many benefits to clinical supervision, not only for the supervisee

---

Mark is a registered nurse for the mentally handicapped (RNMH) and has worked in the field of learning disability for 10 years. He trained in a large institution for the mentally handicapped and had worked there ever since. When the hospital was closing, Mark successfully applied for the post of resettlement officer for one geographical location. He shared an office with a social worker who had part-time in-put into resettlement and together they comprised the 'team'.

Mark was expected to liaise with hospital staff, statutory and voluntary agencies for the purpose of finding appropriate residential accommodation and occupational activities for a significant number of people.

The isolation he at times felt and the pressure he was under to find suitable living arrangements for people, working to a deadline, all led to high levels of stress. When Mark met his supervisor he was able to reflect on his practice, examine his working practices, identify his own development needs, establish priorities and identify possible solutions through the design, with his supervisor, of a 'care plan' for Mark.

Box 2 Case study

themselves, but also for the service for which they work.

Benefits to be gained by the supervisee

- It provides regular space for the supervisee and supervisor to reflect upon the content and process of their work.
- It facilitates the development of understanding and skills within their work.
- It allows the nurse space and time to receive information and another perspective concerning their practice.
- The nurse can be validated and supported both as a person and as a colleague.
- In a stressful occupation, or at stressful times, it helps to ensure that as a person and as a practitioner, one is not left to carry, unnecessarily, difficulties, problems and projections on their own.
- It gives the nurse the opportunity to explore and express personal distress, transference and counter-transference that have been brought up by their practice.
- It may facilitate interactions that help nurses to better plan and utilize their personal and professional resources.
- It encourages nurses to be proactive rather than reactive.
- It will allow the nurse to use self-appraisal in respect to the quality of their work.

Benefits to the service

The service needs to be committed to the provision of clinical supervision, which requires time and energy to be effective. Planning, implementing, monitoring and evaluating a system of professional supervision in learning disability service provision is justifiable if it brings the following benefits:

- Clinical supervision, as part of a staff development and support programme, could allow a sustained and detailed exploration of professional issues with a view to increasing job satisfaction, enhancing sense of colleagueship and corporate purpose.
- The client's needs being met through improvement in the quality of care provision.
- It would provide opportunities for valuing colleagues' strengths and identifying ways in which their professional needs could be met.
- It would encourage colleagues at all levels, across disciplines and agencies to become more confident in exploring their professional input at work in an open way, thus helping to build a climate of trust in which professional development could take place.
- It would involve practitioners working on a common problem or weakness or issue to create a greater sense of effective team work.
- It would provide a formal support system through periods of professional stress, crisis and confusion.
- Clinical supervision could be professionally empowering for nurses working within multidisciplinary teams.

Models of Supervision

Earlier in the chapter I identified the mechanisms by which learning disability nurses may be receiving some sort of supervision, other than identified sessions. It is fair to say that these opportunities may be more available to practitioners working within community support teams. For nurses working in residential or occupational/recreational settings, this type of supervision may not be available.

The most popular way of using supervision is for the supervisor and supervisee to meet regularly on a one-to-one basis, although supervision can be undertaken in many ways. Cooke (1992) identifies four methods of undertaking clinical supervision, of which the most frequently used is the one to one method. Cooke contends that one to one supervision is often undertaken by the nurse manager. The potential problem with this is the unequal relationship that exists between the supervisee and the supervisor. Most community nurses now have to complete periodic records of their activities. These are usually submitted to their manager to provide information for future service planning. There exists therefore the potential danger that managers as supervisors may slip into their management role whilst being involved in supervision. The need for trust and mutual respect is therefore paramount in this type of supervision setting.

A method identified by Cooke (1994) that is perhaps exclusive to the role of the community nurse, as opposed to nurses working in residential settings, is supervision of the home visit. Whilst this may allow the supervisor to see at first hand the relationship that the nurse has with their client and family, the stresses that this may put on that relationship may outweigh the benefits of this type of supervision.

Using role play to 'act out' situations that the nurse may find themselves in, for example dealing with uncooperative family members, either within the supervisor, supervisee meeting alone, or with the involvement of other staff, may help the nurse to develop the required skills. Video playing these role-play situations can provide the nurse with visual evidence of responses and methods of dealing with issues that are stressful or problematic. The supervisor and supervisee can examine together methods of developing the requisite skills.

The model Cooke (1994) refers is only one of several models. I will now describe four main types.

One-to-one: the supervisor and the supervisee

This form of counselling has been discussed in the previous paragraph, but it is important to note that within supervision models, the UKCC position statement on clinical supervision (1996) is quite definite in its stance as to what clinical supervision is. It argues that

Clinical supervision is not a managerial control system. It is not therefore:

- the exercise of over managerial responsibility or managerial supervision;
- a system of formal individual performance review;
- hierarchical in nature.

The role and function of supervision must therefore be very clearly identified by the practitioners involved in this relationship.

This model of supervision involves a supervisor providing supervision to a supervisee. It is probably the most common model of supervision utilized. The supervisee is usually a less skilled practitioner than the supervisor.

One-to-one co-supervision

This model involves two practitioners providing support for each other. The method used is to alternate the roles. This tends to presuppose equal, if different, levels of skill and expertise. Typically, the supervision session is divided equally between the two.

Group supervision with an identified supervisor

There is a continuum of methods for providing this form of supervision. At one end of the continuum of supervision the identified supervisor will be responsible for appointing the times between the supervisees, and then concentrate on the work of the individuals in turn.

At the other end of the continuum, it is the supervisees who organize their clinical supervision times, using the supervisor as a resource. Between these two alternatives, many different ways of working can operate.

Peer group supervision

This model of supervision takes the form of three or more supervisees providing supervision for each other within a group context. They are likely to be of equitable status, degree of training and experience. An example of this model could be that of three members of the multidisciplinary team providing support and help for each other.

Eclectic methods of supervision

This model is structured around combinations of the above models. Practitioners working in the field of learning disability may need or choose to combine elements of the four models to suit their particular professional working needs.

Within all these models of clinical supervision, Procter's 1986 model should represent the fundamental base on which supervision is premised. Procter perceives supervision as a working alliance between the supervisee and supervisor. This relationship focuses on casework being presented, with feedback and guidance then given. Procter sees the dimensions within this relationship as educational, supportive and managerial. The model for supervision she has devised has normative, formative and restorative elements. Rafferty and Coleman (1996) suggest that effective clinical super-

vision is a combination of normative, formative and restorative functions.

The normative element is concerned with professional and organizational standards of professional practice. They provide the quality in supervision. In this aspect the supervisor focuses on values, beliefs, evaluation of care, issues of caseload management and professional accountability.

Kim is a registered nurse working in a residential facility for young people with learning disabilities. Kim is concerned about some staffs' negative and punitive behaviour towards some of the young people who live in this particular house. Kim takes this concern to the supervision session, where it is suggested that staff development across the range of staff should be provided. Kim's response to speak out about unacceptable practices and attitudes is acknowledged, and Kim's decision to speak out is supported.

Box 3 Case study

The formative aspect of supervision is concerned with the identification and the development of skills, and with the integration of theory into practice. For many nurses their training was hospital based and they have had to adapt to changes in the care provision for people with learning disabilities with little or no training. The demands that such care provision often places on practitioners working in this field means that they require both specific and generic skill development. Box 3 provides an example of this.

The third aspect or function of this model of clinical supervision, the supportive function, aims to provide supportive help for professionals. The practitioner will reflect on and seek to develop or improve personal coping strategies, and how to provide both high levels of support and challenge. This element of the model should also provide the opportunity to explore the stresses unique to their work environment, highs and lows of their work, and how to introduce, maintain and end (where necessary), supportive relationships.

Role of the Supervisor

The role of the supervisor is characterized by two key features:

- commitment on the part of the supervisor to the facilitation of growth, both educational and personal of the supervisee;
- an acceptance of the voluntary nature of the contract.

These two features are fundamental to effective, safe, supportive clinical supervision, if the three elements or function of supervision as described by Procter (1986) are to be met.

Clinical supervision should be:

- enabling not dominating
- encouraging not judgemental
- valuing not belittling
- exploratory not dogmatic
- open not defensive
- developmental not restrictive
- accepting and yet challenging.

Skills and Methods

Farkas-Cameron (1995) has identified some of the concerns nurses raise about clinical supervision. There may be a concern about the nature and purpose of clinical supervision – questions such as 'What is the purpose of clinical supervision?' may in fact be about feelings that their practices are being questioned in a negative manner. There may also be concern that supervision is about management and it is here, as has been mentioned previously, that the importance of the clinical supervision relationship being based on trust and being non-judgemental is of paramount importance. Fowler (1996) suggests that the first question that needs to be asked when planning clinical supervision, whether at the individual or organizational level, is 'What is the aim of the clinical supervision?'.

Davies (1993, p. 52) contends that 'Supervision should be "for" the practitioner. It is not an audit of practice'. The aim of clinical supervision is to support, assist and facilitate the practitioner in the delivery of high quality care, but it is also about supporting and helping the practitioner to manage the demands of their professional working life.

The introduction of clinical supervision into a service may meet with some initial resistance due to lack of understanding about the purpose of clinical supervision, fears about criticism of professional practice and a resentment that supervision will remove the autonomy of the practitioner. These fears and anxieties have to be allayed and it is in the methods and skills adopted in the introduction and implementation of clinical supervision that this can and should occur. For many people, the possibility that their professional practices may be criticized would be threatening. However, clinical supervision can assist practitioners to continue to develop existing good practice and learn new skills. Most practitioners informally discuss their clients' needs and ask for advice, clinical supervision puts this into a framework that supports the practitioner and allows for the acknowledgment that in many instances the work that they are undertaking is difficult and that this difficulty needs to be recognized and shared.

To facilitate a supportive, trusting and

therapeutic relationship within clinical supervision requires particular skills and a clear understanding of the purpose of the supervision. Supervision allows for:

- focusing directly on the practitioner case load;
- focusing on the skills, interventions and evaluation of clinical/therapeutic interactions with the client and/or carers;
- self-evaluation and self-awareness;
- guidance/advice on clinical practice and interventions;
- validation of the practitioner's positive clinical/interpersonal practice;
- discussion of events and how the practitioner coped;
- exploration of coping mechanisms and how harmful/beneficial these are (Davies, 1993).

If supervision is to be supportive, challenging, professional and effective the supervisor needs to have high levels of key skills that are used consciously in the supervision. The key skills are:

Clarification – Exploration – Progression – Appraisal.

Butterworth (1994) has identified the need for supervisor training to ensure that supervisors have a knowledge of and sensitivity to the interpersonal processes that can occur between individuals and groups and may impede the therapeutic nature of practitioner/client, supervisor/supervisee relationships. Key skills that facilitate effective communication are therefore vital.

Key skill – clarification

This skill involves identifying clearly a number of aspects of the style and methods that the practitioner uses in their everyday working life. The supervisee will be encouraged to explore their 'style of work', the effects that it has on clients, carers, collea-

gues and their understanding of the efficacy of this style. The skills that the supervisor will need to use here include listening, questioning, summarizing, paraphrasing and checking out.

Being a good listener is not easy and the supervisor should be aware of the difficulties that may arise. The supervisor also needs to be aware of any skill development they may need in listening to others.

Key skill – exploration

This phase of the supervision is a logical progression from clarification. It may involve the supervisor asking 'now that your ideas about your practice have been clarified, can we now explore one of your ideas that you currently manage the least effectively?'.

A possible consequence of exploration is that it may seem threatening and it is therefore vital that this skill is carried out in a supportive manner, which sets the supervisee at their ease and does not make the supervisee feel inadequate.

Exploration may well sound neutral, but it is in fact difficult and value-laden. This skill involves coping with confusion – exploring options, considering different ways of working and examining the possibility of changing attitudes. This skill also requires the supervisor and supervisee to deal with conflict. The range of options suggested by the supervisee may not be options the supervisor would themselves consider using. Whether this conflict is acknowledged and dealt with could affect the relationship.

Exploration involves challenging and this can result in the supervisee feeling inadequate. For the act of challenging practice, beliefs, etc. to be positive it must therefore be perceived by the supervisee as supportive.

Exploration within the supervision session can provide information, identify goals and aspirations, perceived and actual difficulties and can improve skill awareness.

Key skill – progression

This is a generic skill which will be used throughout the supervision session. It is about avoiding going round in circles, becoming blocked down blind alleys and working only at the superficial level. This stage of the session involves identifying relevant action. It is necessary to identify and discuss problems and to discuss goals. This in turn should lead to greater clarity of actions, goals and aspirations. Part of identifying actions must include the exploration of resource availability. Learning to use colleagues as resources is important, seeing their skills and knowledge as useful and supportive can be the first break in the barriers that can often exist within multidisciplinary teams.

Key skill – appraisal

This skill is required in what is perhaps the most sensitive area involved in supervision. Assessment of professional practice can appear very threatening and produce high levels of anxiety. Appraisal is not only sensitive, it is also complicated. This skill involves and necessitates several subsidiary skills: the encouragement of self-assessment in which the supervisee analyses their own strengths and weaknesses, aims, criteria, strategies, etc. It involves being critical in a supportive way. Being critical involves making judgements, but the way in which those judgements are made will significantly affect how they are received.

The previously mentioned skills of clarifying and exploring are important – they will assist in the identification of future action, which assists motivation and continuation of good practice. This skill should

be used to help the supervisee – to use reflective and evaluative practices and to identify the preferred styles of learning for continuous professional development.

Summary and Recommendations

What then is the benefit of clinical supervision? In this chapter I have identified the benefits to the service and to the clients with learning disabilities. The benefits to the practitioner can be numerous and include

- providing space for the supervisee and supervisor to reflect upon the content and process of their work;
- facilitating the development of understanding and skills within their work;
- allowing the practitioner space and time to receive information and another perspective concerning their clinical practice;
- the practitioner can be validated and supported both as a person and as a colleague;
- in a stressful occupation, it helps to ensure that as a person and as a practitioner, one is not left to carry, unnecessarily, difficulties and problems on one's own;
- facilitating interactions that help practitioners to better plan and utilize their personal and professional resources;
- encouraging practitioners to be proactive rather than reactive;
- allowing the practitioner to use self-appraisal in respect to the quality of their work.

It would appear therefore that the implementation of clinical supervision into services for people with learning disabilities would be of benefit to all involved. For practitioners in particular, the implementation of clinical supervision may provide them with the essential support mechanism that they need to care for people with learning disabilities. It would be well to heed the words of Reg Pyne (1987):

To care for and about our colleagues is to care for and about standards of patient care. Our consciences should not rest if we renege on that responsibility.

In order to ensure quality supervision, certain criteria need to be met. The following section provides a list of actions that will assist in the facilitation of quality clinical supervision. Practitioners working in the field of learning disability may find that this action list can provide a basic structure from which they can devise and implement their own systems of clinical supervision.

Actions to Support Benchmarks for Good Clinical Practice

- Time and place for clinical supervision to take place.
- Respect and confidentiality.
- Opportunity to attend training sessions for clinical supervision.
- Clinical supervision arrangements to form part of an individual practitioner's regular review.
- Managers should have clinical supervision.
- A record of clinical supervision should be maintained.

Discussion Questions

- How might supervision improve the partnership of practice in the workplace between parties who do not have equal power or influence?
- Consider the relationship between formal appraisal and clinical supervision and what strategies may be adopted to assist resolution if the supervisory relationship breaks down.
- Identify your local policy and practice which addresses the expected standards, status and content of records of supervision.
- What do you consider essential to be contained in contracts or supervision?
- How does the concept of clinical supervision fit into the strategic aims and established policies of your work situation.

Potential concerns – likely to be identified by discussion

- Who supervises the supervisors?
- Clear expectations needed in the negotiated contract.
- Too busy for regular and uninterrupted supervision
- Can I trust the supervisor to use authority constructively?
- My contribution to the record of supervision.
- Do I really have the rights to learn from my mistakes?
- Do I really have the rights to an opinion and to disagree?
- Am I permitted to have feelings?
- Is the supervisor respected in role and as a person
- Will the supervision climate be genuine, congruent and safe?
- Does the manager or supervisor respect my views with regard to appropriate boundaries?

Further Reading

Butterworth, T. (1997). *It is Good to Talk. An Evaluation of Clinical Supervision Mentorship in England and Scotland*. The University of Manchester, Manchester.

Farrington, A. (1994). Defining and setting the parameters of clinical supervision. *International Journal of Psychiatric Nursing Research*, **1**(2), 34–40.

Freedman, S. and Marr, J. (1995). A supervisory model of professional competence: a joint service (education initiative). *Nurse Education Today*, **15**(4), 239–44.

Kohner, N. (1994). *Clinical Supervision in Practice*. Kings Fund Centre, London.

References

Booth, K. (1992). Providing support and reducing stress – review of the literature. In *Clinical Supervision and Mentorship Nursing* (eds T. Butterworth and J. Faugier). Chapman & Hall, London.

Butterworth, T. (1994). Preparing to take on clinical supervision. *Nursing Standard*, **8**(52), 32–4.

Cooke, P. (1994). Mental handicap nursing. In *Clinical Supervision and Mentorship in Nursing* (eds T. Butterworth and J. Faugier). Chapman & Hall, London.

CPNA (1986). *Guidelines for Supervision*. Unpublished short report on one day workshop and questionnaire about supervision.

Davies, P. (1993). Value yourself. *Nursing Times*, **89**(4), p. 52.

Department of Health (1993). *The Nursing, Midwifery and Health Visiting Contribution to Health and Health Care*. HMSO, London.

Farkas-Cameron, M.M. (1995). Clinical supervision in psychiatric nursing. *Journal of Psychosocial Nursing*, **33**(2), 31–7.

Faugier, J. (1992). The supervisory relationship. In *Clinical Supervision and Mentorship in Nursing* (eds T. Butterworth and J. Faugier). Chapman & Hall, London.

Fowler, J. (1996). Clinical supervision: what do you do after saying hello? *British Journal of Nursing*, **5**(6), 382–5.

Goldberg, C. (1986). *On Being a Psychiatric Nurse. The Journey of the Healer*. Gardner Press, New York.

Hawkins, P. and Shoet, R. (1989). *Supervision in the Helping Professions*. Open University Press, Milton Keynes.

Johns, C. (1993). Professional supervision. *Journal of Nursing Management*, 1, 9–18.

Jukes, M. (1994a). Development of the Community Nurse in learning disability: 1. *British Journal of Nursing*, **3**(16), 779–783.

Jukes, M. (1994b). Development of the Community Learning Disability Nurse: 2. *British Journal of Nursing*, **3**(16), 848–853.

National Development Team for Mentally Handicapped People (1982). *Third Report*. HMSO, London.

Procter, B. (1986). Supervision: A co-operative exercise in accountability. In *Supervision in the Helping Professions* (1992) (P. Hawkins and R. Shoet). Open University Press, Milton Keynes.

Pyne, R. (1987). Confronting stress. *Nursing Times*, **84**(33): 30–1.

Rafferty, M. and Coleman, M. (1996). Educating nurses to undertake clinical supervision in practice. *Nursing Standards*, **10**(45), 38–41.

Thomas, B. and Reid, J. (1995). Multidisciplinary clinical supervision. *British Journal of Nursing*, **4**(15), 883–5.

UKCC (1992). *Code of Professional Conduct for Nurses and Midwives*. UKCC, London.

UKCC (1996). *Position Statement on Clinical Supervision for Nursing and Midwifery*. UKCC, London.

Part Three

Challenges for User-Centred Practice

Chapter 13

Active Contributors: Service Users, Advocates and Support Networks

Andy Stevens

Key Issues

- Labelling
- Barriers to choice
- Empowerment ideology
- Forms of advocacy
- Effective communication
- Planning accessible consultation

Introduction

Health and social care professionals during the second half of the twentieth century have enthusiastically adopted a variety of new concepts in order to improve services for people with learning difficulties within a changing environment of care. Application of concepts such as normalization or social role valorization, community care and empowerment have become so much part of the principles of good practice for nurses, social workers and other professionals operating within health, social services, housing and other community services that they may be considered 'dominant ideologies' (Cullen, 1991).

The success of these concepts has been due to a variety of factors. Three influences relate to the increasing focus on the requirements of the individual user of services. These are:

- the context of changing structures of service delivery which appears to be shifting from maintenance of disabled people in large segregated institutions to individuals living with support in their local community;
- Government policy of a mixed economy of care based on consumerism, in which 'value for money' and user-led services have central importance;
- developments of carers lobby groups for disabled people, such as MENCAP and SCOPE from the early 1950s and organizations of disabled people such as British Council of Organizations of Disabled People and the network of People First self-advocacy groups since the 1970s.

Organizations such as MENCAP and

SCOPE have initiated significant improvement in the range and quality of services since the war. However, service-user perspectives do not necessarily correlate with those of service providers or carers. Disabled people's groups are presenting legitimate challenges to the way the care service provision is currently organized. Self-advocacy groups and other organizations of people with learning difficulties have developed beyond individual self-advocacy towards a broader representation of disabled people through effective collaboration with agencies engaged in planning and delivery of services. Care workers engaged in the identification of the needs of individual people with learning difficulty or in the planning and delivery of services are now confronted with the necessity to work collaboratively with service users, carers and community networks in partnerships that are more equal.

It is necessary for all those assisting people with learning difficulties to be effective in facilitating service user's articulation of their individual needs and collective requirements from a service. This may involve a degree of advocacy on their behalf. More likely workers in care agencies, particularly care managers, will be involved in negotiation and possibly dispute with people with learning difficulties and their supporters over the forms and quality of services available or already provided.

Patients, Clients, Service Users or Contributors?

An assessment and provision of health and social services will involve people occupying different roles such as agency worker, carer or service user. Consider the following list of 'labels' by which someone could be identified in an assessment for services:

- service user
- patient
- colleague
- friend
- contributor
- partner
- advocate
- customer
- client
- protagonist
- carer
- neighbour.

Each of these roles indicates different levels of responsibility or authority, but would you consider that any would not be a legitimate role for a person with learning difficulties? Care professionals can often reduce a person to a passive receiver of services; that is, patient, client or service user.

Research indicates that women with learning difficulties will often be perceived in positions of dependency. Professional care workers often disuade them from motherhood, but this does not mean that caring roles are not an important part of their lives. This has either been unrecognized, or exploited by service professionals, but in either circumstance a false dichotomy of care or dependence often denies the complexity of relationships between people and the need for people to have a choice of roles (Warmsley, 1993). People's perceptions of each other vary (see Figure 13.1).

Lindow and Morris (1995) have identified

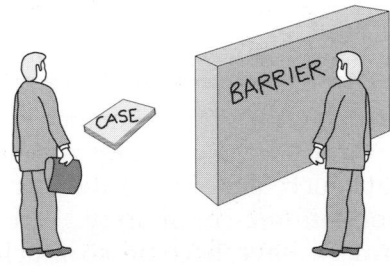

Figure 13.1 Care worker's view of service user/ service user's view of care workers

from research studies common assumptions and behaviour of community care workers that can prevent people from making choices regarding their preferences about support services. You may find it useful to reflect on what these might be before you look at their list summarized below. I have numbered these for reference purposes.

1. A focus on impairment, not on support for independence.
2. Professional assumptions – of expertise and of the nature of independence.
3. Racist attitudes or cultural insensitivity which can stop people's wishes from being heard.
4. Assumed inability of people to make choices.
5. Workers' disagreement with the choices made.
6. Workers not managing to communicate with people.
7. Workers do not always behave as if people have rights.
8. The way services are organized makes it difficult for people to say what they want or for action to be taken to give them what they want.
9. Divisions between health and social services, and between public, private and voluntary sector, do not reflect the reality of people's needs and lives.
10. The way that statutory and voluntary agencies divide people up into service-user groups may reflect the reality of people's needs and lives.
11. The organization of finance has priority over giving choice.
12. People in organizations may do things in certain ways because they have always done them that way.
13. Sometimes the only kind of help that is offered is that which the community care organization already provides.
14. Pressures on community care workers

can make it difficult for them to help people make choices.
15. People can find it difficult to make choices.
16. People may not have the information they need in order to make choices.
17. Sometimes people do not feel able to make the choices about the support they need.
18. Sometimes people do not feel able to complain.
19. Compulsory service use can prevent all choice.
20. Sometimes people face prejudice within the community.
21. Sometimes poverty gets in the way of making choices.

I have grouped these factors into three categories:

- the personal perspective of the care professional (1–7);
- the organizational constraints of the service in which they work (8–13);
- the social barriers on disabled people and other service users (14–21).

Personal perspectives of professionals are influenced by their life experience, their professional knowledge, skills and values and their role within the agency in which they work.

It is common practice for health and social care professionals to identify people in terms of their impairments, their problem or a particular category of service available. Workers define their tasks in particular ways and due to the nature of service jobs this tends to define people. However, there are dangers that any 'professional shorthand' that is used between workers will stereotype and objectify the people that they are working with rather than seeing them as whole individuals living within complex and diverse relationships. This is less of a problem for service users in trans-

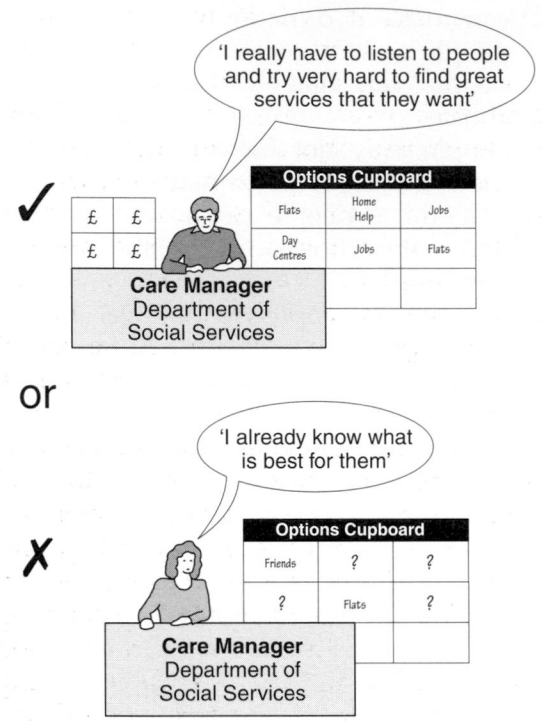

Figure 13.2 Who is this care manager? A care manager is the person who will work with you to try and make sure that you get the things you want and the support you need. Some are more helpful than others. (From People First, 1993a, p. 8, with kind permission of People First London.)

explaining the role of care manager (see Figure 13.2).

Some care workers have supported disabled writers' critiques of the 'medical model' professional approach which emphasizes the pathology, vulnerability and dependency of an individual service user, implies racial/cultural homogeneity and denies the sexuality of service users, and can result in false assumptions about care needs. Another reaction to the disability rights movement is the construction of new ideologies and areas of expertise. Professional support for normalization and social role valorization has been interpreted as a means by which the role of professionals can be sanctioned in the light of changing service delivery from institution to community-based care (Chappell, 1992). Empowerment, like normalization, can degenerate into a superficial 'bandwagon' term and the statements and actions of individual service users can be re-interpreted rather than represented by care professionals. Critics of the current enthusiasm for 'empowerment' among professionals point out the lack of distinction between different uses of the term by some professionals and by service user organizations.

> Because it [empowerment] creates a vogue image and an aura of moral superiority, it affords protection against criticism. Yet the term lacks specificity and glosses over significant differences. It acts as a 'social aerosol' covering up the disturbing smell of conflict and conceptual division.
>
> (Ward and Mullender, 1991, p. 21)

The relationship between health and care service workers and service users is inevitably affected by an unequal distribution of power. Professionals provide access to information and resources as well as individual expertise. Ward and Mullender draw our attention to issues of oppression and power underlying the professional/

actions with a waiter or shop assistant than it is with the provision of nursing assistance or assessment of care needs. The reduction of an individual to the needs of worker is particularly oppressive when the service user is in a potentially vulnerable situation. It is not possible to engage in effective communication in such circumstances and care workers are left with direct observation and assumption to direct their actions. The guide to community care published by People First (1993a), a self-advocacy group of people with learning difficulties, stresses the importance of listening, and access to adequate resources is emphasized in service-user relationship. They suggest that care professionals can develop anti-oppressive practice through what they term 'self-directed groupwork'. However, it might be argued that care professionals have no role at all in developing service-users' empowerment. Adams defines empowerment as:

a process by which individuals, groups and/or communities become able to take control of their circumstances and achieve their own goals, thereby being able to work towards maximising the quality of their lives.

(Adams, 1990, p. 43)

If it is up to groups of people with learning difficulties to define the basis by which they will engage with care professionals, then this is an issue of self-determination rather than empowerment. At an international conference of People First groups in 1993 the following issues were considered at a workshop on power and making decisions:

- having others take our power away and make our decisions;
- becoming powerful and making our own choices;
- having our rights taken away and doing something about it;
- having people abuse and punish us;
- making local groups stronger;
- making People First bigger with more members;
- making sure that People First stays separate from other groups and organizations;
- teaching supporters about what they should and should not do (People First (1993b)).

Employees of care service agencies rarely operate autonomously. They are constrained by the policies and structures of that agency. Organizational constraints and the social barriers existing in care services are often not within workers' control, but this does not mean that such issues should not be recognized and addressed within their work. Empowerment is therefore dependent on a shift in organizational culture which involves managers having an ability to listen to staff with full concentration on their feelings as well as content, a friendly approach, appropriate openness and a capacity to level with others . . . 'The atmosphere they create will be one of partnership rather than fear' (Stevenson and Parsloe, 1993, p. 11).

Health and social care professionals also have a responsibility to listen to and respond to the statements and actions presented to them and provide unambiguous, relevant and accessible information in return. They also have a role in promoting change within their own organization through facilitating access and supporting opportunities for the involvement of service-users' organizations in the planning and quality control of service delivery and training of staff. Some examples and guides to providing support and facilitation are given below.

Summary

People with learning difficulties have diverse roles and responsibilities in society but care professionals have often reduced these to that of a passive recipient defined by the service. Effective contributions by service users require a change in the distribution of power between professionals and service users, but in order for this to happen professionals need a change of perspective which involves acknowledging that the service user is able to determine their own needs. Empowerment ideologies may be a useful way of encouraging professionals to develop more equal partnerships with service users or an attempt to redefine their own power. For the latter activity I offer my cynical definition of empowerment:

Empowerment: the process by which professions procure power from service users then give it back to them in order to enhance the professional's status.

The issue of power ownership is a common problem where someone is representing another's interests.

Advocacy

Service users may need some help in expressing their views. An advocate is literally 'one who pleads for a cause or on behalf of another' (*Oxford Dictionary*, 1984). The term 'advocacy' is being applied to such a variety of support work with people with learning difficulties for equally various motives that it is reminiscent of the evangelist zeal associated with 'counselling' in the 1960s (Halmos, 1965). There are a wide range of approaches that have become established in the past 25 years which can also involve representatives, facilitators and supporters who assist in presenting a person's viewpoint. Brandon (1995) identifies seven forms of advocacy:

- independent professional (lawyer, ombudsman);
- service professional (nurse, social workers, occupational therapists);
- advocacy by families;
- self-advocacy;
- citizen advocacy;
- peer advocacy (support from people with similar experience);
- collective advocacy.

The distinction between these forms is not so clear in practice. Groups such as Advocacy in Action, based in Nottingham, and People First would regard themselves as self-advocacy groups, but could also be identified as offering peer or group advocacy and collective advocacy to their membership. A more practical separation can be made for our purposes between 'speaking for yourself' (self-advocacy as an individual or a group) and where someone else speaks on behalf of another (paid or unpaid advocacy).

Speaking for ourselves – self-advocacy

The current self-advocacy movement can be traced back to development in Sweden in the 1960s when groups of people with learning difficulties – generally in institutional care – began to raise questions about the way they were treated by society. Groups were started in other countries, including Britain, largely as a result of two international conferences in the early 1970s.

People First is an organization of local self-advocacy groups that developed initially in Canada and the USA. Their approach tended to be more strident, with an emphasis on civil rights (access to real homes, proper jobs and voting), than the earlier Scandinavian groups who looked for society to value the different contribution that disabled people could make to the world (Stevens, 1992). The first groups in Britain were started after the first People First International Conference in the USA in 1984. Accounts of the early development of these groups indicate the close association that they had with supportive groups of care professionals such as Values into Action (then Campaign for People with a Mental Handicap) and parental organizations such as MENCAP (Hersov, 1992; Whittaker, 1996). In recent years the self-advocacy movement has become increasingly independent of these groups.

Dowson (1991) identifies four different forms of self advocacy:

- as a very specific individual act;
- during a process such as information-giving or decision-making in care planning;
- as a group activity including members representing their peers;
- campaigning as a group for people with learning difficulties as a whole.

Self-advocacy groups have become involved in a wide range of activities that involve engagement with professionals on a more equal basis. These activities include:

- advice and support to individuals and groups unable to get appropriate services or appropriate recognition of their achievements;
- representation of service users' interests at local, national and international events;
- training of support workers, care professionals and others in disability issues (Advocacy in Action in Nottingham, Skills for People in Newcastle and People First);
- publication of information and training materials in print, tape and video and developing of materials in collaboration with other agencies, such as the Open University (1997) and CCETSW (1994);
- campaigning and lobbying Local and National Government agencies and voluntary agencies for changes in policy and on issues of equal rights and access to services (Black People First and Young People First).

The role of paid or unpaid supporters or advisors to self-advocacy groups is not that of a professional advocate although some similar skills are needed. Supporters assist with information and interpretation with individuals or groups. This role involves both respecting a group's ability and responsibility to make their own decisions and advising them about the implications of making particular decisions. Trust on both sides is essential for supporters to work effectively. There are dangers that in expressing a personal opinion a supporter will unduly influence or suppress legitimate views of individual self-advocates. Service professionals have unfairly dismissed self-advocacy groups as merely representing the views of a supporter. Self-advocates are generally aware of when their views are being unfairly represented by supporters (see Figure 13.3).

A bad supporter

- people who try to make decisions for you
- somebody who treats you like a child or a baby
- people who do not listen
- people who tell you what to do
- somebody who does everything for you
- people who do not teach you how to do things for yourself
- people who decide what to talk about at meetings.

A good supporter

- somebody who really listens to you
- somebody who will not take over and do everything for you
- somebody who believes in what you are doing
- somebody who treats you like an adult
- somebody who will help you and the group to learn to do things for yourselves
- somebody who will not make decisions for you.

Advocacy by families

The most active advocates for people with learning difficulties are their families and friends. Families have always provided the

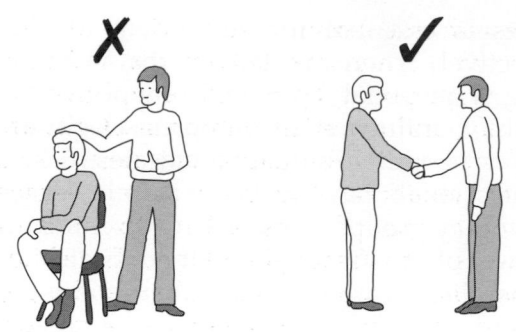

Figure 13.3 Speaking for other people (People First, 1993c)

majority of support for their relatives even when incarceration in mental deficiency institutions was a national policy during the inter-war period. Negotiating with care service workers over access to support services on behalf of their relative or neighbour is seen as part of the care tasks of families and friends (Brandon, 1995). The situation is complicated by family emotional involvement. They may know their relative better than the care manager assessing his or her needs, but they are still 'people on the outside' to self-advocates as they have not usually experienced what it is to be a person with learning difficulties. The perspectives of parents and self-advocates particularly conflict over safety/risk-taking decisions and sexuality. It is often unrealistic for someone with severe learning difficulties, multiple impairments or communication difficulties to compromise the support they receive by challenging their relatives. Support by some parents for village settlements and perpetuation of special hospitals through lobby groups such as RESCARE does not generally represent the views of people with learning difficulties who generally prefer to live in their local communities.

However, care professionals should also consider the role that individuals, such as Phillipa Russell (Russell, 1995), or groups of relatives have also played in promoting or

developing better services. My first professional involvement with advocacy for people with learning difficulties in the mid-1980s was as co-ordinator of one of the first shared care schemes in England, developed by an innovative MENCAP group in Colchester which included Ken Jupp. Jupp suggests that there is no reason why family support when well advised cannot be as effective as any other form of advocacy (Jupp, 1994).

Citizen advocacy

The concept of citizen advocacy is another system of representation that was imported from the USA in 1981 through the organization Advocacy Alliance (later National Citizen Advocacy). O'Brien and Wolfensberger (1978) were responsible for framing the principles of operation of the system which emphasized valuing people with learning difficulties in the community through an advocate.

A citizen advocate is a valued citizen who is unpaid and independent of human services who creates a relationship with a person who is at risk of social exclusion and chooses one or several of many ways to understand, respond to, and represent that person's interests as if they were the advocate's own thus bringing their partner's gifts and concerns into the circles of ordinary life.
(O'Brien in Brandon, 1995)

These relationships are individual and often long-lasting. Citizen advocates are usually recruited and matched with people requiring their support through local management groups. Groups are sometimes funded by health or social care agencies and may be managed by care professionals.

There are some advantages to this method of advocacy as more time can be given to assist people who find it difficult to communicate or who have difficulty in forming relationships. The integrity of the citizen advocate is essential in these circumstances as it can leave some people open to exploitation. The independence of the citizen advocates is maintained through their unpaid status and the influence in their training and support on the values of citizen advocacy.

There is a wealth of literature written by the promoters of citizen advocacy which shares an ideological perspective with normalization or more particularly social role valorization. Brandon (1995) expresses concern for the degree of evangelistic religious flavour and fervour of some citizen advocacy literature. Warmsley addresses the relationship between the matched couple:

It illustrates well the ideological spectacles through which people with learning difficulties are seen as takers, in need of one-sided relationships. Citizen advocates are seen as 'bringing their partner's gifts and concerns into the circles of ordinary community life' (Butler et al., 1988). The use of the word citizen is interesting here. It is open to debate whether the Citizen Advocate is enhancing his or her own citizenship by taking on the role, or that of the person advocated for. In some senses the Citizen Advocate is the very model of the New Right's Active Citizen.

(Warmsley, 1991, p. 228)

The implications of citizenship on people with learning difficulties in the future is discussed below.

Professional advocacy

Advocacy is considered by nurses and social workers to be an important aspect of their work. The UKCC Code of Professional Conduct indicates that nurses should 'act always in a way as to promote and safeguard the well-being and interests of their patients'. Social workers should 'assist children and adults to represent their own interests' and 'advocate directly with and on behalf of children and adults' (CCETSW, 1995, p. 26).

Health and social care workers are in a good position to offer advice and assistance to service users. They will often have had training and experience in counselling, and have access to information and networks of useful contacts. When I was a specialist social worker I was asked to re-assess families with disabled children. The child's behaviour, regarded as attention-seeking or bizarre, had been considered as indicating possible abuse by child protection workers. My knowledge of the implications of environmental problems on disabled people and their families enabled me to advocate effectively on their behalf and intervene to provide more appropriate support services.

However, in Britain most care workers are not in independent positions. They are usually employed in agencies responsible for service delivery, either a purchasing authority or in an agency contracted to supply services. The interests of individual service users will often conflict with agencies over assessment criteria, allocation and distribution of resources. Agencies will constrain care workers' actions where there are issues of complaint. Workers often work in teams where they are dependent on colleagues' support or within other professional constraints which can compromise their independence as an advocate. 'Whistle-blowing' has proved damaging to the careers of professionals who have made public the deficiencies in their services (Dobson, 1996).

Independent professional advocates such as lawyers are occasionally involved with people with learning difficulty – particularly in issues of complaint. Local Authorities in Britain are required to set standards of service delivery in which an effective complaints system is an important component. Where service users regard their complaint has not been properly considered this can involve representation by a legal advocate. Legal challenges by people with learning difficulties may be more common in the future.

Mark Hazell, a young man with learning difficulties, and his family successfully challenged a Local Authority assessment of his needs. In a High Court judgment in 1993, it was considered the Local Authority should have considered more seriously Mark's psychological need to live in a home of his choice. The 2-year dispute had involved five different forms of advocacy: Mark (self-advocate), his mother, Sue Hazell (family advocacy), Richard Mills (an independent advocate), his legal representatives (professional advocates) and social workers (service professional advocates). In my discussions with Sue Hazell and Richard Mills, it was apparent that Mrs Hazell's views generally coincided with those of her son, but an independent advocacy was needed to assist them. Some social workers and other care professionals involved with the dispute were not insensitive to Mark's point of view, others would appear to have had difficulties relating to Mrs Hazell, but they all had other responsibilities to their own agency which restricted them responding to Mark's individual needs.

Summary

Nurses, social workers and other care workers represent the interests of service users in a variety of ways. This may involve providing advocacy support, but there are circumstances when service users and their families do not consider this appropriate. It is therefore also important for care workers to consider appropriate ways of supporting service users' own self-advocacy, and respond appropriately to family, friends, groups of disabled people, citizen advocates, and other advocates assisting service users to present their point of view. All forms of advocacy have some disadvantages, but care agencies and their staff will have to acknowledge the legitimacy of an independent point of view expressed by the advocate on the service user's behalf.

Supporting Communication

Skill in the process of communication is often taken for granted by care professionals. Nevertheless, many disabled people find that their views are not being acknowledged. Failure to listen or inequalites in power between care professionals and service users are contributory factors, but there are also problems about professionals' ineffective communication. Nursing and social work training considers the complexities of the human condition in complex language. Attention given to the development of these elaborated codes and knowledge of the psychology of human interaction can be contrasted with the relative ignorance of the range of spoken and manual languages and other formal systems used for communication by disabled people within a multicultural society. A recent handbook on communication skills makes virtually no reference to minority languages or sign systems (Hargie, 1997). Effective communication with service users can be dependent on an awareness of these forms of communication.

The provision of information by care services is generally constructed on the basis of written or spoken English. Where documents are translated into other languages these may not be accessible to the target local population because of cultural or dialect differences to the translator or problems of literacy. There is no point in producing a leaflet in Gujerati for older women if many of the target audience cannot read.

Understanding the meaning of communication requires knowledge of the language used and knowledge of the real world or context (Leech, 1981). Translation is a poor substitute for consultation to find out which information is relevant to the population you are trying to assist. People with learning difficulties will have cultural, contextual and language differences to care workers. Abbreviation, jargon and local dialects arise from institutionalization (special schooling, residential and day centres) as well as through professional training.

It is good practice to use clear simple and direct statements in a variety of forms where a preferred method of communication is not known. People with learning difficulties and a sensory impairment can be limited in their choice of communication not only as a result of their impairment but also due to the language systems available in the schools they attended, which in many cases are not mainstream schools.

Research into the most common forms of non-vocal communication taught in schools indicates that three sign systems predominate in England, Wales and Scotland (Keirnan *et al.*, 1982). People with learning difficulties may be exposed to more than one system as new systems sometime become 'fashionable' with staff or because they may learn communication in different settings. The research indicated that the most popular taught communication was:

1. British Sign Language (including the use of the Makaton vocabulary)
2. Paget Gorman
3. Blissymbolics.

British Sign Language (BSL) is the preferred language of the deaf community. Makaton signs is a restricted vocabulary derived from BSL signs but not synonymous with them. It is often used to support communication in spoken English in the same way as deafened people may use sign to support lip-reading skills. Paget Gorman is a complex manual code rather than a language and is not derived from BSL. Other manual systems identified in

this research included Amer-ind (based on signs developed by native Americans) and Meldreth Mime (a system developed at Meldreth Manor special school).

Blissymbolics is non-manual sign system based on simple drawn images and includes compound symbols made up of other symbols (e.g. the symbols for electric, sound, vision and box together comprise the sign for television). Rebus is similar system commonly in use. Other mechanical communication aids have also been available. Since this research has been undertaken, computer-assisted systems of communication have been used more extensively. A version of Rebus has been developed within a word processing programme that enables 'translation' of written English into symbols. Semantic problems arise in simply converting English in this way. This program known as WIDGET is used in education centres and has been used as a communication support in large conferences by MENCAP and other groups (see Sutcliffe, 1990 for more on the importance of communication and education).

Drawings used in this chapter are similar to those used by People First groups. The use of drawings may not convey as precise a meaning as formal sign systems, but rather act as an aid to understanding the written text which may have been read out by a supporter. Drawings have some advantages for self-advocacy groups over copyrighted sign systems such as Bliss or Rebus. Some people find the shapes more recognizable than the stick people in symbol systems. They can be drawn easily on paper by most people in a group. Artistic competence is not the important issue if the intended meaning is conveyed.

Environments have an impact on the effectiveness of communication. Poor lighting or standing by a window make lip-reading, manual sign and other visual communications difficult to interpret. A noisy environment is difficult for people who use hearing aids or who have tinnitus. Loop amplification systems can reduce the interference of background noise. It is beyond the scope of this chapter to address these issues in any detail, but information can be obtained from organizations such as SENSE, RNID, RNIB and RADAR with regard to accessible communication and suitable environments for people with sensory impairments, which is also useful to people with learning difficulties. Some other features that facilitate communication with people in groups are identified in the checklists below.

Summary

Most people use a range of systems to communicate and it is important that care service staff are sensitive to the range of communication media that anyone can use to put their point of view across.

Forms of Collaboration

Collaboration between service agencies cannot provide appropriate services where there are inadequate resources, but it can offer innovation and produce services that are better value for money for service users and support agencies. Consultation can be on a one-to-one basis. The involvement of advocates, interpreters and/or other facilitators should not essentially affect this individual communication, as much as the willingness of both parties to work with each other. In situations where staff from various services meet with service users and carers, the involvement of advocates or other supporters is often required for proper acknowledgement of the contribution of most people with learning difficulties.

There are other meetings that are arranged by local organizations of disabled people where service workers may be invited or collaborative events between agencies and self-advocacy or similar organizations. It is important for service staff to be prepared to clearly represent the views of their agency, to seek clarification if they do not understand the issues raised and to fairly support the views of a particular service user if they are acting as their supporter or advocate. Health and social care staff may be asked to facilitate or assist in planning an event that involves consultation of service users or their organizations. Consultation of people with learning difficulties will be required by local agencies and service staff should be able to use their experience of working with people with learning difficulties and other disabled people to facilitate the active contribution of service users through good organization and sensitivity to the participants' access and other support requirements.

Boxes 1–3 list some practical information that might be of assistance in running consultation events.

Information after the event

The results of the consultation exercise should be collated and circulated to the people involved for their comments. It is important to consider that clear statements, drawings and symbol systems are used in written material and that the material is also available in tape and other formats. It is also important to inform participants of the final use of the collaboration – either for a report, publication or service development.

Partnerships in the Future

Recent Government policy in Britain has emphasized citizenship as well as consumerism. This has tended to identify that

- Check if anyone wants to be consulted. Consult with groups of service users or service agencies seeking advice about who might attend. Collaboration in planning events will make it more relevant and support more likely.
- Funding effective consultation exercises can be costly, but where agencies have a requirement to consult and provide appropriate services it can save wasting money on services that are not wanted. All consultants are giving a service so financial support for transport, interpreters/translators and supporters' expenses should be considered as a minimum. Costings should include an appropriate venue, catering, information production, and other incidentals.
- Identify people who can help you facilitate an event. For anything other than the smallest group you will need help. People with learning difficulties may have their own supporters but you might need people to act as group facilitators, note-takers, receptionists and general assistance.
- Check the accessibility of the venue. If display equipment is not provided you will probably have to arrange this.
- Communication needs to be in a format appropriate for everyone concerned to understand the purpose of the event. This may mean direct personal contact, but where letters are sent then clear statements should be used, supported by symbols or drawings. Ask what you need to know, which is usually not medical information. For example:
  Is there any food you don't like to eat?
  Will you need someone to help you at the meeting?
  Do you need any help with arranging transport?
- Send a time table early as it often helps people to know what will be going on. The planning of the time table should take account of the mobility needs of participants – particularly with regard to catering and toilets – and adequate arrangements for explanations and comments – best done in small groups at large events. An example of a time table and briefing notes is shown in Figure 13.4. I used this for a large consultation event for 100 people which involved different groups of disabled people.
- Only send information that is helpful. People with learning difficulties should be given the same information as other participants but in an accessible form as far as possible. Sufficient time must be given for them to work through this with supporters. Massive documents are inaccessible to everyone. Summary documents that accurately reflect the content of larger official documents are necessary if consultation is to be effective rather than tokenistic. Large documents should be evaluated by professional advocates acting for service users.

Box 1 Preparation checklist

individuals have responsibilities as well as rights. People with learning difficulties who are likely to require support at exercising their rights will also need support in addressing their responsibilities as citizens. Warmsley (1991) cautions that there is a long way to go before people with learning difficulties can be regarded as active citizens. Paternalistic welfare systems which reinforce dependency will probably be further challenged by both service users and Government policy.

The rights of families and other informal carers may conflict further with the rights of

Central Council for Education and Training in Social Work

SERVICE USERS AND PARTICIPATION IN SOCIAL WORK EDUCATION
CONSULTATION CONFERENCE

Venue:

Date:

10.00 Coffee, Reception and Choosing Session Groups

12.30 Lunch

10.30 Introduction

2.30 Second Group Session

10.45 First Group Session

3.30 Afternoon Tea and Final Comments from Participants

4.00 End

BRIEFING NOTES

The conference

The purpose of the conference is to develop ideas that can be used to compile a set of guidelines for social work trainers. They will assist in the involvement of service users and their carers in social work training.

The workshops

These are an opportunity to raise issues that they feel ought to be included in the guidelines. Each workshop will last up to one and a half hours. This will give people time to put their points across. There will be an opportunity to attend two workshops, one in the morning and one after lunch, as well as a chance to make comments outside the groups.

Each will have a person leading the group discussion and a scribe writing comments down on flipchart paper. Anyone can add any comments, drawings or diagrams if they feel this would get their point across better. It would be helpful if the main scribe could put an explanation of the drawing underneath with the name of the person drawing it, if they are agreeable to this for ease of reference. There are to be drawings, pictograms and diagrams in the publication.

It is suggested that the group leader introduce the group to the main starting point of the group. Some group members will have had bad experiences, others have not been involved in training. Theses are as follows:

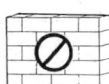

1. Personal barriers

What things put people off from assisting in training of social workers and other welfare professionals? What should be organized? Examples: access, expenses, introductions and explanations.

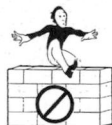

2. Overcoming the barriers

What needs to be done to assist people to participate in training students? Examples: planning together in advance, access, information.

Continued opposite

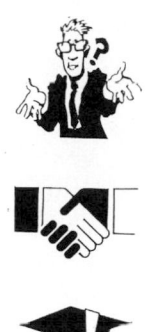

3. Who is representative?

How do trainers choose who to invite? Is this really an issue? How can service users and carers put the views of people who have different difficulties to themselves?

4. The value of partnership

What is the value of trainers and service users working together in training students? Who does it benefit?

5. Student expectations

What do students think about service users training them? What do service users expect from them?

Figure 13.4 Conference details (CCETSW, 1994, pp. 87–9)

■ If you are responsible for the event, walk through all the areas of a building that can be used yourself rather than rely on recommendation. Clarify with the manager of the facility the range of activities and support required.

■ Catering – arrange for a choice of drink and food suitable for those with different diets to be available, appropriately labelled with symbols and in separate categories – vegetarian, halal or kosher separate from meat or fish.

■ Check ramps, doors, toilets, lifts and seating arrangements are appropriate for wheelchair users and others with particular mobility needs.

■ Check parking and dropping off areas to the building and access to the venue – through the kitchens or service lifts is not advisable!

■ Check signage, lighting in corridors and rooms. Make sure that the main speakers or display areas are facing rather than silhouetted against window areas.

■ Check the loop systems that are installed or available are in suitable positions for the groups or presentation sessions. Test amplification and projection equipment if computer, slide or other visual aids are used.

■ If you are concerned about particular issues, raise these formally with building staff. Make sure all arrangements are clarified in writing – you will need this when you claim a discount for something that has gone wrong!

Box 2 Access to buildings

- Bring prepared display and other material, attendance list, trainers/presenters survival kit – including spare information agendas, assorted pens, flip chart and other paper, Blutack, adhesive tape and ohp acetates.
- Arrive early. Give yourself sufficient time to deal with any issues that might arise. Half an hour may be sufficient for a small group – half a day may be essential for a large event.
- Walk through the venue again and check that access issues are adequately addressed. Check leads and other wires are safely taped down.
- Establish reception areas – locate support staff to direct or assist people. Registration requires space and staff as half the people will probably want to register at the same time. People may be sensitive to labels. They can be helpful but should not be imposed.
- Check catering arrangements as far in advance as possible. Catering staff are not always sufficiently briefed and may need to sort out problems.

Box 3 Checklist at the event

disabled people represented through self-advocacy and advocacy. Negotiations over the development of care plans will have to deal with these conflicts. Resolution of conflict may involve additional community support rather than exploit the carer's feelings of responsibility.

Contracting arrangements between service purchasers and providers may more commonly involve establishing with service users their rights and obligations. The three-way contract has been found effective in maintaining quality and consistency where other disabled people are known by service suppliers to be active partners in the agreement (Best, 1994).

Nurses, social workers and other welfare professionals may perceive an erosion of status and autonomy with more active contributions from people with learning difficulties. As direct payment schemes become more established, it will become more likely that people will be more active in running their own services. This may eventually mean service professionals could be employed by them (e.g. contracted to plan or organize services in a similar way to service brokerage).

Individuals and groups of self-advocates have developed roles as service providers – as consultants for service agencies in the planning and inspection of services; in training of care staff and other advocates; and in research. It is also likely that the demand for these services will increase as agencies and their staff recognize their effectiveness. The current benefits system is too restrictive for self-advocates in part-time employment. If they are to become active citizens the reform of the benefits system is essential.

Proposals and Recommendations

- Health and social care professionals should develop more effective methods of working with service users which recognize the legitimacy of people speaking for themselves and planning their own services.
- Service users should be encouraged to become more involved in choosing, planning and managing their own services

and evaluating the quality of the services they receive. This includes recruitment of staff and evaluation of staff performance in training and in practice.

- Development of service users' active collaboration is also dependent on better recognition and support of self-advocacy groups and other forms of independent advocacy. Health and social care workers should be able to identify the limits of their abilities to represent the interests of the service user and the agency that employs them. Service agencies should assist in identifying more often where independent advocacy is appropriate and support its development.
- Training of health and social care professionals should be more sensitive to the legitimacy of a variety of forms of communication used by disabled people, including the use of sign languages. Organizational skills relating to more effective communication and collaboration with service user groups and community support networks should be considered as relevant to professional competence as clinical/individual therapeutic interventions.
- Legislative reform is needed if people with learning difficulties are to become active citizens in the community. The reform of the welfare benefits system which restricts disabled people from benefiting from part-time work and more effective anti-discrimination legislation which protects them from being discriminated against in employment, housing, transport, etc. is particularly necessary.

Discussion Questions

- Imagine you are asked to write a policy guidance document about the appropriate use of advocacy. Draw up a list of scenarios and identify the type of advocacy you consider most appropriate. If your manager or a disabled service user were to do this exercise – how far would their conclusions differ from yours?
- Draw a graphical representation of the *actual* process of your agency's complaints procedure. How far is this process comprehensible to a person with learning difficulties?
- Identify suitable accessible venues for consultation with disabled service users in your area. Who would you ask to check out that they are really suitable?

References

Adams, R. (1990). *Self Help, Social Work and Empowerment*. Macmillan, London.

Best, D. (1994). *Purchasing & Contracting Skills Improving Social Work Education & Training No. 8*. Central Council for Education and Training in Social Work, London.

Brandon, D. (1995). *Advocacy: Power to People with Disabilities*. Venture, London.

Butler, K., Carr, S. and Sullivan, F. (1988). *Citizen Advocacy: A Powerful Partnership*. National Citizen Advocacy, London.

CCETSW (1994). *Changing the Culture: Involving Service Users in Social Work Education*. Paper 32.2. Central Council for Education and Training in Social Work, London.

CCETSW (1995). *Assuring Quality in the Diploma in Social Work – 1: Rules & Requirements for the DipSW*. Central Council for Education and Training in Social Work, London.

Chappell, A.L. (1992). Towards a sociological critique of the normalisation principle. *Disability Handicap & Society* 7 (2), 35–54.

Cullen, C. (1991). Experimentation and planning in community care. *Disability Handicap & Society* 6 (2), 115–28.

Dobson, R. (1996). Gagged! *Community Care*, **1114**, 18–19.

Dowson, S. (1991). *Keeping it Safe: Readings on Self Advocacy Groups by People with Learning Difficulties*. Values into Action, London.

Halmos, P. (1965). *The Faith of the Counsellors*. Constable, London.

Hargie, O.D.W. (ed.) (1997). *The Handbook of Communication Skills*, 2nd edn. Routledge, London.

Hersov, J. (1992). Advocacy – issues for the 1990s. In *Standards & Mental Handicap* (eds T. Thompson and P. Mathias), pp. 284–92. Baillière Tindall, London.

Keirnan, C., Reid, B. and Jones, L. (1982). *Signs & Symbols: A Review of Literature and Survey of the Use of Non-vocal Communication Systems*. Heinemann, London.

Jupp, K. (1994). *Living a Full Life with Learning Disabilities*. Souvenir, London.

Leech, G. (1981). *The Study of Meaning*. Pelican, London.

Lindow, V. and Morris, J. (1995). *Service User Involvement – Synthesis of Findings and Experience in the Field of Community Care*. Joseph Rowntree Foundation, London.

O'Brien J. and Wolfensberger, W. (1978). *CAPE: Standards for Citizen Advocacy Program Evaluation*. Canadian Association for the Mentally Retarded.

Open University (1997). *Learning Disability: Working as Equal People*. Open University, Milton Keynes.

People First (1993b). *Newsletter* Summer 3. p. 17. People First, London.

People First (1993a). *Oi It's My Assessment*. People First, London.

People First (1993c). *Self Advocacy Starter Pack*. People First, London.

Russell, P. (1995). Supporting families. In *Values and Visions: Changing Ideas in Services for People with Learning Difficulties* (eds T. Philpott and L. Ward), pp. 20–42. Butterworth-Heinemann, Oxford.

Stevens, A. (1992). Independence 92 – A report of the Vancouver conference. *CMH Newsletter*, Autumn.

Stevenson, O. and Parsloe, P. (1993). *Community Care and Empowerment*. Joseph Rowntree Foundation, London.

Sutcliffe, J. (1990). *Adults with Learning Difficulties. Education Choice & Empowerment*. NIACE, Leicester.

Ward, D. and Mullender, A. (1991). Empowerment and oppression: an indissoluble pairing for contemporary social work. *Critical Social Policy*, **32**, 21–30.

Warmsley, J. (1991). Contradictions in caring: recipro-city and interdependence. *Disability, Handicap & Society*, **8** (2), 129–42.

Whittaker, A. (1996). The fight for self-advocacy. In *Changing Policy and Practice for People with Learning Disabilities* (eds P. Mittler and V. Sinason), pp. 86–97. Cassell, London.

See also

O'Brien, J. and Tyne, A. *The Principle for Normalisation: A Foundation for Effective Services*. CMH Publications, London.

Contact Addresses

Amer-Ind
Mrs Maggie Cooper, Colchester General Hospital, Turner Road, Colchester, Essex CO4 5JL

Blissymbolics
Ena Davies, The Blissymbolics Communication Resource Centre (UK), Thomas House, South Glamorgan Institute of Higher Education, Cyncoed Centre, Cyncoed Road, Cardiff CF2 6XD

Makaton
The Makaton Vocabulary Development Project, 31 Firwood Drive, Camberley, Surrey

Paget Gorman
Stewart McKenna, City Lit, Keeley Street, London WC2B 4BA

People First
Instrument House, 207–215 Kings Cross Road, London WC1 9DB

RADAR
12 City Forum, 250 City Road, London EC1V 8AF

RNIB
224 Gt Portland St, London WC1N 6AA

RNID
19–23 Featherstone St, London EC1Y 8SL

SENSE
11–13 Clifton Terrace, London N4 3SR

Widget
Widget Software Ltd, 102 Radford Road, Leamington Spa, Warwickshire CV31 1LF

Chapter 14

Competency in Diversity: Providing Care in a Multiracial Society

Carol Baxter

Key Issues

- Racial discrimination within services
- Origins of racism
- Double discrimination
- Current reforms
- Anti-racist practice

The message to all who choose to care for others is that, unless their actions are guided by a sense of importance of every human being, their competence and professionalism will remain questionable.

(Nzira, 1986)

According to the 1991 Census, 5.9% of the British population describe themselves as being black or from a minority ethnic group. However, national information about the prevalence of learning difficulties amongst this section of the population is very sparse indeed. Over the past two decades there has nevertheless been growing concern about the disproportionate numbers of ethnic minority children assessed as having moderate learning difficulties and placed in special schools (Coard, 1971; Tomlinson, 1982). Similar anxieties have also been expressed regarding the over-representaton of ethnic minority children in schools for those with severe learning difficulties. Local studies have also provided some useful information. A study in Camberwell demonstrated that children with severe language impairment were significantly over-represented among children born to parents from the New Commonwealth (Wing, 1969). In 1986 it was reported over 40% of the Bangladeshi children with special needs in Tower Hamlets were in these schools, yet the overall figure in inner London was only 17% (Chaudhury, 1986). Data from the north of the country are particularly revealing. In Rochdale, for example, black and ethnic minority children comprise 40% of all children attending a Development Therapy Unit and 35% of children receiving Portage (S. Whitfield, pers. comm.). A Manchester study revealed more of each type of severe disability (Akinsola and Fryers, 1986). In Oldham it was reported that babies born to South Asian mothers made up 18% of births yet over a third of children (double the expected rates) had severe learning difficulties (BASW, 1987).

Despite the limited nature of the available data there are indications that there will be an over-representation of young adults from black and minority ethnic communities with learning difficulties within services, well into the next century. Competency in the delivery of services can only be achieved if service providers possess the appropriate knowledge, skills and attitudes required to meet the needs of this diverse clientele.

This chapter identifies ways in which racial discrimination can operate in services and makes suggestions for development of services which challenge its existence and which are more likely to be responsive to the needs of individual black or minority ethnic service users.

Racial Discrimination within Services

The needs of people with learning difficulties from black and minority ethnic groups are often viewed as special, when in fact they are not dramatically different from those of their white counterparts. There are, however, differences in life experiences and culture, which means that some needs have to be met in different ways. In addition, the added factor of racial discrimination means that black and minority ethnic service users will be amongst the most vulnerable of client groups; addressing the issue of racial discrimination should therefore be viewed as a moral responsibility for those who provide them with support and care.

The origins of racism

Black and other ethnic minority people are more likely to be in semi-skilled and unskilled jobs, to be disproportionately affected by unemployment and are economically worse off than their white counterparts (Balarajan, 1996). There is also evidence that black people have poorer health experiences and less access to appropriate health care (Balarajan and Raleigh, 1993; Health Education Authority, 1994). Black people consistently receive less than their entitlement in benefits or services (Gohil, 1987). These inequalities have their roots in racism. It is an ideology and an institution developed out of imperialism. Westerners needed to see African and Asian people as inferior and even subhuman in order to rationalize slavery and colonization and the furtherance of economic wealth and gain. Racism is therefore based on the myth of the superiority of the white race. Stereotyping is one way in which racism is perpetuated.

If you think back to your childhood and identify images you have learnt about white and black people (images from family, school friends, literature, radio, television and newspapers) it will become apparent that the words that are used to describe white images often reflect what you have learnt about the British Empire. They are generally positive images such as discoverers, Christians, powerful, inventors, scientific researchers, responsible, civilized and intelligent. Words that are used to describe black images are generally negative in contrast to the images of white people – poor, needy, savages, primitive, unreliable, helpless, incompetent, aggressive and subservient. These sterotypical views are still prevalent in our society. Black people who live in Britain today continue to be seen through this myth and continue to be discriminated against socially, politically and economically. This is reflected in all institutions, including health and social welfare services.

Racism operates at both individual (or personal) and organizational (or institutional) levels. Incidents of personal racism within services may well be rare since most people in the caring professions would not deliberately withhold care or treat people differently on the basis of their colour. However, institutional racism within services is the more pervasive and damaging and occurs in a variety of ways. First, it often happens by default where the way things are done within organizations do not take account of the needs of black people. For example, despite the multilingual nature of our society, services are on the whole provided through the English medium only, with limited language support for those who do not speak English. The second way in which racism operates within services is where service planners and managers base their decisions on assumptions and stereotypes. An example of this is the assumption that black people do not need services because 'they prefer to look after their own'. The third dimension to institutional racism is where the rules and regulations of the organization apply equally to all, but they have the effect of excluding black and ethnic minority people while maintaining the privileged position of white people. An example of this is the fact that doctors, nurses and other health professionals trained abroad (particularly in developing countries) find it difficult to have their qualifications accepted in Britain.

Racial discrimination in hospitals

McNaught (1985) from his analysis of a variety of reports and accounts by black and ethnic minority people summarized that racial discrimination against black and minority ethnic patients in hospital had the following characteristics:

- *Patient reception and handling.* Where ethnic minority patients are kept waiting unnecessarily; and where staff make racist comments in earshot of the patient and address them in a derogatory manner.
- *Clinical consultation.* Poor or no explanation is offered to ethnic minority patients. There is also often the assumption that they are 'faking' or hypochondriacs. Black and ethnic minority patients also receive inadequate or no examination before diagnosis and prescription of treatment. Treatment is often delayed or inappropriate and suspected of being experimental.
- *Patients' consent to medical procedures.* The procedures that the patient was advised are often exceeded without further consultation. Concerns have also been expressed about unnecessary procedures which are said to be racially motivated.
- *Nursing care.* There were accounts of off-hand treatment and racist slurs or comments made to patients. The issue of unnecessary medication, particularly of the mentally distressed was also seen as racially motivated.
- *Health surveillance/diagnosis.* The use of parameters and behavioural models that are culture specific to white British people (e.g. in mental health diagnosis, child health surveillance, social and medical assessment for special education) are viewed as inappropriate policies and practices which are racist in their effect.

Double discrimination

As with discrimination against people with learning difficulties, racism is also a form of devaluation and oppression.

To be black and have a learning difficulty as well therefore means double levels of discrimination. Wolfensberger (1975) identifies eight social role perceptions that are particularly damning to people with learning difficulties. As the following discussion demonstrates, there are clear parallels between these social role perceptions and the way in which black people are evaluated in British society (Baxter, 1987).

As subhuman

People with learning difficulties are viewed as subhuman and therefore not having the same human needs, for example for the ordinary comforts of a home. One of the largest documented areas of discrimination against black people and people with learning difficulties is the area of housing. People with learning difficulties living in the community are more likely to live in poor housing or a poor-quality environment (Flynn, 1989). This experience is also true for many people from black and minority ethnic groups. Figures from the 1991 Census suggest that for the larger proportion of people from this section of the population housing conditions, available space and amenities are worse than for whites (Balarajan, 1996).

As sick

Despite resettlement from large institutions into the community, many services for people with learning difficulties are largely the responsibility of Health Services and involve medical and nursing staff. There is also a tendency to view black people as the source and means of the spread of diseases. There is a tendency to associate black people with unsocial diseases such as tuberculosis and now AIDS.

As a holy innocent

As Williams (1985) points out, in some cultures mentally handicapped people are revered as holy 'children of God' being regarded as without original sin. He stresses that this image is one that also still exists to some extent in Britain and draws the reader's attention to a newspaper article (*Daily Mail*, 3 May 1982) in which people with learning difficulties were referred to as 'these truly lovely innocents'.

Media portrayals of black people in situations of natural disaster, such as famines in Third World countries, present images of them as innocent victims of a divine plan. This kind of emphasis inevitably serves to focus attention away from the exploitative relationship between the Western nations and these Third World countries.

As an eternal child

The paternalistic relationship between people with learning difficulties and those who care for and support them is well established. Like small children, people with learning difficulties do not have a choice about where they live and what they eat. The relationship between black and white people is still one of patronage. Adult black people are denied the economic resources and political and social power to determine their own direction. Black adult people are often referred to in endearing terms such as 'boy', 'girl' or 'sunshine'.

As an object of pity and burden of charity

Rather than their rights to an ordinary life, people with learning difficulties are often presented as victims in need of charity. Some charities have, in the past, used the 'evoking of pity' as a means of fundraising. Very rarely are we presented with images of rich, famous black people. We are, however, all familiar with pathetic media images of black people – the classic appearance of the naked bodies, protruding ribs, distended abdomens and fly-swarmed mouths of black children being the most prevalent.

As an object of ridicule

Williams (1985) also points out that the mentally handicapped person as a jester is a well-known historical image. Even today, people with learning difficulties find themselves associated with silly images, such as clowns and funny monkeys. Many people, service providers included, when talking with people with learning difficulties often make jokes or funny remarks. Such experiences are also familiar to black people. Their chances of success are largely limited to the performing arts, entertainment and sport – areas where they are constantly on display. The 'simple, fun-loving people' image is as prevalent today as it was in the 1920s and 1930s.

As a menace

Even today people with learning difficulties are viewed as a threat. Attempts to establish community living are met with objections based on the notions of dangers to local people, children, pets, property and property values. Petitions to help black people out of white neighbourhoods are commonplace.

The National Association for the Care and Resettlement of Offenders (NACRO, 1984) highlighted that black people are more likely to be locked away in mental institutions and to receive custodial sentences and imprisonment.

As an object of dread

The birth of a child with learning difficulties is still largely seen as a dreadful misfortune. As Williams (1985) points out, most handicapped people today will have experienced people crossing over the road rather than meet them. Black people are seen as socially undesirable and unattractive and are dreaded by some people in white society. Many will admit to fear and anxiety when there are large numbers of black people around. Much of the dread is as a result of

their supposedly predominant sexual orientation. This racist stereotype of black people's strong and uncontrolled sexual drive parallels with the popularly held belief about people with learning difficulties.

Unusually physically endowed

Another very prevalent image of people with learning difficulties and black men is that of being unusually physically endowed. The characteristics of this image include being unusually tall, muscular and possessing a surplus of physical strength.

Interviews with 30 nurses across the country revealed, among other things, that stereotypes influenced the way in which male nurses from these communities are deployed within the health service. Their supposed physical strength is often viewed as their sole attribute to the profession. Consequently, they are frequently placed in specialisms or work situations in which the emphasis is on physical containment rather than therapeutic nursing (Baxter *et al.*, 1990; Beishon *et al.*, 1995). This may in part be responsible for the over-representation of black male nurses in areas such as psychogeriatrics, psychiatry and learning difficulties.

When the off duty was being made out, Sister would often say, 'X is on today so we won't need many nurses. He is big and strong'.

Given this double level of discrimination and disadvantage, it is no wonder then that there is serious concern that the needs of people with learning difficulties from black communities are not being met. Athwal (1990) identified that services to this section of our community leave much to be desired. It is often assumed, for example, that black families prefer to 'look after their own'. However, experience has shown that they *do* want to use services. Migration may have severed their traditional networks of support and many black people may there-fore have a greater need for support than their white peers. Black women carers are often extremely isolated but may not use existing support groups because they are inappropriate to their needs or seem unwel-coming. Many worry about the type of care their relative will receive. Others may not be aware of what is available.

Current reforms

Even within the present climate of reform in services, it is still very questionable as to whether the very philosophies which under-pin these changes will not in reality further work against black users of services. One change which has a great impact on people with learning difficulties is the move towards care in the community. It is now expected that voluntary organizations will play an increasing role in providing services. However, mainstream white voluntary organizations do not cater adequately for the needs of black people (Dungate, 1984). The service is mainly based on the needs of the majority of people who are white. However, the few black voluntary organizations that exist are too grossly under-funded and resourced to take on this role. There will therefore be an increased burden on black families.

Criticisms about other concepts and philosophies are based on these very same principles. For example, the primary pur-pose of the normalization philosophy is to promote the social value of people with learning difficulties by encouraging people in society to see them in a more valued way. Service providers are urged 'to enable peo-ple with learning difficulties to enjoy pat-terns and conditions of everyday life which are as close as possible to the norms and patterns of mainstream society'. This has been blindly welcomed as revolutionary to the lives of people with learning difficulties.

However, for black people with learning difficulties, it is not all good news. One aspect that is of particular concern is the fact that, although the normalization theory recognizes that black people are a devalued group in society, it fails to help services to recognize and address the effects of racism on the users and providers of services. More generally, since service planners and man-agers are largely white, there is concern that the normalization principles will not be interpreted in ways that are beneficial to black people with learning difficulties. It is possible that it is only these needs, wants and wishes of the white society which will be considered as 'normal' or 'valued' experiences. A simple exercise carried out by a community mental handicap team in Harlesden, for example, demonstrated that what white staff would value for them-selves would, in many cases, conflict with what black service users valued (Baxter *et al.*, 1990).

People with learning difficulties often have to rely on others to plan their lives. Accordingly, individual programme plans enable service providers to recognize and meet individual needs. As the name implies, individual programme plans have the individual primarily as their focus. However, in many black communities the family and community collectively may take precedence over the more self-centred individualism encouraged in British families. This difference in emphasis may be very important when working with adults with learning difficulties from black communities.

Assessment of an individual's abilities is often based on white British norms which bear little relationship to the everyday life of black people. This is particularly apparent when applied to black children with learn-ing difficulties. Many standard test proce-dures and equipment involve images based on white middle-class lifestyle and experiences. A clinical psychologist who was herself from the Asian community expressed these concerns as follows:

One well known test has a picture of a couple involved in a Western style wedding ceremony. Hindu, Sikh and Muslim wedding ceremonies bear no resemblance to this. I know that Asian children would have difficulty in recognising this one.

There is a major concern that children for whom English is a second language are being disproportionately placed in schools and units for children with severe learning difficulties. In Tower Hamlets, Bangladeshi parents felt that if Bengali was used to assess their children instead of English, their children would have achieved a more positive result (Chaudhury, 1986).

Black and ethnic minority staff

A likely conclusion is that black and ethnic minority staff would be able to assist services in becoming more ethnically sensitive. Black staff, especially those from backgrounds similar to service users, are indeed vital in providing services to a multi-racial clientele. Experience shows that employing staff who can communicate with people in their own languages can result in a dramatic increase in the take-up of services by potential clients who are non-English speaking.

However, staff from this section of the population often feel that their particular perspectives, experiences and skills are not valued and that initiatives and approaches which they develop to respond to needs are seen as unprofessional by their colleagues and managers. Others feel that they are viewed as the 'expert' in caring for black service users and that black clients are 'dumped' on them to relieve white service providers of their professional responsibility. Furthermore, since service providers all undergo the same white-client-oriented

training, not all ethnic minority service providers will therefore have the necessary skills or feel confident and supported to work from an anti-racist perspective. The majority of this staff group tend to occupy low-grade positions and their presence in services is not reflected at a managerial level. Very rarely, therefore, are they in a position to become involved in informing decision-making (Beishon *et al.*, 1995).

Anti-racist Practice

The rationale

Despite their primary intention to care and support people, as we explored in the early part of this chapter, as products of a culture in which racism is a feature, service providers will have unwittingly accepted some of its negative attitudes. We cannot change the past, but by recognizing its effects, we can work towards developing higher professional standards in our future practice.

The needs of black and ethnic minority service users should therefore not be considered as an afterthought or as additional or special, but should be enshrined within the concept of good professional practice. Conelley (1988) puts forward the following arguments as to why the implications of services to black people should be considered:

- We all share a common humanity. To preserve this, all people should be given the opportunity to work for and enjoy all improvements in our society. Taking account of individual, racial and cultural diversity of needs is part of this process.
- As tax and rate payers, black and ethnic minority people have a right as a matter of course to expect equal access to services that are appropriate and relevant to their needs. Planning and policies to enable this are crucial to social justice.

- To maintain professional integrity, the competence of service providers hinges on their readiness, willingness and ability to apply existing and increasing knowledge to new situations.
- Statutory and voluntary organizations have obligations under the Race Relations Act of 1976 to eliminate racial discrimination in employment and the provision of services.
- Providing services that are appropriate to the needs of the population is making efficient and effective use of scarce resources. The multi-racial society is indeed itself a resource and an opportunity to be utilized and cherished.

An approach to practice which focuses on the situation of the most severely handicapped people from black and minority ethnic groups is advocated, since competence at this level will undoubtedly lead to general improvement in services for *all* users.

First and foremost, the issue of human rights should be addressed. *All service users will need assistance in exercising their rights*. For black users, attention will need to be paid to their right to be treated with dignity and respect as equal human beings. Service providers will need to reflect on the following:

- Is your relationship with black service users influenced by unhelpful racist stereotypes?
- What measures have you taken to learn about and understand the nature of racism and how it affects your work practice?
- Do you challenge racist jokes or slurs from patients or colleagues?
- What type of policies are there to ensure that where the client's rights are violated, the appropriate action takes place?
- Black clients will need assistance to minimize destructive self-criticism and focus on their positive self-worth.

Freedom of choice is an integral part of the client's rights. However, as professionals, we have the tendency to make assumptions about people's wants and wishes. This is particularly true for people with learning difficulties from black communities where white professionals are less likely to take the time or feel confident to get to know them as individuals. Even where there is some appreciation of the need to provide more individual and culturally specific forms of care, service providers often have difficulties in gaining information relating to a person's culture or racial origin. Most people tend to shy away from these topics, having been brought up to consider such conversations impolite. There are others who may wish to ask questions, but do not know where to start or what questions to ask. Further difficulties can arise when the service providers and service users do not speak the same language.

If freedom of choice is to become a reality for black service users, then it is important that the options and range of wants and needs are recognized and found out. A priority must be to develop a closer working relationship and partnership with families. Included in this approach will be a greater priority and confidence in working and taking on board the views of a wider range of people – balancing the individuality, the position of the family and the long-term relationships between them. Below are some ideas which will help to pave the way in developing a good partnership.

Most black and ethnic minority people in this country are British citizens by birth so it is important not to be blinded in your search for differences. Build up a rapport by acknowledging that you have things in common. Build up a mutual trust and liking by reassuring the service user and family members that you do not see their differences as a problem and that their differences will not detract from your ability to plan appropriately for their care. Questions based on some existing knowledge indicate your interest and professional competence and will increase the client's and their family's confidence in you. For example, 'I know you are of the Muslim faith. Is there anything I need to know about how this will influence the care needs of your relative?' Do not rely too much on cultural information books you have read because this could stereotype your clients. Use such information as a guide to asking questions. Everyone has difficulty analysing what is second nature to them unless they have a lot of experience in doing this. It may be helpful therefore to ask yourself the same question first to make sure that you are not asking questions that are difficult to answer. There should be access to good interpreter services in those situations where there are language differences.

Physical care – hygiene and grooming

Personal hygiene, hair and skin care are very important to a person's feeling of well-being and it is important that workers should be able to give the appropriate attention to these areas. Workers should follow personal care and hygiene routines adopted at home.

- Choice of either showers or baths should be available as not everyone would feel happy sitting in a bath.
- Support workers of the same sex may be preferred when carrying out intimate forms of care.
- Close attention should be paid to grooming the client's hair to their preference.
- Differences in skin colour also have implications for routine physical care procedures. To use white skin as the norm is dangerous. Appropriate hair and skin care is still an area of gross

neglect for black clients. Support workers and care assistants will need to appreciate that some people require their skin (and hair) to be moisturized, especially after procedures that deplete hair and skin moisture, for example swimming or a bath. Where such procedures are neglected, this could lead to damage to hair and skin.

Religious and cultural requirements

Black service users need assistance in maintaining and developing their religious and cultural identity. Service providers should consistently work to the following criteria:

- All clients should be addressed by their preferred name. Attempts should be made to accurately pronounce and record clients' names. These should not be changed to more English-sounding ones.
- Clients should have the opportunity to have personal possessions which reflect their culture.
- Appropriate and preferred dress is important in helping service users to maintain personal appearance. For example, a support worker should be able to help Asian girls to wrap their saris or a young man to wrap his turban if this is their wish and that of their family.
- Service users should be encouraged and assisted to join organizations or attend events in their own communities. A support worker should be able to be involved with service users if this is necessary.
- Celebrating such events as Dwali, Hanuka and Christmas will be an important part of many peoples' lives. Very little adjusting of services is needed to achieve this.
- Wall-hangings, toys (such as dolls), books, television programmes and other

artefacts should reflect a multi-racial society. Videos from most ethnic minority communities are now widely available and would be helpful. Golliwogs and books and other artefacts that portray negative images of black people should be removed.

- The service-user's religious beliefs (if any) should be established and respected. Assistance to make available places for those who may wish to practise their religion should be given. Mosques, Afro-Caribbean churches and Sikh gudwaras and temples are welcoming to anyone who wishes to support members of their communities.
- Catering arrangements should ensure the availability of choice and range of foods to suit individual preferences. This should include those normally eaten at home. For example, vegetarian, halal and kosher meals should be available if required.
- Service users should be encouraged to speak in their first language and be assisted in finding situations where this is possible.
- Play and learning experiences and other daily routines in the case of adults should be of sufficient variety to promote positive identification with their own racial and cultural background.

Discussion Questions

Voluntary sector

- Make a list of local community organizations with which your service is in contact.
- Identify in what way these organizations make efforts to address specific needs of black and ethnic minority users.

- How many of these organizations fall within the black voluntary sector?
- What efforts are being made by your organization to work with black voluntary sector?

Black staff

- When providing services for black clients, are the particular knowledge and skills of black staff drawn upon?
- Are black staff seen as having sole responsibility for protecting the interests and rights of black clients?
- What support are black staff given to enable them to carry out this aspect of their role?

Cultural needs

Think of a service user who is black or from a minority ethnic group.

- How well do you think their cultural and religious needs are being met?
- What efforts have you taken to find out what such needs might be?

Attitudes

- Is the way you relate to black and ethnic minority service users influenced by racial stereotypes?
- Are there policies in place in your service to protect black and ethnic minority clients from racist jokes and slurs from other users or staff?

Acknowledgements

Some of the material contained in this chapter is based on information which first appeared in *Double Discrimination – Services* for People with Learning Difficulties from Black and Ethnic Minority Communities by C. Baxter, K. Poonia, L. Ward and Z. Nadirshaw and published by the Kings Fund, London in December 1990. This publication is based on a research study project carried out from the Norah Fry Research Centre at the University of Bristol and funded by the Kings Fund Centre and the Commission for Racial Equality. The project, which ran from July 1988 to November 1989 was established in response to the concern about the lack of information on good services for people with learning difficulties from this section of our communities. The primary aim of this chapter is to provide practical suggestions and improvements in services.

References

Akinsola, H.A.A. and Fryers, T. (1986). A comparison of disability in severely mentally handicapped children of different ethnic origins. *Psychological Medicine*, **16**, 127–33.

Athwal, S. (1990). A special case for special treatment. *Social Work Today*, **8 February**, 12–13.

Balarajan, R. (1996). *The Ethnic Minority Dimensions: Result from the 1991 Census*, Vol. 1. National Institute for Ethnic Studies in Health and Social Policy, London.

Balarajan, R. and Raleigh, S.V. (1993). *Ethnicity and Health. A Guide to the NHS*. Department of Health. HMSO, London.

BASW (British Association of Social Workers) (1987). Special Interest Group on Services for People with Mental Handicap. *Newsletter*, No. 7, January. Available from John Smith, Treasurer, BASW, 46 Chilton Way, Hungerford, Berkshire RG17 0JE.

Baxter, C. (1987). Parallels between the social role perception of people with learning difficulties and black and ethnic minority people. In *Making Connections. Reflecting the Lives of People with Learning Difficulties* (eds A. Brechin and J. Walmsley), pp. 237–246. Hodder & Stoughton, London.

Baxter, C., Poonia, K., Ward, L. and Nadirshaw, Z. (1990). *Double Discrimination Issues and Services for People with Learning Difficulties from Black and Ethnic Minority Communities*. Hodder & Stoughton, London.

Beishon, S., Virdee, S. and Hagell, A. (1995). *Nursing in a Multi-Ethnic NHS*. Policy Studies Institute, London.

Chaudhury, A. (1986). *ACE Special Education Advice Service for the Bangladeshi Community*. Advisory Centre for Education, London.

Coard, B. (1971). *How the West Indian Child is Made Educationally Subnormal in the British School System*. New Beacon Books, London.

Connelly, N. (1988). *Care in a Multiracial Community*. Policy Studies Institute, London.

Dungate, M. (1984). *A Multiracial Society. The Role of National Voluntary Organisations*. Bedford Square Press, London.

Flynn, M. (1989). *Independent Living for Adults with Mental Handicap: A Place of My Own*. Cassel, London.

Gohil, V. (1987). DHSS service delivery to ethnic minority claimants. *Leicester Rights Bulletin*, **32**, 7–8.

Health Education Authority (1994). *Black and Ethnic Minority Groups in England: Health and Lifestyles*. Health Education Authority, London.

McNaught, A. (1985). *Race and Health Care in the United Kingdom*. Occasional Paper 2. Health Education Council, London.

NACRO (1984). *Black People and the Criminal Justice System: Summary of the Report of the NACRO Race Issues Advisory Committee. Organisations*. Bedford Square Press, London.

Nzira, V. (1986). Race: the ingredients of good practice. In *The Residential Opportunity? The Wagner Report and After* (ed. E. Philpot). Reed Business Publishing/Community Care, Wallington.

Tomlinson, S. (1982). *Educational Subnormality. A Study of Decision Making*. Routledge and Keagan Paul, London.

Williams, P. (1985). The nature and foundations of the concept of normalisation. In *Current Issues in Clinical Psychology. Clinical Psychology 2* (ed. E. Kracos). Plenum, New York.

Wing, L. (1969). Prevalence of different patterns of impairments in immigrants. In *Recent Research in Social Psychiatry* (ed. J.K. Wing), MRC Social Psychiatry Unit, Institute of Psychiatry, London. Unpublished Report.

Wolfensberger, W. (1975). *The Origin and Nature of our Institutional Models*. Human Policy Press, New York.

Further Reading

Bardsley, J. and Perkins, E. (1983). Portage with Asian families in Central Birmingham. Parents as Partners. *Proceedings of the National Portage Conference held in London*. Nelson/NFER, London.

Baxter, C. (1985). *Hair Care of African, Afro-Caribbean and Asian Hair Types*. National Extension College, Cambridge.

Baxter, C. (1994). Sex education in the multiracial society. In *Practice Issues in Sexuality and Learning Disability* (ed. A. Craft), pp. 81–92. Routledge, London.

Baxter, C. (1995). Confronting colour blindness: developing services for people with learning difficulties from black and minority ethnic communities. In *Values and Visions* (eds T. Philpot and L. Ward), pp. 204–217. Butterworth Heinemann, London.

Brown, B. (1989). Race: needed – policy and practice. In *The Residential Opportunity? The Wagner Report and After* (ed. T. Philpot). Reed Business Publishing/Community Care, London.

Commission for Racial Equality. (1976). *Afro-Caribbean Hair and Skin Care and Recipes*. Commission for Racial Equality, London.

Contact-a-Family (1989). *Reaching for Black Families? A Study of Contact-a-Family in Lewisham and the Relevance of Services for Black Families who have Children with Disabilities and Special Needs*. Contact-a-Family, London.

Duncan, D. (ed.) (1989). *Working with Bilingual Language Disability*. Chapman & Hall, London.

Fryer, P. (1978). *Staying Power. The History of Black People in Britain*. Pluto Press, London.

Katz, J. (1978). *White Awareness*. University of Oklahoma Press, Oklahoma.

Mares, P., Henley, A. and Baxter, C. (1985). *Health Care in Multiracial Britain*. National Extension College/Health Education Council, Cambridge.

Celestin, N. (1986). *A Guide to Anti-Racist Childcare Practice*. Voluntary Organisation Liaison Council for Under Fives, London.

Nzira, V., Phillipson, J. and Sugden, M. (1986). Race: a faltering first step. In *The Residential Opportunity? The Wagner Report and After* (ed. T. Philpot). Reed Business Publishing/Community Care, Wallington.

Open University (1990). *Mental Handicap: Changing Perspectives*. Course K668. Department of Health and Social Welfare/Open University, Milton Keynes.

Poonia, K. and Ward, L. (1990). Fare share of the care. *Community Care Journal*, **11 January**, 16–18.

Shackman, J. (1985). *The Right to be Understood. A Handbook on Working With, Employing and Training Community Interpreters*. National Extension College, Cambridge.

Woolley, A. and Dhanoa, B. (1985). *A Study of Asian Families with Handicapped Children in Smethwick*. ICAA, London.

O'Brien, J. (1986). A guide to personal futures planning. In *A Comprehensive Guide to Activities Catalogue – An Alternative Curriculum for Youth and Adults with Severe Disabilities* (eds G.T. Bellamy and B. Wilcox). P.H. Brookes, Baltimore.

Resources

Black. A BBC film (1983: 50 minutes) which examines the history of black and white relations and features young people talking about their experience of racism. Concord Films Council, 201 Felixstowe Road, Ipswich, Suffolk IP3 9BJ. Tel 01473 715754.

Physical and Mental Handicap in the Asian Community – Can My Child be Helped? A VHS video (with supporting booklet) available in five languages of the Indian subcontinent (Urdu, Punjabi, Gujurati, Hindi, Bengali) and in English. It is for use by Asian families with a young disabled child. Produced by the Voluntary Council for Handicapped Children with support from the Department of Health. Purchase £29.50, Hire £10.50. Available from: CFL Vision, PO Box 35, Wetherby, West Yorkshire LS23 7GX. For further information, contact: Philippa Russell, Voluntary Council for Handicapped Children, 8 Wakley Street, London EC1V 7QE. Tel 0171 278 9441.

Asian Parents of Children with Special Needs. A booklet produced by the King's Fund, which aims to give parents of children with special needs information and advice about a number of issues covering the following:

- finding out your child has a disability
- finding out exactly what is wrong
- understanding what help is available (such as services and benefits)
- education

The Right to be Understood. A video about working with interpreters. Available from the National Extension College, 18 Brooklands Avenue, Cambridge CB2 2HN.

Black and In Care. A video in which children talk about their experiences of being in care and how they have and are trying to overcome their difficulties. Available from Black and in Care Steering Group, c/o Children's Legal Centre, 20 Compton Terrace, London N1 2UN. Tel 0171 359 6251. Cost £32.50, plus 50p postage.

Being White. A video (35 minutes long) in which white people from different backgrounds talk about their understanding of the roots of racism and how they take account of it in their daily lives and work situations. Available from Albany Distributions, Battersea Studios, Television Centre, Thackery Road, London SW8 3TW.

Chapter 15

Risk Management

Marc Saunders

Key Issues

- Risk
- Risk management
- Likelihood
- Consequence
- Risk variables
- Risk and value
- User involvement
- Benefit/harm

Introduction

There can be few developments that so reflect the mood of an era than the increasing interest in risk and risk management. Significant changes in the structure of Health and Social Services allied to an increasingly litigious society have clearly indicated to care workers and managers that they can ill afford to ignore the existence of risk because in doing so they miss the opportunity of effectively managing those risks.

Risk management in human services has two distinct focuses. First, as a tool for direct care staff where risk assessment and risk-management processes are actively pursued as part of the care-planning process. Second, as an approach used predominantly by service managers to identify broad areas of risk within an organization followed by appropriate action. This chapter focuses on the former: the use of risk management in direct care settings.

How relevant is an understanding of risk management to people with a learning disability and service providers? If risk management was purely a method by which professionals and their organizations sought to avoid the legal consequences of their decisions and actions then risk management would be of little relevance. However, imaginatively implemented approaches to managing risk have very clear benefits for those who use our services and can be considered to be closely associated with good practice in service provision. For example, good risk-management systems will involve the service user, support multiprofessional and multi-agency working and will operate from a clearly visible service philosophy. This chapter is concerned with the origins of risk management as well as the practical application of risk assessment and risk-management procedures in services for people with a learning disability.

Understanding Risk and Risk Management

On a very superficial level, many people would feel that they are perfectly well qualified to articulate what is meant by the term 'risk'. Service workers will be very familiar with service structures such as 'at-risk registers' and will find themselves using terms such as 'high risk', 'low risk' and 'acceptable risk'. Yet unless we are able to place these in a useful context they remain highly subjective.

For clarity, 'risk' is defined as:

Supporting a service user to identify a course of action in order to realise one or more beneficial outcomes in the knowledge that there are consequences or outcomes that would be perceived as negative or harmful in nature should they occur.

Once risk has been defined, the term 'risk management' can also be defined:

The identification and analysis of risk combined with explicit plans to manage this risk which might include action to increase the likelihood, impact or frequency of beneficial outcomes as well as action to prevent or decrease the likelihood of harmful consequences and action to reduce or eliminate the extent of harmful consequences should they occur.

Risk and Services for People with a Learning Disability

Throughout this book there is consistent evidence in support of the changing nature of services provided to people with a learning disability. Hopefully, these changes will reflect the real hopes and wishes of clients and their carers. Such developments are manifest in an ever-increasing variety of innovative and imaginative service models.

High-quality risk-management procedures might therefore be considered a necessary development in the face of services that, quite correctly, focus ever more on the specific needs of the individual. Twenty or thirty years ago services for people with a learning disability tended to be based around an institutional model of care, whether that was hospital-based services or large-scale community facilities. People working in those services at the time would have been enthusiastic to testify to their quality and effectiveness. Progress and hindsight has taught us to reconsider what benefits were derived from this type of provision in favour of a wider range of models such as shared living, family placements, small group homes, sheltered accommodation and many variations on these. Respect for the needs of the individual compels us to acknowledge that where people are encouraged to exercise their rights this cannot happen in isolation from society in its widest sense. People with a learning disability, like anyone else, will be exposed to risk, will be familiar with risk and will occasionally experience unpleasant or even harmful outcomes from everyday situations.

Arguably, the desire to develop effective services for all people with a learning disability is reaching a critical point. Institutional services have, for a number of years, managed resettlement programmes designed to facilitate community living opportunities for all people with a learning disability. In many cases, the process of resettlement, albeit inadvertently, has selected those people for whom community care represents a relatively small number of challenges. The consequence of this is that many people with the most complex needs and who require the most sophisticated services have tended to remain in long-stay, segregated services. The risks associated with developing services for this group of people are many and varied where the focus of the risk may be the individual service user, the local community or the direct carers.

Changes in society, whilst in themselves not necessarily risk laden, have impacted upon services. They have required people with a learning disability and service providers to consider more carefully the risks associated with everyday living. For example, public attitudes towards Health and Social Services, the perceived increase in violent crime against the person and the media representation of people with mental health needs as well as the rise in consumerism and the increasingly litigious nature of society have all served to heighten the awareness of risk and, therefore, the need for managing risk effectively.

Finally, changes in services and public policy have also focused provider's minds on risk and risk management. In public services, the publication of the *Patient's Charter* (DOH, 1991) and community charters has shifted the emphasis of service provision toward the service user. This is not a criticism. However, services have to be ready to respond to increased expectations. Equally, the high profile given to the need for effective systems of handling complaints might also have had a similar effect.

The Origin of Risk Management

Some of the factors that have encouraged service providers to look closely at risk and risk management are explored here. Above all else, risk management is about providing good quality services. Risk-

management procedures should effectively be absorbed into the fabric of a service to become an implicit part of the care planning and care management process. In short, good risk management is about good practice.

The terms 'risk' and 'risk management' have increasingly become part of our working vocabulary and may well have foundations in industry (Roy, 1996). Whilst this would clearly be risk management as seen from an organizational context the terminology has nevertheless begun to permeate our language at a number of levels.

Changes in services driven by the NHS and Community Care Act (DOH, 1990) has also concentrated service providers' minds. The loss of Crown immunity in Health Services means that provider units have been required to purchase insurance cover for their services. Premiums are often based on claims experiences and neither the service nor the insurer wishes to pay for unnecessary claims against the organization. As an additional incentive, many insurance companies now employ risk managers who provide advice to services and will even train staff to manage risk, although this tends to be very much from an organizational perspective.

In services provided directly to people with a learning disability risk management is a term given to a group of processes, many of which have been implicit in service policies and approaches to care for some time. However, the 1990s have witnessed the drawing together of these ideas and principles into what we now understand as risk management. Risk management has been well received by many professional groups and is one of those rare developments which may be of equal benefit to service users, direct care workers and service managers.

The legal context

It is important to be very clear that the implementation of risk-management procedures does not render services, or professionals working within them, immune from legal action. Equally, it is important to consider risk management from a legal perspective. If asked, a group of service workers would be able to describe a number of situations relevant to people with a learning disability that might be considered risk laden. There would be a number of relatively unique scenarios reflecting the high level of individuality of service users. There would also be a number of situations to which many people would be able to relate. Typically, access to community facilities by someone with many behavioural challenges, supporting someone to embark on a new relationship or helping a service user to start up their own home away from recognized support centres would all be familiar.

One of the most powerful elements of risk management is the necessary and explicit involvement of the multiprofessional team in the decision-making process. These discussions should, wherever possible, constructively involve the service user. The process is also very logical in sequence and transparent to those who wish to look again at how a decision was made. Finally, risk management is ideologically explicit, which means the values of the multiprofessional team are clearly reflected in the decision-making process, the documentation and the outcomes.

Consider, for example, a situation where a person with a learning disability is learning to use local shops before moving to their new flat. There are a number of risks associated with this activity. Imagine that the unthinkable happens and the service user is knocked down by a car and badly injured whilst on a trip to the shop. The accident is very regrettable and the family is very angry because they felt the service was there to protect their family member from the outside world. They decide to take legal action. The decision made by the staff team and the service user is possibly more effectively defended because the court is able to see the processes the staff team has gone through in an attempt to increase the service user's independence whilst minimizing the possibility and severity of harmful consequences.

Good risk-management procedures will not prevent legal action from being taken, nor will it compensate for poor practice or poor-quality care. To deny a person with a learning disability and their families access to the legal system would not be in their interests. However, good risk-management procedures, carefully implemented, will demonstrate the thought processes behind a decision and will clearly show what actions were taken to minimize the possibility of harmful outcomes.

The Value of Risk

So far, the connection between good risk management and high-quality services has been explored. The basis for this relationship deserves further investigation.

Services for people with a learning disability have, for many years, attempted to focus on the rights and needs of individual service users supported by a strong ideological framework. Concepts such as normalization, ordinary life principles and social role valorization represent variations on this ideological theme. These themes have been organized into manageable ideas by a number of writers, for example, the King's Fund (1980) published *An Ordinary Life* whilst O'Brien (1987) described the five accomplishments. By looking at these more closely it is clear that access to opportunities and, therefore, to situations that might be risk laden, is fundamental to service users who wish to exercise their rights based on these principles.

O'Brien (1987) described five service accomplishments which are well known to those who provide services to people with a learning disability. These are:

- community presence
- community participation
- competence
- choice
- respect.

Arguably, there is risk explicitly associated with four of the five accomplishments and implicit in the fifth. Both community presence and community participation contain clear elements of risk. Equally, the client may make *choices* to develop new skills (competence) which also contain an element of risk.

Further investigation of the association of risk with value will show that as individuals we clearly measure our personal development through all the stages of our life on a number of factors; one of these factors is risk. We make comparisons over time in terms of the nature and severity of the consequences related to the risks we take. For example, as children we derive personal value and satisfaction from being trusted to manage increasingly risk-laden situations such as crossing the road, making hot drinks and so on.

As adults we feel our growth is recognized if we are given work roles of increasing responsibility; that is, with an increased level of risk. It would be arrogant of us to assume that people with a learning disability would not wish their growth to be acknowledged as powerfully as we would wish for ourselves. Shirtliffe (1995) suggests that harm is being inflicted if service users under-achieve and questions which is more negligent: over- or under-protection?

In addition, many people, not satisfied with the levels of risk they experience on a day-to-day basis, choose to pursue pastimes that might be considered of high risk. Examples such as mountaineering, motor racing and parachuting are good illustrations of this. These high-risk pastimes are also associated with high value. Once we begin to organize our thoughts in relation to risk we begin to understand that in working to manage risk it is not desirable to eliminate it completely. A no-risk occupation generally has little associated value.

Therefore, if services are to effectively infer the value that people with a learning disability have a right to expect, it should be anticipated that their plans will include exposure to a degree of risk. The role of the service is to support the user to experience the benefits associated with any risk situation whilst attempting to ensure that the possibility of harmful or negative consequences is minimized.

Risk Assessment and Risk Management

The following sections outline a systematic approach to managing risk. This approach was originally described by Carson (1988). An effort has been made to relate this approach directly to services for people with a learning disability and to raise some of the issues that emerge from the process of risk management when it is used in this context.

Developing a proposal

Regardless of the personal circumstances of an individual, the discussion of risk taking will mean that the service user or the care team are considering one of the following (and in some circumstances more than one where the risk activity has a variety of components):

- to pursue a new activity/a new course of action/a new approach;
- to discontinue an activity/course of action/approach;
- to continue with the current activity/ course of action/approach.

The proposal will be dependent upon a number of factors, for example:

- progress made by a service user;
- views of the service user;
- the service user's strengths and abilities;
- areas where skills need to be developed;
- the age of the service user;
- previous experience of both the service user and the care team.

The term 'proposal' is used throughout the rest of this chapter and refers to the course of action to be followed should it be agreed by the service user and the care team. It is important that such a proposal is clearly understood. For example, a proposal to increase the service user's access to community leisure facilities is insufficiently clear. The proposal must be specific. 'The service user will make use of the local public swimming bath without direct staff support' is more helpful and clear enough for the service user and the care team to consider from a risk-management perspective.

It is important to remember that risk management is not conceptually isolated; it has to be used as a device alongside other approaches to the management of care. For example, care planning, the Care Programme Approach, life planning and so on. On this basis, risk management is used only in tandem with an established decision-making process. In short, it is unsatisfactory to develop plans to expose a service user to risk situations merely because there are risk-management models in existence. It is far more appropriate for decisions to be made relating to the development of the individual using established means to achieve this, and risk-management procedures are then applied when they are required.

The critical views of the service user

Despite the alarm stimulated by the popular media, a meaningful contribution by users to the everyday co-ordination of their care is almost universally welcomed. As such, service users will hopefully have a significant degree of control over their own future and this is viewed by many as a fundamental precondition of service delivery. In terms of risk management this contribution is critical for a number of reasons:

- users are able to obtain an insight into the risks involved;
- users are able to contribute to, agree to or reject a particular proposal;
- a clear message is given to those involved that the views of the service user are essential.

Working with people with a learning disability creates some very particular challenges in this respect. By its very nature a learning disability can prevent people from understanding the full complexities of any proposal and this is especially true for those people with very complex needs. This does not preclude involvement in the decision-making process. However, the care team will need to be especially imaginative in its approach. Where the skills and approaches to involving people with complex levels of need are insufficiently developed or are technologically beyond our scope, then the care team need to be clear with themselves, the service user and their family, what the philosophical drivers are behind a particular proposal.

This approach is not without its challenges – not least the possiblity of conflict between the service user's right to influence their own destiny and the care team's established view on the degree of risk it feels the service user might realistically be exposed to. Yet these dilemmas have always been there. Risk management is an opportunity to explore them with the service user and others who are involved.

The mechanics of involving the user in organizing their own care, in contributing to service management and service design, is discussed in more detail in Chapter 15 and in many other books and journals. The approaches needed, by definition, tend to be highly individualized and there is insufficient scope, in this chapter, to go into great detail. However, the message is clear. The service user must be afforded a central role in the risk-management process, wherever this is possible. Where user's needs are exceptionally complex, those involved must do whatever they can to be clear to the service user, and their family if they wish, what decisions have been made and on what basis.

Assessing the risk

Identifying a proposed course of action is the beginning of the risk-management process. Establishing potential benefits and harms is the first stage of the risk assessment. Once again, it is important to involve the service user at this point in the process. The benefits and the harms are experienced, or will potentially be experienced, by the service user. Care should be taken not to assume that our values can be effortlessly superimposed on to other people.

The nature of benefits and the nature of harms

Whilst risk management is largely concerned with the impact upon people, the wider aspects of risk should not be ignored. Essentially, there are three focuses for benefits and harms:

- to the service user;
- to the environment (including accommodation, the community, etc.);
- to third parties (including paid and unpaid carers, the general public and other service users).

It is interesting to consider briefly the nature of benefits and harms. In effect, the team working alongside a person with a learning disability is attempting to identify avenues for progress on behalf of the service user. Without care, the person with a learning disability will end up living their life by proxy. Yet it is important not to ignore the nature of the potential benefits and harms. There is possibly a tendency to focus on the possible harms and negatives even when the benefits of a proposal have already been identified. Maybe this is because many of the negatives could have legal repercussions that might reflect on the overall quality of the service. Understandably, carers may also feel that they are, by definition, in a position where they must advocate for the service user as best they can and that their objectives are best realized through a protective model of care rather than one that overtly fosters independence.

The nature of benefits, on the other hand, is apt to sound a little benign; for example, the use of phrases such as 'increased independence' and 'increased interaction'. It is difficult to interpret words such as these into more concrete experiences, whereas 'is assaulted while making a withdrawal' requires little further explanation and can easily be understood by all involved.

Therefore, when identifying potential benefits and harms it is important to be specific in as many areas as possible. There is also a temptation for those working with people with a learning disability to take for granted some of the things to which service users aspire. For example, many people take for granted their ability to get from one place to another without having to rely on someone else and perhaps find it difficult to comprehend what it must be like not to be able to do that. Once these factors are combined, there is a powerful energy against people with a learning disability having the opportunity to develop. This is not a charter for the pursuit of unacceptable risks as this is in no one's interest. However, it is a clarification of the notion of benefits and harms so that those people involved in the decision-making process can work towards achieving the most appropriate outcome for the service user.

Risk variables

The potential benefits and harmful consequences identified during this part of the process may be affected by the following variables:

- internal variables
- external variables.

Internal variables include those things that are implicit to the individual yet should be borne in mind when thinking about the benefits and harmful consequences that might be experienced by the service user. These include:

- mental health status
- skills and abilities
- previous experience
- personality/personal qualities
- physical health.

External variables are factors that should be considered by the team and are those things that will be explicit to the service user but will also have some level of impact upon the possible benefits and harmful consequences experienced by the service user. These might include:

- accommodation
- location
- relationships

- access to support
- attitudes of local people
- financial or other resources
- access to a telephone.

Whilst there is a limited number of internal variables, the potential list of external variables is extensive according to the unique circumstances of the service user and the proposed course of action. It is not necessary to document those variables relevant to the service user as part of the risk-management process. However, it may occasionally be worthwhile focusing on these variables in order to ensure that an effective overall picture has been developed prior to making a decision.

Identifying possible benefits and possible harmful consequences

Those undertaking the assessment should consider what the potential harmful consequences to the service user are, how often the person is likely to experience those harms as well as a view on how severe the impact of that experience will be upon the service user. Equally, there should be a view within the team, which will include the service user, on what benefits will be experienced, the likelihood that the client will experience those benefits (will they be ongoing, frequent or infrequent?) and a view on just how much of a benefit this will be to the service user. These are complex considerations and need careful thought because at the end of this process the service user and the staff team will decide whether, having examined the benefits and the harms, the suggested proposal remains one worthy of pursuit.

It is critical that whilst undertaking this stage of the process that great care is taken in order to document this. This demonstrates that the process is very transparent and accessible to service users. This also clearly identifies for the user and the care team what issues must be taken into account in the decision-making process. Having the potential benefits and harmful consequences clearly articulated will also help to ensure that the subsequent stages of the process are effectively managed.

Once the team has completed this part of the exercise, a decision can be made. On the balance of the potential benefits and harms that have been identified should the service user and the team continue to pursue the proposal? It may be clear that the possible benefits significantly outweigh the possible harmful consequences and that what potential harms there are do not impinge on the health and well-being of the service user. In these circumstances a decision in favour of pursuing the proposal is easily made. However, the picture may not be quite so clear and the team may not agree on whether to pursue the proposed action or not. Should this be so, the risk-management process should be allowed to continue.

Managing the risk

So far, the service user and the team have considered what benefits and what harmful or negative consequences might be experienced should the proposed course of action be implemented. At the end of that part of the process those involved make a decision whether or not it is acceptable to continue. If it is acceptable, then the process is complete. However, there will be many occasions when the proposal is unacceptable because the likelihood and/or the severity of the potential harms are not sufficiently outweighed by the likelihood or the impact of the benefits on the service user. The value of risk has also been highlighted. Therefore, it is important not to immediately abandon the proposal but to revisit the possible benefits and harms and to take action to increase the likelihood and the magnitude

of the benefits whilst decreasing the likelihood and magnitude of the potential negatives or harms.

As an example, consider how this might be achieved with a service user who currently lives in the community who is learning, for the first time, to use a bank card to withdraw money from a cash machine. The potential benefits to the service user might include:

- the service user is not limited to gaining access to money inside bank hours;
- the service user does not always have to rely on staff to access their money;
- there is an increased opportunity for the service user to manage their own finances;
- flexibility in paying for items;
- feelings of increased self-esteem for the service user;
- helps the service user develop further money management skills.

The possible negative or harmful outcomes might include:

- the service user experiences financial difficulties;
- is assaulted whilst using the cash machine out of hours;
- someone else learns the service user's personal number;
- the card is lost.

It is possible to list many more benefits and harms in this scenario. It is important the team takes time to make itself aware of as many of the potential benefits and harms as possible.

The benefits of risk taking

In order to make the risk an acceptable course of action the service user and the care team may wish to do one or both of the following. Take action to:

- increase the impact of the benefits;
- increase the likelihood that the service user will experience the benefit.

In the example a number of benefits were identified. From the list it is not possible to identify how likely the person is to experience the benefit or how great a value the service user would place on those benefits. The agenda is beginning to become clear. First, the team may wish to spend time with the service user in order to be sure that the benefits identified are perceived as such by the service user. More specifically, the team may also wish to work with the service user to ensure that those benefits identified will actually be experienced. In the example, one of the benefits highlighted suggests that the service user will have an opportunity to access money when staff are not around. This may mean an extensive programme of skills development for the service user to ensure they are able to interpret the messages on the screen, making sure the service user is able to cope with problems should they arise, making sure the service user knows the routes to the bank, helping the person to be able to calculate whether sufficient funds are available, and so on.

The care team is therefore working towards developing a written plan that can be carried out with the service user. The plan will aim to specify those actions required by the service user or the care team in order to ensure the identified potential benefits will be experienced. The plan may include:

- the need to develop effective systems or procedures;
- the need for environmental changes;
- change to the local support mechanisms within a service;
- any other reasonable action in agreement with the service user.

Once again it is important to remember that the process is effectively underpinned by good documentation.

Avoiding harmful consequences
Perhaps the nature of benefits and harms explains the desire to focus initially on potential harms. When talking of risk there is an acknowledgement that given the right set of circumstances there is a range of harmful possibilities to be avoided in order to access the benefits. Similar to the experience of benefits there are two ways in which to manage potential harms:

- to reduce the likelihood of a harmful experience/outcomes;
- to reduce the impact of the harmful outcomes.

In the example above, there is a number of actions the service user and the staff team can take in order to achieve successful management of the possible harms. The service user and the staff team may consider having an agreement with the bank whereby the person's cash card will not allow withdrawals to be made if there is not enough money in the account. Alternatively, the service user may put aside a few minutes each week in order to ensure that the 'books balance'. The issue of security will be high on the agenda and there are many imaginative and innovative approaches the service user and care team could adopt in order to ensure the service user is not exploited in any way. They may choose a machine that the service user uses regularly that is in a relatively busy street with good lighting. The service user may receive assertiveness training so that they can request any person who is standing too close to them when they are making a withdrawal to move a step away. There are many possibilities within this framework.

This stage of the process is added into the action plan. This part of the plan will contain specific actions to be taken by the care team and the service user to minimize the possibility of harmful consequences or to minimize the impact of those consequences should they occur.

Once this process has been completed the question still stands. Is the risk worth taking? Prior to the action plan being developed this may have appeared to have been an unacceptable risk. The action plan will demonstrate why the benefits are worth pursuing and how the likelihood and impact of these benefits may be maximized. The action plan will similarly describe what action the service user and the team will take to minimize the likelihood of negative or harmful outcomes or to reduce the impact of these consequences should they occur. If at this point it remains unclear whether or not to proceed it may be necessary to revisit the benefits and harms to see if work could be done to further develop the action plan. Alternatively, it may be necessary to review the initial proposal in favour of a completely new proposal for action.

Developing Risk Management in Services for People with a Learning Disability

This chapter has hopefully demonstrated the advantages of good risk-management procedures in services for people with a learning disability. Figure 15.1 summarizes in diagrammatic form the process of risk management for ease of reference. However, much work is required if effective risk-management procedures are to be implemented across services so that they become an accepted part of regular practice. Service providers may wish to consider the following:

- a programme of education on risk management;
- consultation on how risk management interrelates with other local policy;

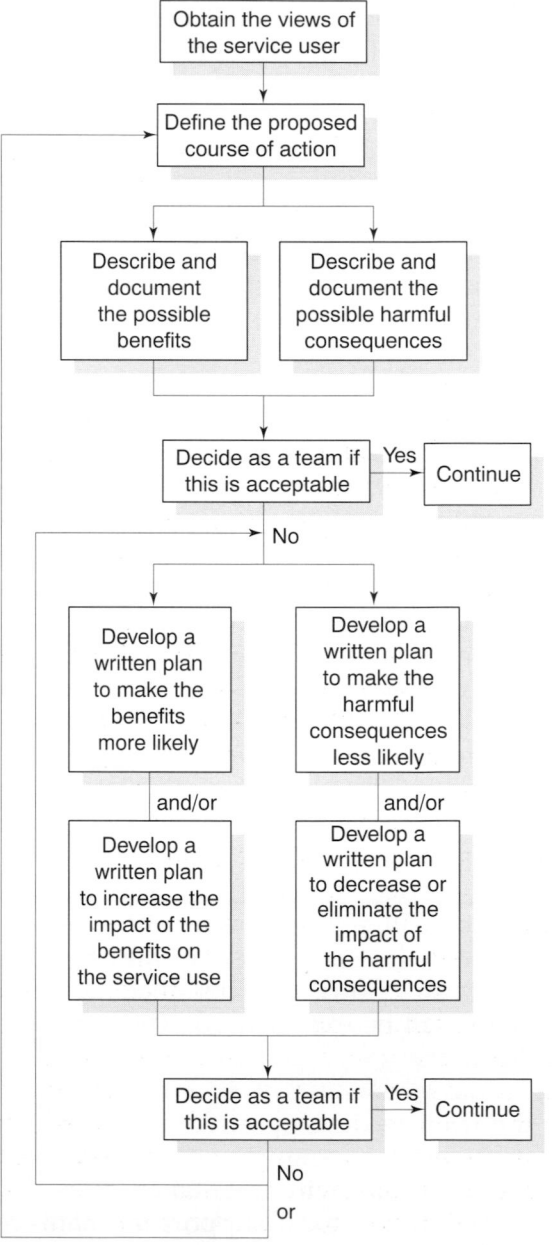

Figure 15.1   Flow chart illustrating the process of risk assessment and risk management

- development of supporting documentation;
- audit of current risk-management practice;
- risk-management awareness for managers;
- obtaining resources that would support effective risk management.

There is often a reluctance to accept new approaches to work. It is important that the opportunity to effectively manage risk for service users is not lost because of hostility to the concept borne out of a lack of real understanding.

Conclusion

Services should be concerned with value. If they are concerned with value then they are concerned with opportunity. If they are concerned with opportunity then they are concerned with risk. For many reasons, service providers are asked to balance the needs and wishes of users with the expectation that this will be achieved with little or no personal cost to those involved. Whether or not this is achievable is open to debate. However, services can do a great deal to ensure that, where there is a risk associated with an activity, careful planning and the involvement of the user will help to ensure that the benefits are experienced whilst the possiblity of harmful outcomes is minimized. Effective risk management will help to achieve this.

Good risk management is not a replacement for good practice. It has to sit alongside tried and tested approaches to managing care. Equally, good risk-management procedures cannot guarantee that legal action will not be taken against a service. However, it can encourage multiprofessional, multi-agency working where the user is explicitly central to the process.

If it is our intention to continue to develop innovative, high-quality services designed to meet the individually assessed needs of people with a learning disability these services have to be delivered against a complex backdrop of diverse pressures and organizational change. Now, more than ever, services and those who work within them could justify a reserved and somewhat protective view on service provision. Yet our philosophies do not fit comfortably with this view. Generally, service users and providers wish to be associated with a supportive culture where the acquisition and accumulation of skills, the making of decisions and the fostering of independence are seen as a high priority. The implementation of good risk-management procedures will significantly contribute to the achievement of this goal.

Discussion Questions

- What is the most efficient way that risk management procedures can be absorbed into the structure of the services you help to provide?
- Where do you feel that there are significantly under-managed risks in your area of work?
- What might you do to change this situation?
- How would you raise the profile of risk management in your area?
- Think about the risks you take in the course of your life. Where is the value in the risks you take? How would these be perceived by others?

References

Carson, D. (1988). Taking risks with patients. *The Professional Nurse*, **April**, 247–250.

Department of Health (1990). *The NHS and Community Care Act*. HMSO, London.

Department of Health (1991). *The Patient's Charter*. HMSO, London.

King's Fund (1980). *An Ordinary Life*. King's Fund, London.

O'Brien, J. (1987). A guide to personal futures planning. In *A Comprehensive Guide to the Activities Catalog* (eds G.T. Bellamy and B. Wilcox), pp. 175–89. McGraw Hill, London.

Roy, S. (1996). Risk management. *Nursing Standard*, **10** (18), 51–54.

Shirtliffe, D. (1995). Risk taking for clients with learning disabilities. *Nursing Times*, **91** (5), 40–42.

Chapter 16

Income and Money

Paul Stafford, Peter Rippon, Giles Blower and Karen Lowater

Key Issues

- Social work and welfare rights
- The importance of money
- Real lives: two case studies
- A guide to benefits: Disability Living Allowance; Invalid Care Allowance; Severe Disablement Allowance; Income Support; Housing Benefit; the Council Tax; the Social Fund loans; Disability Working Allowance; Independent Living Funds; appointees.

Introduction

Money, for better or worse, is central to most of our lives. Without adequate income we cannot participate in activities more widely taken for granted; we cannot deal with very basic domestic problems such as the cooker breaking down, or with more exceptional crises. Inadequate income is at the centre of multiple deprivation. It forces restrictions and exclusions from most aspects of community living.

Social work practitioners and managers have often failed to place policy or organizational emphasis on money issues. There has been considerable debate about the appropriateness and relevance of welfare rights work to professional social work activity (Becker and Macpherson, 1985), and recently by CCETSW (1989). These debates have continued to place distance between what is widely considered as legitimate social work practice, and the pursuit of welfare rights income maximization.

This conflict is the more surprising because almost exclusively those who use social work services are claimants (Becker 1987). Becker and MacPherson's (1986) work shows that 90% of social work clients are claimants of Social Security, and over half are dependent on income support. Only one in ten is in paid employment. More and more people are becoming clients because of financial poverty. This also applies to people with severe learning disabilities. The vast majority of referrals concerning learning disabilities to Social Work

Departments are from claimants of Social Security (Becker and MacPherson, 1986, p. 35).

In this chapter we have modest aims. First, we want to indicate, through two case studies and discussion, the integral and core nature of welfare rights activity in social work practice. As practitioners working with people with severe learning disabilities in a multidisciplinary context, we have no doubts, nor do our clients, that money is central to their lives, their well-being and their futures. Second, we want to provide the reader with a basic 'tool kit' – a guide to the benefits available for people with learning disabilities. We also want to be explicit about our values. We have not rehearsed here the welfare rights/social work debate (readers can refer to this in the texts cited in the references). Our position is that the debate must shift ground, from questioning *whether* welfare rights *should* be part of social work, to *how* welfare rights can best be delivered to vulnerable and poor people.

Real Lives

The range of benefits, their conditions of entitlement and the ever-changing nature of the Social Security system causes much confusion in the minds of professionals, claimants/clients and lay people alike. This is a situation often exploited, for different reasons, by social workers, welfare rights officers and benefits agency staff, who sometimes promote the view that only welfare rights officers have the skill and knowledge to deal with the benefit system and clients' welfare rights needs.

The Dalby family

Our first case example concerns the Dalby family. Mr and Mrs Dalby are a middle-aged couple who live with their 18-year-old son Peter in a two-bedroom council house in a small isolated village. Mr Dalby has spent all his working life employed by a local farmer and Mrs Dalby has been unable to do any paid work since the birth of Peter.

Peter is a person with severe learning disabilities and a physical disability that renders him unable to walk. When Peter was younger his mother welcomed support and counselling from Social Services and the local Health Authority, but after a while she made it quite clear that Peter was her 'problem' and that she would cope with him. Consequently, all professional help was withdrawn. Throughout his school years Peter attended a school which specialized in education for children with severe learning disabilities. The family struggled along financially, never being able to afford even a weekend away from the family home. Peter, although clean and tidy, was always one of the most poorly dressed attenders at his school. When Peter was 16 he left school and started to attend a Social Services day centre. At this stage a 'key worker' was assigned to work with Peter. The key-worker met and talked with Mr and Mrs Dalby and soon became aware that the family were not claiming any Social Security benefits for Peter or themselves.

A referral was made to the County Council Welfare Rights Service requesting a home visit and a full benefit assessment. A welfare rights officer who worked as part of the local multidisciplinary community learning disability team made contact with the family and arranged to visit. During the visit it became clear that Peter qualified for a number of benefits, some from his 16th birthday and one that should have been claimed a lot earlier.

There was also a benefit that Mrs Dalby could possibly claim in her capacity as a carer. Resulting from the home visit, claims for the following benefits were submitted.

Disability Living Allowance (Care Component)

Along with the claim pack a letter from Peter's GP was sent as supportive evidence of Peter's need for care, attention and supervision during the day and throughout the night.

Disability Living Allowance (Mobility Component)

Peter is unable to walk, therefore a claim for the highest rate of the Disability Living Allowance (Mobility Component) would be successful.

Severe Disablement Allowance

Peter is under 20 years old, therefore two medical certificates needed to be obtained from the family's GP. The first a 'Med 5', needed to state that Peter had been unfit for work for 28 weeks prior to his 16th birthday and the second, a 'Med 3', needed to state that Peter would be unfit for work for the foreseeable future.

The welfare rights officer wrote a letter requesting that the Benefits Agency consider backdating any award of benefit to Peter's 16th birthday. In the letter the welfare rights officer argued continuous good cause for the late claim by nature of his severe learning disabilities and therefore fell within the scope of Regulation 19(2) Social Security (Claims and Payments) Regulations.

Income Support

A claim for Income Support was also submitted again with a letter from the welfare rights officer and using the same argument for backdating as was used for Severe Disablement Allowance.

When the claim for Disability Living Allowance (Care Component) was finalized, if Peter was awarded either the middle or the highest rate then his mother will qualify for Invalid Care Allowance.

During the initial home visit the welfare rights officer was able to discover that some 9 years previously Mr Dalby had a period off work due to sickness and had claimed Sickness Benefit with a top up of Supplementary Benefit. When the claim was submitted Mr Dalby informed the local Benefits Agency office about Peter's disability and consequently received the appropriate additional requirements, for example laundry addition (because of Peter's incontinence), bath addition, heating addition and an addition for wear and tear of clothing.

Since the birth of Peter, Mr and Mrs Dalby have struggled along in often desperate financial poverty. When all the claims for benefit were finally processed the family income *increased* by approximately £170.00 *per week*; there was also the possibility of backdated benefit for Peter and his mother in the region of £18 000.

Some months later the welfare rights officer visited the family again and was amazed in the transformation in the family's life. Peter was dressed in modern colourful clothes and his mother 'appeared to be 10 years younger both physically and mentally'. Mr Dalby had used the Disability Living Allowance (Mobility Component) to purchase a new car using the Motability Scheme, which enabled the family to get out and about for visits to the coast, etc. Mrs Dalby had acted upon the advice of the welfare rights officer and renewed contact with Social Services to request social work input.

Resulting from this approach a new social worker was allocated to the family and plans were made for Peter to have periods of short-term care three or four times a year. The social worker and the welfare rights officer worked together in planning Peter's spells of short-term care. This needed careful planning so that Peter's entitlement to Disability Living Allowance (Care and Mobility Components) was not affected. Peter was able to have a total of 28 days short-term care without his entitlement to Disability Living Allowance being affected. Once Peter had accumulated 28 days of short-term care he had to then spend at least 29 days in the family home, otherwise he would have lost his entitlement to Disability Living Allowance for the period of short-term care he was having. When calculating the 28 days it should be remembered that the day he left home and the day he returned both count as days in the family home; for example, as Peter went into a Health Authority establishment on a Monday returning home on the Friday evening, only Tuesday, Wednesday and Thursday count as days in care. This pattern could be repeated for 9 weeks, then Peter would need to spend at least 29 days at home after which the cycle of 28 days care would start again.

When Peter's claim for all the benefits was processed his mother was appointed to act on his behalf. Each time Peter went into any short-term care setting the onus would be on Mrs Dalby to notify the Benefits Agency about the period of short-term care. The family recognized that the breaks that Peter had away from the family home were of great benefit to him and also enabled his mother to 'recharge her batteries'. An occupational therapist also visited the family to make an assessment of Peter's need for aids and adaptations; this resulted in an application being submitted for an extension to be built on to the house. The extension included a downstairs bedroom and a fully equipped bathroom to cater for Peter's personal needs. Once the work was completed it was possible to apply for a Community Care Grant from the Social Fund to cover the cost of decoration/refurbishment of the new bedroom/bathroom.

The intervention of the welfare rights officer profoundly affected the living conditions, stability and opportunities of the Dalby family. The family income was increased by nearly £200 per week and with renewed social work intervention and careful planning the family and Peter were able to have more choice and direct control over their lives.

Brian Yorke

Brian is 37 years old. He has a moderate learning disability and partial physical disability caused by hemiplegia. He originally lived with his elderly mother in the community, but sadly, she died when he was 23 years old.

Unfortunately, Brian was unable to remain in the community. His brother Colin (his only living relative) was at that time away at university and unable to care for him. Brian, therefore, went to live in a local learning disability hospital where he has remained for the past 14 years. Whilst a resident at the hospital, assessments were undertaken with a view to Brian's eventual return to community living.

Colin is now married with two small children and although he lives some 40 miles away from the hospital he tries, whenever possible, to visit his brother at least once a month, for a 2-week holiday every year and for occasional weekends. The number of visits had to be limited because despite Colin's good job and relatively reasonable salary he and his wife found it increasingly difficult to meet the cost of visiting Brian at the hospital and of having him home.

Despite this extra financial burden Colin insisted on maintaining contact and trying to provide Brian with the best possible 'family life' he could.

Brian received only the hospital rate of

Severe Disablement Allowance which was paid on a quarterly schedule by the Benefits Agency to the hospital. Whenever Brian visited home he was given £3 per day by the hospital, out of his account. This amount could, of course, in no way cover all cost of travelling or the extra food to be provided. Brian smokes, enjoys a drink and a game of darts at the local pub.

Additionally, he would want to be able to spend some of his money on his brother Colin. On a number of occasions Colin approached the hospital for increased financial support but each time he was told not to be 'greedy'. If Colin wanted his brother home he was told he should finance the visits.

It was at about this time that the hospital started to have access to the services of the welfare rights officer based with the local multidisciplinary community learning disability team. The first task the welfare rights officer undertook was to determine the level of support that residents and staff need. For the staff this largely took the form of trying to make them aware of the welfare benefit entitlement of the residents through a series of training courses and user-friendly leaflets. During one of the training sessions a staff nurse made the welfare rights officer aware of Brian Yorke's case.

The welfare rights officer was able, through feedback from hospital staff, to pinpoint the main areas of possible take-up of benefits for residents as a whole. These areas included helping residents claim their full entitlement to benefits when away from hospital and staying with relatives; and helping some of the families claim Community Care Grants from the Social Fund to cover the cost of travelling expenses to visit the hospital.

To claim help with travel expenses to visit someone in a hospital, the visitor must be in receipt of Income Support. They may apply for a Community Care Grant from the Social Fund to help cover the cost of travel. These grants are discretionary and applications therefore have no guarantee of success. Brian's brother Colin was employed full-time and not on Income Support.

In Brian's case the main area that the welfare rights officer was able to help with was in claiming his full entitlement to benefits during the time that he was at his brothers. The 'out of area' nature of Colin's address meant that a meeting had to be held at the hospital with Brian and Colin. *The increased benefit entitlement arises because periods spent away from the hospital do not count as in-patient treatment and therefore benefits are payable at the full community rate. It is important to remember that the days of travelling to and from hospital count as days at home.*

The Benefits Agency will only allow one appointee (official representative for benefit purposes) per claimant and as the hospital's administrator was responsible for the claims of Severe Disablement Allowance it is they who were required to submit the claims on Brian's behalf. In Brian's case the application for extra benefit comprised of three separate elements. First, a letter was sent to the local Benefits Agency office covering the hospital area asking for Severe Disablement Allowance to be paid at the full rate. Proof was needed confirming the dates of Brian's home visits. The hospital appointee would therefore pay Brian out of his account the daily rate of one seventh of Severe Disablement Allowance. This would then be recouped into Brian's account at a later date as payments are made retrospectively by the Benefits Agency.

Second, the Welfare Rights office was also able to help Brian claim a top-up of Income Support. This would add an extra £18.45 per week for each week Brian spent at his brothers, paid on a daily basis of one-seventh. The Income Support Claim Form A1 was submitted to the Benefits Agency local office covering the area where Brian lives. This benefit was also paid in arrears to Brian via the hospital.

A third benefit claim for disability living allowance was also made. This claim was processed and payments made by the Disability Living Allowance Unit at Blackpool for the days Brian was away from the hospital.

For Brian the efforts of the welfare rights officer meant that the extra benefit payments removed the financial strain on Colin and his wife and encouraged them to have Brian home more frequently. After a long period of time it was decided by the hospital consultant and nursing staff that Brian was ready to move back into the community. It was suggested that he would be able to live independently in a small house with two other former hospital residents, supported on a daily basis by community care assistants who would provide budgeting and domestic assistance. Throughout Brian's return to community living the welfare rights officer was consulted at each step. Most of the larger household items were provided by the Health Trust, but Brian was badly in need of new clothes, bed linen and personal items of furniture in order to allow him the best possible start.

It was important to check Brian's hospital bank account to see what savings he had as they would affect benefit claims on leaving hospital. At that time he had only £327 in his account so this would not affect his entitlement to Income Support on leaving hospital nor his ability to apply for a Community Care Grant from the Social Fund. An application to the Social Fund was submitted to the local Benefits Agency office 6 weeks prior to him leaving hospital.

On discharge, a claim for Income Support was sent in to the local Benefits Agency office. A letter confirming the date of discharge and new address was also sent to the Disability Living Allowance Unit in Black-pool and a further claim was submitted to the local District Council for Housing Benefit and Council Tax Benefit (to help towards the rent and Council Tax).

On leaving the hospital Brian's weekly income increased from the hospital rate of Severe Disablement Allowance to full-rate Severe Disablement Allowance topped up by Income Support including the Disability and Severe Disability premiums and also an additional amount for Disability Living Allowance Care Component at the middle rate and mobility component at the lower rate, *a total weekly income of £150 per week*.

Once Brian had become fully established in the community it was felt important to ensure he had plenty to occupy his time. Whilst at the hospital Brian had 'worked' at a horticultural unit within the hospital grounds and he had expressed a desire to continue in this work.

The local community learning disability team together with Brian drew up a varied programme of day activities. Brian would spend 2 days a week at a Social Services day centre, one day at the local College of Further Education improving his literacy skills and 2 days community experience in the local Council's Parks and Gardens Department.

Brian naturally hoped to be paid for his efforts but unfortunately this could have a detrimental effect on his benefit entitlement. His social worker and welfare rights officer had a meeting at the local Benefits Agency office to discuss Community Experience placements in general. After negotiations it was accepted in Brian's case that until such time as his job became of a more permanent nature he would be better off working voluntarily so as not to affect his benefits. For Brian, paid employment could result in his Disability Living Allowance being re-assessed if the Benefits Agency believed his care needs had diminished. His Severe Disablement Allowance could also stop if he were deemed capable of work unless therapeutic earnings could be accepted but any payment over £15 per week would be deducted from Income Support. For Brian the voluntary nature of the placement and full support provided by Social Services enabled the Benefits Agency to ignore the benefit implications. The welfare rights officer was also able to advise Brian and his social worker on possible charitable payments and helped them get a greenhouse to allow Brian to develop his gardening hobby on the land at the back of his home. It is hoped that in the future the job may become more permanent and at that time a claim for Disability Working Allowance could be made to top-up his wage.

The ever-changing nature of the benefits system make it essential that regular contact be maintained between Brian and the welfare rights officer in order to update him on any amendments to regulations and check on possible changes in circumstances.

Brian Yorke's case clearly demonstrates the central role that welfare rights can play in improving the financial well-being of a resident in a long-stay hospital, and during the transition to community living. This help also has a beneficial effect on the overall finances of the claimant's family and on improving the community care planning by Social Services, the Health Service and other multidisciplinary staff. For Brian Yorke community care was only possible because his finances and income were sorted out. Social Security provision was used to support rehabilitation, semi-independence and empowerment.

A Guide to Benefits for People with Learning Difficulties

In this section we concentrate on the most important benefits that people with severe

Birth
- Child Benefit
- Health benefits (e.g. prescriptions)
- Parent or carer can claim Family Credit or extra Income Support for dependent child.

3 months
- Disability Living Allowance (Care Component) for baby with an obvious need for attention and supervision due to disability
- Carer can claim Invalid Care Allowance if the disabled child receives either the high or middle rate of Disability Living Allowance (Care Component)
- Carers can claim extra Income Support or receive Housing Benefit and Council Tax Benefit
- Family Fund.

2 years
- Vaccine damage payments.

5 years
- Disability Living Allowance (Mobility Component).
- Mobility passport benefits (e.g. Orange Badge exemption from road tax).

16 years
- A young person can claim Social Security benefits in their own right, for example Severe Disablement Allowance, Income Support and Housing Benefit.

Box 1 The benefits available for people with severe learning disabilities from birth to 16

learning difficulties can claim. Naturally, the descriptions given in this section are brief. We hope that many of the points highlighted will give the reader some 'benefit awareness' and help understanding of the two case studies which appeared earlier in the chapter. The case studies themselves illustrate how many of the benefits interact with each other.

Many of the key benefits mentioned in Box 1 are now examined in turn.

Disability Living Allowance

(Claim form DLA 1)
This is the main disability benefit claimed by people with learning disabilities up to the age of 65 years. It is paid to people with a long-term illness or disability which will last at least 6 months. You must have needed help for a 3-month qualifying period before you start to receive DLA (unless a claim is made because of terminal illness). DLA is not taxable or means tested. It is paid in addition to other benefits and often means an increase to some benefits (e.g. Income Support).

DLA is divided into two parts: the Care Component and the Mobility Component. Both components can be paid independently of each other.

Care Component
The Care Component of DLA is paid to people 'who make a claim before' the age of 65 years who need help with personal care. In order to qualify the claimant must be so severely disabled that they require from another person:

■ attention in connection with their physical care, for example help with dressing, bathing, eating, taking medication; and/or
■ continual supervision in order to avoid substantial danger to themselves or other people. This covers help required by people who are not aware of common dangers or do not understand the implications of their actions.

The Care Component is paid at one of three rates. The claimant will receive the higher rate if they need help during both the day and the night. Entitlement to the middle rate exists when this care is required during either the day or night. The lower rate is applicable to somebody who requires a lesser amount of care, amounting to over an hour a day, or if the claimant is over 16 years, and they require help to prepare and cook a main meal. If the claim is in respect of a child, they must be assessed as requiring substantially more care than other children of the same age and sex.

Mobility Component
The Mobility Component is designed to help people who have either severe mobility problems or require guidance and supervision out of doors. It can be claimed for children from the age of 5 years and by adults up to their 65th birthday. The Mobility Component is paid at one of two rates.

The higher rate is paid to a person who:

■ is unable to walk;
■ is virtually unable to walk;
■ has had both legs amputated at or above the ankle or was born without legs or feet;
■ is both deaf and blind;
■ is severely mentally impaired and has severe behavioural problems and entitled to the highest Care Component.

The lower rate is paid to a person who:

● requires guidance or supervision out of doors or in an unfamiliar location.

It is anticipated that most people with learning disabilities will qualify for the lower rate. Entitlement to the higher rate for people with learning disabilities is often problematic as many people with learning disabilities can walk perfectly well in terms of putting one foot in front of another, but often this ability is frequently interrupted by unpredictable behavioural problems. In this situation, people could qualify by being classed as either 'virtually unable to walk' or 'severely mentally impaired with severe behavioural problems . . .'.

To qualify for the higher rate via all but the last category the person's walking difficulties *must* be caused by a *physical condition*. A learning disability can, of course, be classed as a physical condition. To qualify via the last category the person must have a severe mental impairment and display severe behavioural problems for which they require restraint. The person must also be entitled to the highest rate of the Care Component of Disability Living Allowance.

Extra help with mobility

Road Tax exemption
Recipients of the higher rate of the Mobility Component are sent a form to apply for exemption from Road Tax (Vehicle Excise Duty). Exemption is granted as long as the vehicle is used mainly for the purposes of the disabled person.

Motability
A voluntary organization established to help people with disabilities use the higher rate Mobility Component of Disability Living Allowance to buy or hire a car or suitable vehicle. Electric wheelchairs can also be purchased.

Invalid Care Allowance (ICA) (DSS claim form DS 700)

Invalid Care Allowance is a weekly benefit paid to people of working age who care for someone receiving Disability Living Allowance at either the high or middle rates.

The benefits can be claimed by men and women, married or single. They must meet the following qualifying conditions:

- be caring for the disabled person for at least 35 hours per week;
- aged between 16–65 years for men and women;
- not in full time education;
- living in Great Britain – resident for 28 weeks out of the last 12 months;
- not earning more than £50 per week from employment (after certain allowance deductions, such as the cost of getting to work and child-minding fees).

The age of the disabled person being cared for does not affect the claim – it does not matter whether the disabled person and their carer are related, nor whether they live in the same household.

Invalid Care Allowance is a taxable benefit and will affect the amount of Income Support, Housing Benefit and Council Tax Benefit that the claimant receives. However, it is still beneficial to claim ICA because it qualifies the carer to the Carer's Premium added to their benefit entitlement. The claimant will not be paid ICA if they receive such National Insurance benefits as Jobseekers Allowance and Incapacity Benefit.

Severe Disablement Allowance (SDA)

(Claim form SDA 1)
Severe Disablement Allowance is intended to provide a basic income for people who are unable to work because of a disability, but who have not paid sufficient National Insurance contributions to qualify for Incapacity Benefit. Many 16 year olds who stay on at school for special education can claim Severe Disablement Allowance as a basic income in their own right.

Severe Disablement Allowance can be paid to a person who:

- is aged between 16 and under 65 years;
- is incapable of work and has been for 28 weeks (196 days) (the 28 weeks can precede the claimant's 16th birthday);
- meets certain residence conditions.

To claim SDA the application form should be sent to the claimant's local Benefits Agency office. The form can be completed on behalf of the claimant if they are incapable of managing their own affairs. The parent or carer should ask the Benefits Agency if they can become the claimant's appointee. The claim form should be accompanied by a doctor's certificate (Med 5) confirming the claimant's incapacity for work for the last 28 weeks and confirming the claimant's ongoing incapacity for work.

Since April 1995, incapacity for work for Severe Disablement Allowance is further assessed under the *all work test*. Certain categories of claimants, including people with severe learning disabilities, are exempt from the new test. The test involves the claimant completing a long questionnaire about their physical ability to perform various work related tasks. Many of these questions will be inappropriate to people with learning disabilities. Instead, information about how their learning disability would affect them in the work place should be stated at the end of the form. In practice, most people with learning disabilities should still qualify for SDA.

SDA is treated as income for Income Support and Housing Benefit, but receipt of SDA will mean that the claimant becomes entitled to extra Income Support.

Income Support (claim form A1)

Income Support is a means-tested benefit which can be claimed by people who do not have to be available for work or 'sign on'. It is intended to bring an individual or family's income up to the minimum level which the Government says they need to live on. If the benefit or income which the claimant receives is less than this level, a claim for Income Support will 'top up' these benefits, raising the claimant's income to their Income Support 'applicable amount level'.

Income Support is made up of a basic Personal Allowance – which is awarded in accordance with the claimant's age, partnership status and whether or not they have dependent children. In addition anyone who receives Disability Living Allowance (Care or Mobility Component) or Severe Disablement Allowance will automatically qualify for a Disability Premium. Parents on Income Support who look after a child who gets Disability Living Allowance will qualify for a Disabled Child Premium. Certain people with learning disabilities who live on their own and receive either the middle or high rate of the Disability Living Allowance Care component, may qualify for a Severe Disability Premium.

To qualify for Income Support most people have to be over 18 years, although special conditions exist which mean that most 16–17 year olds with severe learning disabilities can claim Income Support, even if they stay on in full-time specialist education.

As a means-tested benefit the claimant must have less than £8000 in capital. Savings above £3000 will affect the amount of benefit. However, the claimant's entitlement to Disability Living Allowance is not treated as income when the Benefits Agency compare the amount that the claimant needs to the amount of money they have coming in.

Claims for Income Support should be made direct to the local Benefits Agency office. Claimants who are unable to manage their own affairs should get an appointee (normally the main carer or parent) to complete and sign the form on their behalf.

Housing Benefit

People aged 16 years or over who pay rent for where they live, may be able to receive Housing Benefit from their local council to help with these costs.

The amount of help available depends on the claimant's income compared to their needs and level of housing costs. In most cases the amount they need to live on is calculated in the same way as Income Support:

- Claimants on Income Support may receive the maximum amount of Housing Benefit, pending the restriction introduced in January 1996.
- Claimants not on Income Support and whose incomes are higher than their Income Support level receive proportionally less than the maximum Housing Benefit (see above). For every £1 over their Income Support level, their rebate will be reduced by 65p

If they have over £3000 in savings, this may affect the level of rebate they receive. If the claimant has over £16 000, they will not be entitled to Housing Benefit.

The Council Tax

The Council Tax was introduced in April 1993. It is a tax made up of both a property and a personal element. The amount of Council Tax paid can be reduced in a number of ways, some of which have to be claimed, others are given automatically. People with learning disabilities receiving Income Support living by themselves, do not have to pay Council Tax because they will get maximum Council Tax benefit. If they live with carers, certain other discounts may be applicable.

There are three main ways to receive a reduction of the Council Tax.

The Disability Reduction Scheme

The whole bill may be reduced if a person with a substantial disability predominantly uses one room in the accommodation or if there is enough space in the dwelling for that person to use a wheelchair indoors.

The Discount Scheme

The personal element of the tax assumes that there are two or more residents living in the household. Certain adults can be disregarded as a resident, including people with severe learning disabilities and some carers. This disregard can result in a reduction of the personal element of the tax, which is applied regardless of the income of the householder.

Council Tax Benefit

This helps people on low income to pay their Council Tax. A maximum rebate of 100% can be given, dependent on a means-tested assessment of the liable person's income (which is similar to the assessment for Housing Benefit).

Second Adult Rebate

This is an alternative to Council Tax Benefit based on an income assessment of certain second adults in the dwelling. Claims for benefit and discounts need to be made via the local council, not the Benefits Agency.

The Social Fund

There are two parts to the Social Fund. The first part makes payments to people as a statutory right. This part covers such payments as maternity needs, funeral expenses and cold weather payments. It is not cash limited and claimants have the right to an independent appeal if they disagree with the decision.

The second part of the Social Fund is discretionary and is cash limited. This means that the success of the application is dependent upon how urgent the Social Fund officer considers the application to be in relation to others, as well as the amount of money left in the budget.

While some claimants will receive grants, most will only be offered a loan which they will have to repay via deductions from their weekly benefit. There is no right of appeal against decisions to disallow an application, only a right to an internal review.

There are three types of payment in this part of the Social Fund.

Budgeting Loans

These loans are available to people who have been on Income Support for at least 26 weeks. Savings over £500 (£1000 for claimants over 60 years) will be deducted from the loan.

Claimants must be 16 years or over and working for at least 16 hours a week, and have less than £16 000 in capital – savings above £3000 reduce benefit. Claimants must be receiving on the date of claim, or during the 56 days preceding the claim at least one qualifying benefit (e.g. Disability Working Allowance or Severe Disablement Allowance).

Crisis Loans

These loans are intended to help claimants whose need for assistance has arisen due to an emergency or a disaster, and the loan is the only way to avoid a serious risk to their health or safety. It is unlikely that a loan will be given if the claimant has savings.

Community Care Grants

These grants do not have to be repaid. They are awarded in circumstances where a grant will help a person move into the community from residential care, or the grant will help the claimant to remain in the community, or help a family under exceptional stress.

To qualify you must be getting Income Support (or will receive it once you leave institutional care) and any savings over £500 (or £1000 if over 60 years) will reduce the amount of grant.

To claim a Community Care Grant use form SF 300 and send it to the Benefits Agency office that is currently involved in paying the claimant's benefit.

Disability Working Allowance

This is a weekly tax-free Social Security benefit for people with a physical or learning disability, which puts them at a disadvantage in securing employment.

Disability Working Allowance is calculated by comparing a claimant's weekly income with a set figure similar to the Income Support applicable amount. If applicable a 'top up' of Disability Working Allowance is made. Once in payment, the level of benefit remains in payment for 26 weeks. At this stage a repeat claim has to be made.

If the claimant gives up work within 2 years of claiming Disability Working Allowance (providing they are still incapable of work) the claimant can return to their previous entitlement of Severe Disablement Allowance.

Claim forms are obtainable from the local Benefits Agency office.

Independent Living Funds

The original fund was established in 1988 to provide support to severely disabled adults with the cost of domestic assistance or personal care whilst living at home. Following the introduction of the Community Care Act in April 1993, two new funds were set up to replace the Independent Living Fund.

Independent Living (Extension) Fund

This successor body was established to maintain the payments that were previously being made to beneficiaries of the old Independent Living Fund. It can therefore not deal with new claims, although increases in awards can be considered if circumstances change.

Independent Living (1993) Fund

The Independent Living (1993) Fund is a Government financial discretionary trust. It works in partnership with the Local Authority to enable jointly financed packages of care to be arranged so that severely disabled people can maintain an independent life in the community. To qualify for help from the 1993 Fund, applicants must:

- be aged between 16 and 66 years;
- be receiving Disability Living Allowance high rate Care Component;
- have an income around the Income Support level;
- be receiving services to a value of at least £200 per week from the Local Authority;
- have care needs whose total cost to the 1993 Fund and Local Authority is no more than £500 a week.

To make an application, contact your local Social Services Department.

Appointees

Claimants who are unable to manage their own affairs, due to their disability, can have someone else to deal with their finances. Such a person will become the claimant's appointee, and they will sign all the claimant's forms and cash their benefit for them. An appointee takes on all the responsibilities of the claimant. It becomes their duty to disclose any changes in the claimant's circumstances. If the appointee fails to notify the Benefits Agency of any changes, they will take action against the appointee and not the claimant.

The Benefits Agency will interview the person wishing to act as an appointee. The purpose of this will be to decide whether the claimant is unable to deal with their own affairs and whether the person applying to become the appointee is a suitable and trustworthy person.

Appointeeships when going into care

If the person who is unable to manage their own affairs goes into some form of care the appointee can choose to give up their appointeeship in favour of the owner of the home or the Local Authority.

The arrangement for the Local Authority is very similar to the conventional appointeeship, all of the person's benefits are cashed by Local Authority who have the responsiblity to notify the Benefits Agency of any changes in the person's circumstances.

Conclusions

Professionals working with people with learning disabilities and their carers are only too aware of the essential role Social Security benefits play in providing clients with a financial lifeline. Few people with learning disabilities are in paid employment. Most learning disabled and mentally ill people living in the community are dependent on state benefits for all or part of their weekly income. The average household with a learning disabled adult receives about one-third of its income from benefits.

With the policy of closing down old institutions and the gradual move to community care, it is inevitable that more and more people with learning disabilities will rely on support from the Social Security system. The reality of community care for the majority of people with learning disabilities is the care provided by their families at home. Welfare benefits advice is central to the 'maximization of income'. Many vulnerable people who fail to claim their rightful entitlements are forced to live in dire financial poverty. Welfare rights advice and advocacy are central in a strategy of empowerment. It is inevitable that there will be increased pressure on social workers to deal with Social Security issues as a result of legislation changes, including the Children Act, the Disabled Persons Act and the NHS and Community Care Act. Welfare rights work needs to be fully integrated into the services provided to people with learning disabilities. Multi-disciplinary approaches have benefited from the presence of welfare rights officers. In Nottinghamshire, for example, the community learning disability teams each contain a welfare rights officer. Their work is largely proactive, seeking out 'need' and maximizing income, as part of a considered and multifaceted process of case assessment and care planning.

There are many issues, however, that need further discussion amongst managers and practitioners. It is clear that money is central to all our lives, not just for people with learning disabilities. For most people, if the weekly or monthly pay cheque fails to materialize, or the travelling expenses are delayed, instability is the result. This may be at a personal or family level; whatever the results, choices and opportunities are constrained and, in some instances, crises follow. This is the same for people with learning disabilities. Inadequate incomes restrict opportunities for participation – they compound the disadvantages already experienced.

There are a number of key, and yet unresolved issues, namely:

■ What level of welfare rights knowledge and expertise is expected of social workers and other care staff, including case managers, who provide casework and development services for people with learning disabilities?

■ What level and kind of specialist welfare rights support is expected – caseworker, development worker, trainer, facilitator, consultant, etc?

■ As part of the assessment and case management process, who will maximize the incomes of people with learning disabilities and their carers? What skills, knowledge and training will be needed?

The future opportunities of many people with learning disabilities rely on the answers to these questions.

We believe that welfare rights is an essential core activity for social workers and other groups. We are realistic in our expectations of what 'non-specialists' may achieve, but it is our view, borne out by experience of multidisciplinary work, that the skills and knowledge of welfare rights officers are central to effective social work intervention. The case studies demystify the subject by looking at two case studies. One is a client living with his family while the other is a long-stay hospital resident moving into the community. The case studies demonstrate the successful, rewarding and core nature of welfare rights work. Maximizing the incomes of people with a learning disability and their carers, and helping them to make the most of opportunities and life changes, is an essential part of their assessment and case management process. It is central to the notion of empowerment and client self-determination.

Discussion Questions

■ What efforts are made in your professional area to ensure that service users are receiving their correct entitlement to Social Security benefits?

- Is there potential for collaboration between agencies to ensure that benefits maximization is achieved?
- Consider what the impact would be on the community care planning process of welfare rights involvement with service users.
- Now check the benefits of someone you are working with to see if they are receiving their correct entitlement.

References

Becker, S. (1987). *Responding to Poverty, The Policies of Cash and Care*. Longman, London.

Becker, S. and Macpherson, S. (1985). Scroungerphobia – where do we stand? *Social Work Today*. Also, cash council – the art of the possible. *Social Work Today*. See also Finister, G. (1986). *Welfare Rights Work In Social Services*. Macmillan, London.

Becker, S. and Macpherson, S. (1986). *Poor Clients Benefits Research Unit*, Nottingham. See also Becker, S. and Macpherson, S. (eds). (1988). *Public Issues, Private Pain: Poverty, Social Work and Social Policy*. Insight Books, London.

CCETSW (1989). *Welfare Rights Education in Social Work*. Report of a Curriculum Development Group. CCETSW, London.

Chapter 17

A Lifetime of Caring

Joan Vagg

Key Issues

Experience of parents and families in relation to:

- Community care policies
- Life-stage changes
- Professional activity

Learning disabilities are for life! If modern trends concerning the life expectancy of people with learning disabilities continue, it could indeed be a very long life!

Professionals, along with their ideas, fads, whims and fashions, hand-in-hand with a baffling array of insider jargon, come . . . and go, leaving in the wake of their well-intentioned bursts of enthusiasm, the parents and families of people with learning disabilities. It is with parents and families that the ultimate responsibility for the provision of that essential day-to-day, night-by-night, unwavering care often rests. They cope year after year, with varying degrees of frustration, disappointment, despair, anger – but also with love and, in many cases, laughter.

'Care in the community', that most recent, much-heralded and already well-worn and over-used expression, describes, for the majority, nothing new. It has always been with us. Most people with learning disabilities have always been and will continue to be, cared for by parents and families in the community, from the cradle to the grave.

Parents, especially those who are older and who have already given a large proportion of their own lifetime to caring, will smile ruefully and say 'care in the community? That means with Mum and Dad'. One parent said recently 'When I was younger I used to say "I hope you're not going to expect me to be looking after her when I'm 60!" I'm now 62 and I still have her at home'. Learning disability is indeed for life, for everyone concerned.

For some families the professionals have a vital part to play in offering support and advice but how many can realistically offer that long-term commitment so necessary for a long-term problem.

Most families do not have a social worker on a regular basis – some do not want one. However, every now and then some change in the local Social Services office or the appointment of a new 'team leader' will result in a sudden urge to visit all families with a learning disabled member. In fact, there might be three or four visits within a short period of time. There is a sudden concern about how carers are managing and whether they have considered what lies ahead. Questions like, 'What do you see as the future for your son/daughter?' are likely to be met with answers bordering on cynicism or even sarcasm.

In this modern age of financial cutbacks and dwindling resources, questions such as these, which are often asked irrespective of facilities actually available, can only receive hypothetical answers accompanied by a wistful look or weary sigh. Of course, parents have thought about the future, but to dwell on what is, in reality, a future depressingly empty of the ideals for which parents yearn on behalf of their learning disabled offspring, is a futile exercise.

Parents are, not surprisingly, irritated when, after years of looking after their sons or daughters to the best of their ability and with very little help, they receive a somewhat patronizing metaphoric pat on the head for having done a good job; or, conversely, a metaphoric rap on the knuckles for apparently having done it all wrong.

It can only be insensitivity and ignorance which prompts professionals to utter such throw-away remarks as, 'It's hard to think of her as an adult when she wears such unfashionable shoes'. A statement such as this simply hasn't given any thoughts to the efforts of the parent who has combed the shops looking for shoes that actually fit, never mind look fashionable. How infuriating for the parent of a typically overweight learning disabled woman, after years of experimenting to find clothing that is practical and appropriate, comfortable and hygienic, to be told by a visiting social worker that surely her daughter, as an adult, should be wearing tights and not

socks. The implication is always that the carers are deficient in their judgements. Would not an overall assessment of the situation, based on a thorough and informed understanding of *all* the circumstances be more supportive?

Of course there is a place for challenging the practices of ageing parents who are becoming out of touch with what is appropriate in a modern setting for their learning disabled sons and daughters, but it takes time to build up the kind of relationships with families which eventually allow for the giving of advice, even criticism. Time and consistent support are two necessary elements which are usually in short supply. It is not surprising, therefore, that the advent of a new social worker is viewed by parents with an understandable degree of scepticism. 'Social workers come and go all the time. They call – put in their two penn'orth – and then they are gone', said one father recently.

All the qualifications and theories in the world cannot equip people to face life in all its realities. A true understanding of learning disability begins with an experience of the disability itself. Most of us will be thankful that we will never personally encompass this as part of 'life's rich tapestry'. The next best thing must be to live alongside someone with a learning disability for 20, 30 or 40 years from birth through to old age; sharing their life in its minutest detail; facing their problems with them, sometimes for them, sometimes because of them.

Many professionals have little idea of learning disabilities, except that which they have managed to glean from books or videos and maybe the occasional brief placement – a 'hands on' experience.

What is learning disability? The experts seem to find it difficult to agree on an adequate definition. It is after all a term which covers such a wide range of ability from the profoundly mentally and physically handicapped, who rely on others to meet their every need, to those who are able to lead independent lives. We all have a place along the continuum formed by the full range of intelligence and there is no sharp distinction which separates the person who is normal from the person who has a learning disability.

We have come a long way from the days of 'idiots, imbeciles, and moral defectives' but we still seem to have difficulty, even in the 1990s, in fully understanding and adequately meeting the needs of those who, in the modern vernacular, experience learning difficulties. The fact of the matter is that whatever the fashionable jargon of the day nothing will ever alleviate the effect to the family of having a learning disabled child. The birth of a baby with a disability completely changes the way of life for parents – nothing is ever the same again. There is not one period when life is normal.

Parents vary in their ability to cope but everything they do in future will be governed by the fact that they have a handicapped child who will (as things are at present) almost certainly be living at home long past their own childhood and their parents' retirement, at a time when other siblings will have left home and be living independent lives.

To begin with, there is the grief, devastation, despair and sometimes rejection that overwhelms people when they discover that their longed for baby is handicapped. For the rest of life there is grief for the child who might have been; the child who would have grown up normally, left school, got a job, brought their boy-friends home, got married, had children, etc. On a personal level I often wonder how different our family life would have been had two of our four daughters not been learning disabled. We would not necessarily have been happier because we have worked hard to make the best of the situation, but certainly

we would have had more freedom. In recent years, particularly, we have had to contend with the constraints imposed by always having to be there.

Forty years ago when my eldest daughter was born, things were very different in terms of public awareness, medical diagnosis and prognosis, attitudes, Local Authority services, provision for education, etc. – all of these were to undergo immense upheaval and innovation over the next 40 years. Forty years is a long time in one person's lifetime. My daughter has changed very little in that time – her needs certainly haven't diminished and she is as dependent now as she was at 6 years old. Times may have changed; public awareness may have been heightened; expectations greater; attitudes of professionals much improved; education a right, and yet there still remains a dearth of services available to support parents stuggling to cope with dependent learning disabled adults still living at home.

So, how can those professionals whose objective it is to provide an appropriate effective service for the learning disabled and their carers, fully understand the problems encountered by their clients? The realistic answer is that probably they can't. What they can do, however, is to tread carefully and with sensitivity, assume nothing, approach each situation with an open mind uncluttered by preconceived, ill-informed ideas, show interest without being patronizing, offer a listening ear without feeling under pressure to offer advice, show support without being judgemental, be realistic about the application of modern theories and parents' response to them, help where help is possible, and stop short of making empty promises.

Parents of a learning disabled child will probably experience feelings of guilt; parents may feel that it is their fault – that they are in some way responsible for their child's disability. Other members of the family – brothers, sisters, grandparents, other relatives – may find it difficult to accept that the child is different. If there is acceptance by relatives, then parents may have to contend with opposing advice as to what should be done with the child. There is greater public awareness of learning disability nowadays but this does not prepare people for the possibility that their own child might be disabled, or make it easier to explain to the neighbours. Other siblings may begin to exhibit behaviour problems – their peers at school have the capacity to be very cruel, particularly on the subject of learning disability. This will doubly burden the parents of a new baby who has arrived with a puzzling array of its own problems. As time goes on parents will find that this child *is a child* and needs the same care, love and encouragement as any other child.

In the first years the professional most likely to be encountered is the health visitor but there may be many others – paediatricians, GPs, Portage workers, specialist teachers for the under 5s, perhaps speech therapists and physiotherapists – who will be around to give help and advice. Sometimes there may be many callers, sometimes very few. Sometimes a child will be able to attend a playgroup, sometimes this is not possible or appropriate. Parents need to be given optimistic but realistic ideas of what the future is likely to hold for the child and of what facilities are available. They also need very practical advice regarding the various benefits which can be claimed by parents of children with disabilities. Guidance may be needed regarding the filling in of forms.

Being put in touch with other parents in the same situation can sometimes help. Often a local society or other voluntary support group can help but parents do not always want this in the first few weeks or months. The kind of support that the family needs is moral support, whole family support, social support and information support.

Once the child starts school, whether a 'special' school or in the form of integration into an 'ordinary' school there may be (but not necessarily) more help, support and advice available. At least the child nowadays attends a school run by the Local Education Authority and not, as was the case 20 years ago in a centre run by the Health Authority. At least the child born in the 1990s is not in danger of being classified 'unfit for education', as was the case with my own two daughters.

But the child who attends a special school presents to its parents a whole host of problems not experienced by others in normal circumstances. The school will probably be some way away from where the family lives and certainly not within walking distance. This necessitates a school bus calling twice daily to transport the child to and from school. Some families find this public drawing of attention to their specific problems every day very difficult to cope with.

The daily contact with other parents at the school gate is denied to parents of children who travel by school bus. The useful incidental contact between parents and other parents and parents and teachers when the child is collected in person from the classroom does not occur when a child is transported to and from school by others. If a problem or anxiety arises then a specific effort must be made to go to the school; an appointment must be made to speak to the teacher. Informality and spontaneity are lost. Many parents feel that their concerns do not warrant this formal action – they do not visit the school and their 'molehills' become the proverbial 'mountains'; minor issues become major tragedies. Ultimately other professionals may be called in to mediate, analyse, advise, or offer support.

Some schools in London used to have

attached social workers who were able to build up a good three-way relationship between social worker, school and family. Unfortunately, this service has largely disappeared.

It must never be forgotten that families do not actually *want* to have a member with a learning disability. Every parent hopes that their child will be perfect in every way; given that sometimes a child is born less than perfect, many parents learn to suppress or come to terms with their disappointment. They will make the best of a difficult situation by endeavouring to ensure that their child reaches the very best of its potential. The situation is born out of necessity and not of choice. There is great danger nowadays, when there is so much emphasis on the positive aspects of learning disability, of overlooking the fact that many people with learning disabilities still need a great deal of love, care, tolerance, patience and sometimes skilful handling. The media will often emphasize what the learning disabled *can* do, and rightly so, but let us also remember that there is an enormous amount that learning disabled people can't do for themselves. It usually falls to their families to do it for them.

Problems do not end or even diminish when the child with a learning disability becomes an adult – he/she simply becomes an adult with a learning disability. Indeed for many parents and families this is probably the worst time, when further problems present themselves. It may also be the time when most disagreements with professionals occur.

With the changes in thinking on the way adults with a learning disability are cared for – with more emphasis on 'normalization', 'independent living', 'community placements', 'sexuality' and 'sexual fulfillment' – the more objective opinions of the professionals differ widely from those of parents,

which are naturally of a more subjective nature.

Although most parents welcome the gradual disappearance of the old subnormality hospitals and even of local hostels, in favour of smaller houses and homes (with a small 'h'), not so many embrace the more extreme ideas that are prolific in current thinking. Most carers will regret the apparent loss of the 'care' element in the more modern trends.

Many of us, having looked after our sons and daugters for 20, 30, 40, or even 50 years, feel that we know them pretty well – we know what they are capable of and what their needs are. Parents are accused by professionals of being restrictive, over-protective and not letting them 'make their own decisions' (a phrase which is like a red rag to a bull to many). There is some truth in these accusations of course. Parents are often restrictive and protective – experience has proved it necessary.

My 39-year-old daughter, who has the additional disadvantage of poor eyesight, will fall over the kerb, bump into lampposts or trip over uneven paving slabs unless she takes my arm when walking in the street. To the observer I am being protective; in my opinion I am attempting to protect her from the indignity of falling over in public and from possible injury. A professional who accompanied my daughter on a shopping expedition, determined to allow her freedom of movement and measure of independence free from the usual restrictions, complained of the embarrassment caused by my daughter constantly bumping into people and objects. To me the remedy is simple – hold her arm. Protective but practical (for all concerned)!

Parents often find it difficult to allow their sons and daughters to make their own decisions. This is not always due to overprotection but often the result of years of experience of having to make judgements on behalf of someone else. One of my daughters is very fond of food. There are times when I decide, against her own opinion, that she has had enough to eat. One of my daughters is very fond of watching television. Her wealth of knowledge obtained through this medium is rich and varied. She would sit in her bedroom all day every day glued to the television, left to her own devices. Against her will, there are times when I persuade her to do something else – to interrelate with other members of the family, to join us for a meal, to accompany friends on an outing. To the casual observer this might well seem unreasonable, constituting the loss of free will and the right to make her own decisions. I beg to differ!

To be realistic, it must be admitted that at times parents have been surprised to find that the dependent adult for whom they have cared for so long, is capable of more than they gave them credit for. Conversely, some professionals have been surprised to discover that some adults with a mental handicap are able to do less than they assumed at first glance.

An issue that often proves to be a bone of contention is that of independent travelling. Parents are often urged to give their consent to 'travel training'. Of course there are many people with a learning disability who can and do travel on their own. Their lives must have been enriched by their ability to do so. Many, however, are very vulnerable, they are often very trusting of everyone in spite of warnings to the contrary. There is no certainty that they will know what to do in an emergency. Of course parents are protective. If my 30-year-old daughter is functioning at the level of a 6-year-old, I am as protective of her as if she were 6 years old. The fact that she is in reality a 30-year-old adult is relevant only in that it provides a guide as to what she would be capable of if she were 'normal'. She isn't!

The majority of the parents I know believe that their offspring need 24-hour support and supervison – even the most able. At best, even if they are able to cope satisfactorily with all the ordinary tasks of everyday living, they can be isolated and lonely. Much of their time will be spent alone in bedsits, flats, etc. At worst, they can live in really deplorable conditions, dirty and uncared for and badly fed. Those defending this standard of living on behalf of the people concerned claim that this is how they have chosen to live! Undernourished, and in squalor but all in the cause of independence!

When voices of parents are raised in concern regarding the issue of loneliness, we are told that we all have to get used to being alone. That when we first leave home we all have had to learn to manage money, learn to cook, learn to care for ourselves and make our own decisions. After all, we learn from our mistakes. That's where the comparison ends, however. People with a learning disability often do not have the capacity to learn from their mistakes and are often further hampered by a lack of basic skills in other areas, for example by an inability to read complicated instruction manuals (e.g. on how to work a washing machine) or read a recipe in a cookery book. Of course, we want to encourage people to live independent lives but let's be realistic by acknowledging that independence without a high level of support or supervision is, at best, impractical, and at worst, disastrous.

People with a learning disability living alone can be very isolated. They may not have the language, the social skills, the confidence, even the motivation to talk to their neighbours or to initiate an active social life. Perhaps they have no money to spend. Modern thinking demands that such people must not be grouped into 'ghettos'; instead they must live in isolation amongst those with whom they share no interests – all in the cause of independent living.

Parents worry when they see the unkempt state that some learning disabled people are living in. One mother said 'You struggle for years to dress them nicely, to bring them up to be socially acceptable – then you're told it doesn't matter'. Are professionals really surprised when parents wish to acknowledge the rights of their learning disabled dependants to be acceptable socially by ensuring that they are clean and appropriately dressed? My view is that my daughters are disadvantaged enough by factors beyond anyone's control, without adding to their problems by failing those issues that are more easily approached and dealt with. Professionals must not blame parents for wanting the best for their children.

Some social workers and support workers place great importance on what a learning disabled person says. They insist upon seeking opinions regardless of the relevance of the answer or of the ability of the person being interviewed to express him or herself adequately. A learning disabled young man who spent the weekend in a training flat was asked by his enthusiastic but misguided support worker what he got out of the experience. The question thereby displayed openly a complete lack of understanding of this particular young man's level of functioning in both receptive and expressive langauge. Even if he had understood the question, he did not have the necessary language to answer it. No doubt there was a vital evaluation sheet that had to be completed, come what may! Professionals must not be surprised when parents express doubts regarding views apparently expressed by their dependants. We all know how easy it is to determine the answer by carefully phrasing the question.

The issue of sexual relationships is yet another stormy subject about which parents and families often hold views differing from the professionals. Older parents, brought up in a different age and different social climate, see as an alien concept the idea of their learning disabled son or daughter developing a sexual awareness which leads to a sexual relationship and possibly a desire to get married. One of the greatest fears (sometimes perfectly justified) is that these ideas have not been spontaneous but are the result of suggestion initiated by others. Well-meaning and idealistic professionals are quick to defend the 'rights' of the learning disabled to have a sexual relationship; to get married; to have a family. Professionals must not be surprised when parents are quick to defend the rights of their adult children, who do not fully understand the implications inherent in a marriage relationship, to remain single, or the rights of the child who may be born to inadequate parents who may ultimately lose their parental role when the child is taken into care.

Parents know that their adult offspring, often still battling with the egocentric features common to childhood, will be unable to make the sacrifices necessary in bringing up a child. Professionals who ignore the views of parents in the initial stages, often turn to those parents when things go wrong. These are the grandparents – of course they are concerned – but they don't want to be landed with bringing up an unwanted child. I know of several instances where this situation has ended in great distress – the child (in some cases more than one) has been taken into care and the learning disabled parents left in total despair and denied access. Often the professionals who have given their blessing to these ideas have long since gone and are spared the experience of witnessing the results of their handiwork. The professionals, usually young themselves, are the strongest advocates of these 'rights' for the learning disabled and have the least patience and tolerance when things go wrong. From the best possible motives I am sure, there is often far too much emphasis on 'rights'; and too little on 'care'. I maintain that the learning disabled have a 'right' to the necessary care and protection needed to lead as good a quality of life as possible.

Another fashionable concept of the modern age is that of 'advocacy'. No-one would deny the need for someone to speak up for learning disabled people who are not equipped to do so themselves. One must be aware of the very real danger of putting words into people's mouths – a warning for parents and professionals alike. How does an advocate realistically speak on behalf of someone so profoundly physically and learning disabled that it is impossible to know what he or she is thinking. Those able to indicate preferences regarding everyday matters – for example whether or not he would like a drink – may not be able to communicate their wishes concerning those bigger issues of relationships or future plans, for example. Even those who are in possession of language skills adequate to express themselves vocally are often vulnerable and easily swayed by the strongly expressed views of others. It is a very brave person who assumes the role of advocate; an awesome responsibility. Don't be surprised when parents are sceptical.

And so we come to the last great worry of families – 'What will happen when we can no longer look after him/her?'. This is a cause of constant and considerable anguish to parents. After a lifetime of living with a person with a learning disability, with all its worries, problems, sorrow, restrictions, and also with compensations, this question could be the most difficult families have had to face. My own feeling is that the worst is yet to come – having to part with my daughters.

The problem is complicated by the fact that in most parts of the country, there is nothing available that parents would be happy with. Parents know in their hearts that the most sensible thing, and really what they want most, is to get their offspring settled happily somewhere while they (the parents) are still around to visit, to keep an eye on things, and have their sons or daughters home for weekends, holidays, etc. However, because of the shortage of all kinds of residential care, it is very rare for this option to be available. Far more often, residential care is offered only when a crisis situation is reached and then there is no choice.

It must be said though that parents have very ambivalent feelings about this. While they would like to see their sons and daughters settled and know this is best, it is a terrible wrench to let this adult 'child', for whom you have cared for so long, go and live somewhere else. This is made more difficult by the fact that the learning disabled people often do not want to go either. Some are content to go and live somewhere else, but most of them want to stay at home with Mum and/or Dad, or possibly live with siblings. The majority of parents do not even ask for respite care because their offspring get very upset at the idea. Professionals sometimes seem to think that the world is full of parents refusing to let their learning disabled adult sons and daughters go and live their own lives, keeping them at home against their will. In most cases the people I know do not have their sons and daughters clamouring to leave home.

It must be admitted, however, that it is often very difficult for parents to make the decision, especially if there is only one parent left. They often rely very much on the learning disabled adult for companionship (limited though that may be) and a justification for their own lives. Sometimes, if the disabled person is fairly able, they are of real help in the home and an elderly parent would find life very difficult without them.

We are, therefore, faced with an impossible situation – on the one hand we want to see our 'children' settled and happy and to know that our other childen will not have to take on the burden. On the other, there is the very real sense of loss that will be felt by the parents and, maybe, by their offspring. I do ask social workers and other professionals to make allowances for and try to understand the very real heartache felt by parents/carers when they have to face up to taking the decision to let their 'children' go.

As I said before, at the time of writing this the question is academic because there is such limited residential accommodation on offer – maybe one day that will change, and we will really have a choice!

Conditions, facilities and attitudes have improved enormously over the last few years. This has been brought about almost entirely by pressure and campaigning from parents – the parents who ignored the advice given 'to put him/her away and forget about them'; but who kept them at home.

What started as a group of parents of backward children in the 1950s has now become the Royal Society for Mentally Handicapped Children and Adults (Royal Mencap), with its affiliated 300 local Mencap Societies. They have campaigned ceaselessly over the years to get the needs of learning disabled people and their families recognized and provided for. Inclusion in the education system was one of their biggest successes. On a local level people have battled with Local Authorities and Health Authorities to get improved services and a recognition of need. In many areas they have had considerable success in getting representation on consultation groups, Social Services groups, joint planning groups, etc. Nor can they relax their efforts. In the present climate they all have to keep up continual pressure just to keep the services they have – never mind increasing

them. It is not uncommon to find that services for which people have fought so hard and so long, and which they thought were safe, have suddenly been cut. It should, however, never be forgotten that parents and families have always been behind every step forward.

Also, these voluntary groups have played, and still do, a valuable part in offering support, advice and information to families. In the early days this was almost the only support available, and many friendships were formed and still continue among parents – particularly older parents who were in at the beginning of the move to get people with learning disabilities recognized and acknowledged as needing services. Help is still given between parents – if you want your learning disabled child or adult looked after for an evening, or in an emergency you will ask another parent, not very often the neighbours or relations.

There is a great deal of talk about integration into the community but very little evidence of it in practice. Learning disabled people live in the community but are not often part of it, and this is where so much difficulty lies when it comes to independent living. The general public may be sympathetic but do not often want to become involved.

And so to conclude this chapter, let me emphasize that professionals working with learning disabled people and their carers are those who bear an awesome responsibility. They deal with a very vulnerable sector of society – both the carers who experience a wide variety of emotional stresses and practical worries, and the learning disabled themselves who deserve to live as fulfilled and satisfying lives as those who possess all their faculties in full working order!

Many of the professionals working within this sphere, and with whom I have had contact, do an excellent job. Many families and their learning disabled dependants have been tremendously supported by those who, through training and experience, are equipped to do just that. My wish, through this chapter, has been simpy to set out some of the doubts, fears and worries of many parents and families, to alert professionals to some of the difficulties that may be encountered in contact with those in a similar situation to myself and to share some of the insights gathered through 40 years of living and working alongside the learning disabled themselves.

was pressure from parents that finally got children with learning difficulties included in the education system.

It is also absolutely essential to maintain Day Services if parents/carers are to continue looking after people with learning disabilities at home. It is the only way we can cope.

Box 1 Advances in community care since 1991

Since I wrote this chapter in 1991 things have got very little better – we are faced constantly with threats to services. Recently, we were faced locally with drastic cuts to our Day Services. We managed to get these partly re-instated but not to the level we had before. Now again, we are faced with a 'chipping away' of the services.

I feel I must mention 'Community Care'. Of course living in smaller homes and units must be better than living in large institutions but there are enormous implications in terms of resources. Day Services are now catering for a very much wider range of ability and need than they used to and the necessary provision in terms of staff, resources and suitable buildings is not being made. There is a new breed of parents coming along whose childen have benefited from the great improvements in education and they are expecting this to be continued in Day Services. Often it is not happening; people with profound and multiple learning disabilities, challenging behaviour and sensory disabilities are not being adequately catered for and the fight by parents and carers for better services has to go on. Maybe one day it will be mandatory for proper Day Services to be provided for adults, as education now is for children. It

Discussion Questions

- *'Parents vary in the ability to cope'* – what might support parents and carers as they look after and support someone with a learning disability at any or all of the following times:
  a) in the early years
  b) in the school years
  c) in making the transition to adulthood
  d) in middle ages
  e) in older ages
- What skills and knowledge do you have/could you acquire to support your practice?
- There have been many changes and improvements in provision for people with learning disabilities, and in public awareness, over the last few years. However, one thing that has not changed is the devastation and grief felt by parents when told that their child has a learning disability.
  How would you help parents to overcome this and to think positively about the future?

- Many parents initially find it difficult to accept the idea that their child may need to go to a special school.
  Do you think special schools are necessary? What are the benefits for the child of going to a special school compared with the benefits/difficulties of integration into mainstream schools?
- The majority of parents find it very difficult to let their son/daughter leave home, especially if this means going into some kind of residential care, either when the time is appropriate or when the parents can no longer cope.
  Do you understand and sympathize with these feelings? How would you try to work with other professionals to make this easier?

Chapter 18

It Doesn't Happen Here!

James Churchill

Key Issues

- Sexual abuse *does* happen – the evidence
- People with learning disabilities are often victims and/or perpetrators of abuse
- There are complex legal issues involved
- Any appropriate response to abuse requires a policy framework within and co-operation between agencies
- The consequences of abuse are far reaching and can be personally and professionally very damaging
- Perpetrators with learning disabilities still need care, support and treatment
- Abuse poses special challenges to the many professionals involved.

Introduction

This is a difficult and frequently distressing topic. For many years sexually abusive acts done by and/or to people with learning disabilities were either tolerated in long-stay institutions or ignored elsewhere. 'It doesn't happen here' would, until recently, have been a very common response to any casual inquiry about sexual abuse of or by people with learning disabilities. Such a response is no longer possible and any learning disability professional must be prepared to acknowledge that it *does* happen and to be able to respond appropriately on discovering it.

'Responding appropriately' involves a wide range of actions from detecting and sensitively handling a victim trying to disclose abuse, through to contributing to an interagency case conference advising a risk manager on a strategy for a known service user abuser. Implicit in all the above is the existence of a coherent framework of policy and practice on abuse which covers all the agencies involved and supports both victims and (where required) abusers. Running through all the actions and options here is the constant presence of the law. If ineptly applied it can interfere with legitimate and fulfilling personal relationships of people with learning disabilities. It does, however, have an important role in affirming to all concerned the illegality and unacceptability of abuse, even if the sanctions it offers may be of limited use to some offenders. The law in this area is not easy to apply, may be seen as 'inconvenient' by some more liberal spirits, but it is the law and must be upheld by professionals.[1]

A key responsibility of the learning disability professional is to promote 'informed vigilance' on the abuse issue, aiming at reducing the likelihood of abuse going undetected and improving the response when it is detected or suspected. There are implications for effective interagency working at a local level as well as for commissioning, purchasing and inspection staff. No-one is left untouched by instances of abuse. Friends, family, other service users and staff are all variously affected and will require support from competent professionals who understand the whole picture and can explain, as far as possible, what is going on.

Sexual abuse of and by adults with learning disabilities is *par excellence* a litmus test of the competence of the learning disability professional. It demands:

- a professional approach, the putting aside of any personal opinions based on what may be firmly held views on sexual or legal issues;
- an understanding of the role and contribution of other agencies;
- a willingness to make interprofessional collaboration work under often very difficult circumstances;
- the need for a long-term commitment to upholding the rights and best interests of service users – even when they have clearly committed abusive and illegal acts and could well re-offend if given the opportunity.

Definitions and incidence of abuse

First, before all else, let us be clear that sexual abuse of adults with learning disabilities *does* happen and that no self-respecting professional in learning disabilities can or should ignore it.

Definitions are important, not least because in matters of sexual behaviour one person's preference may constitute abuse to another. Only a common definition can form the bedrock of any subsequent policy and practice. It can also underpin a coherent understanding by a staff group of what is and what is not seen as acceptable sexual behaviour within an agency or workplace.

Brown and Turk[2] offer the following definition of sexually abusive acts:

When one person exposes his or her genitals or looks at or touches certain parts of another's body (breast, buttocks, thighs, mouth, genital or anal areas) for the purpose of gratifying or satisfying the needs of the first person . . . sexual offence may also include exposing one's genital area to another person and/or compelling that person to look at or touch the above mentioned parts of the first person's body, when a barrier to consent is present for the second person.

As in other areas any one particular act is not, in itself, *always* abusive and every individual instance needs careful consideration of all the circumstances. For example, a vaginal examination by a male doctor of a patient during treatment is not abusive, but a similar examination of a young girl by a male bus driver would be.

In addition to considering the context of the act there is the issue of ability of the victim to give meaningful consent to the act. The law considers that some people (e.g. girls under 13 years) are never capable of giving meaningful consent at all to sexual intercourse and, consequently, any such act must always be illegal. When the 'victim' has mild learning disabilities the law accepts that she (or he) may be able to give meaningful consent to sexual intercourse (though it still prohibits certain relationships). Even so, the normal laws on sexual relationships apply and sexual intercourse without consent is rape. In any one sexual relationship between two service users, making a judgement about whether or not it is abusive or exploitative is particularly difficult and requires great skill, sensitivity, knowledge of those involved and the willingness to involve appropriate others if need be.

Recent research[3] suggests that there are in the region of 1400 new cases of sexual abuse of adults with learning disabilities every year. This means that, on average, in every Local Authority or Health Authority area in the country there is *at least* one new abuse case per month. The research[4] revealed some unpalatable facts about who the abusers and victims were, which scotched the persistent myths of 'stranger danger' as the main source of abuse. It also showed that high levels of disability were no protection against abusers.

Adults with learning disabilities were at most risk of being abused by:

- other service users (42%)
- members of their family (18%)
- other known adults (17%)
- staff/volunteers (14%)

Only 5% of alleged perpetrators were not known to their victim and the perpetrators were overwhelmingly male (97%). The victims were usually female (but a large number of male victims were noted)[5] aged mostly between 21–30 years old and in 60% of cases with a severe/profound learning disability, often with communication problems. Abuse normally occurred in:

- staffed homes (36%)
- at home with the family (31%)
- in hostels (15%)
- unstaffed accommodation (9%)
- hospital (7%)

In summary, abuse is most likely to happen to the most vulnerable clients in an area supervised by staff or family by a male almost certainly known to the victim. Such shocking statistics should give every learning disability professional pause for thought. It is just not possible to assume that abuse is not happening in your service and *no-one is beyond suspicion*. (In 1996 one Director of Social Services was jailed for indecently assaulting a young male.)

It follows that close attention must be paid by staff to all the relationships a client has and especially those where sexual activity is known or suspected. Additionally, the circumstances under which intimate bodily care is provided must be carefully controlled, particularly when service users are not able to communicate and would be vulnerable to abuse in extended one-to-one contact. The implications for staffing levels, care routines and the gender balance of shifts are considerable. The implications for the way staff behave, observe, reflect and report on what they (think they) see are even more far-reaching.

The law

Space does not permit a full examination of the complex legal issues relating to the sexual activities of people with learning disabilities.[6] However, every competent learning disability professional needs to know the basic legal issues and where to find out about the wider picture.

People with learning disabilities are subject to and protected by the same laws that govern the rest of society. So, for example, a father having sexual intercourse with his learning disabled daughter is committing incest (even if she 'consents'). In addition there are a number of other laws which are intended to provide more protection for learning disabled adults, particularly women. Section 8 of the 1956 Sexual Offences Act makes it unlawful for any man to have sexual intercourse with a woman who is a 'defective'[7] – which has been defined as someone with 'a state of arrested or incomplete development of the mind which includes severe impairment of intelligence and social functioning'.[8] There is a possible defence in which the man can argue that he did not know that the woman was severely mentally impaired or had no reason to suspect she was.

Additionally, Section 128 of the 1959 Mental Health Act makes it an offence for sexual intercourse to occur between staff and patients (either in- or out-patients). The definition of a 'patient' here is wide enough to cover many people with learning disabilities living in the community, in nursing or residential homes. It is also an offence to 'procure' (i.e. to arrange for her to have sexual intercourse with a man) a woman who is a 'defective' in any part of the world.[9] There are a number of other specific laws protecting people with learning disabilities against abusive behaviour by those who are supposed to be caring for them.[10]

Finally, there is the law relating to indecent assault, which covers acts of a sexual nature which fall short of sexual intercourse. This is an important area of the law because staff may well become involved in more (or less!) well-intentioned efforts to facilitate the wishes of their clients in having a sexual relationship or experience. Any such action in this area is fraught with potential legal pitfalls for staff, who could be charged with indecent assault. Actions such as assisting a client who has difficulties with his/her sexuality (e.g. by teaching him/her to masturbate) should

only be undertaken under strict supervision and after careful consideration by a multi-disciplinary team. Such actions may be legal under such carefully controlled and recorded circumstances, but 'freelance' initiatives by lone members of staff are certainly not!

Consent

Central to all issues relating to sexual relationships is the issue of consent. Where consent is lacking then serious problems arise. Sexual intercourse without consent is rape and other actions may well constitute indecent assault. Yet staff are often called upon to make complex judgements about the sexual or physical content of relationships of their clients. When one (or both) of the partners is learning disabled this requires that all learning disability specialists understand how to consider the issues involved and who else may usefully need to be consulted.

Remember that learning disabled adults may well pick up on the general workplace culture and reflect back to staff the standards and behaviour that they observe in staff relationships. In this context all staff need to understand that they themselves are powerful people in relation to service users. Their behaviour, dress, demeanour and language sends powerful messages to clients. It should be clearly understood by all that not only are all sexual relationships between staff and users illegal, but also that sexual teasing and sexual harassment at the workplace is not allowed.

This should be clearly stated in the agency's Code of Practice on sexuality and sexual abuse. Actively supporting the implementation of this Code (whether as manager, deputy or team member) is the clear duty of all learning disability professionals, even though it may take time to change the 'culture' of a workplace.

There are many barriers to consent which need to be considered.[11] Not the least of these is an evaluation of the relative power of the two partners in a relationship. It requires sensitive and sustained intervention to prevent one service user abusing another, without damaging the independence of either party. This means not only evaluating and monitoring relationships between service users, but also fostering the kind of atmosphere within a service that respects individual autonomy and the right to say 'no'.

Also, amongst staff, service users and families there has to be an understanding that any disclosure of abuse or expression of concern *will* be properly investigated, the outcome properly recorded and that well-intentioned allegations subsequently found to be untrue will not be held against the discloser. In other words, there is an organizational culture of openness and a willingness to be vigilant in the battle against abuse in all its forms.

This will not happen by accident and requires active promotion amongst staff, families and other local agencies with whom a service works. In particular, it requires explanation and regular reinforcement to all service users. Learning disability specialists should be able to contribute to and reinforce the service user's ability to understand what constitutes acceptable sexual behaviour, the need to respect the wishes of others and their own rights.

Agency policy

All staff work within the twin frameworks of the law of the land and the operational policies laid down by their employer. It will be clear by now that the issues of sexual abuse cannot be dealt with in isolation from the wider questions of sexuality and sexual relationships which confront anyone working with people with learning disabilities. Reference has already been made to an agency's Code of Practice which should cover both these areas. Such a Code needs to be endorsed at the highest level within the agency and be actively implemented, with appropriate explanations and reinforcement to all staff and clients. It should make clear what behaviour constitutes abuse and what should happen when abuse is reported/alleged. All staff and clients should be clear about who they can go to, both inside and outside the agency, to report their concerns and there should be clear links to the police and Local Authority responsible for investigating and monitoring allegations of abuse.

If such a Code does not yet exist or is only in draft unadopted form, then it is the clear duty of any learning disability professional to press for one to be introduced. This is not only good professional practice but it also makes sound operational sense. Any lack of clarity over policy, roles and responsibilities can contribute to abuse going undetected or being seriously mishandled when reported. It can also increase the chances of a successful legal action for negligence against the agency or a staff member.

There is also a pressing practical need for such a Code because everyone (staff, clients and their families) needs to know where the boundaries of acceptable behaviour lie. Staff, in particular, may regularly face situations where they must exercise judgement about behaviours they observe. Do they intervene? Do they report it – if so, to whom? Will they be supported and listened to?

The Code is needed not only to prevent abuse occurring, it is also needed to avoid the opposite danger – that of an oppressive 'policing' of behaviour of clients which denies them the legitimate expression of their own sexuality. In all such matters consistency of approach is vital if there is to be any hope of empowering clients to assert their own individuality and rights within the law. There is no room here for staff to impose on others their own personal views. A refusal to comply with agency policy should (ultimately) be a sackable offence.

Consequences of Abuse

There are often profound consequences for anyone involved in abuse cases. The focus of attention is usually rightly on supporting the victim (sometimes termed the 'survivor') and 'dealing with' the alleged abuser. This is frequently easier said than done, since in many situations no quick resolution is possible, and, in circumstances of doubt about the allegations, they can be traumatic for many beyond the victim and alleged abuser.

Supporting the victim

Immediate appropriate action upon disclosure should come from any staff member who should act in accordance with the agency's Code of Practice. This will vary with circumstances but, as a priority, the victim will need immediate support and to be kept safe.[12] When the disclosure does not involve any immediate re-occurrence (e.g. where the abuse happened many years ago in childhood by someone now dead) a different procedure can be followed as Figures 18.1 and 18.2 demonstrate.

Figures 18.1 and 18.2 were written with managers in mind, but they contain all the principles which should inform all the actions of staff. Equally important is the fact that 'who does what' is clear to all. There can be no doubt about the following key questions:

- Who calls the police and under what circumstances might this change from (say) the manager to a member of staff?

- Who may speak to the victim?
- Who may speak to the (alleged) abuser?
- Who informs the Registration Authority?
- Who informs the owner/director/Trustees?
- Who speaks to the family?
- Who speaks to other service users?
- Who speaks to the media?
- Who needs to know what?

The Code of Practice should provide answers to these questions. Any evidence should be kept and the scene of crime (if appropriate) preserved. The possibility of forensic evidence should also be considered. It is not the role of the staff or manager to start an investigation of the incident; leave that to the police or the Local Authority/ agency investigating officer.

After the inital rush of interviews by police and the investigating officer,[13] there will need to be a decision about how and where to keep the victim safe beyond the initial (say) 72 hours. It is important to remember that, when all other things are equal, it is the abuser not the victim who should move or change service. The victim may well suffer from fear and/or self-loathing and does not need the additional 'punishment' of being made to move away whilst the abuser stays. Victims will need to be allocated a specialist support worker to support them through the post-abuse period to recovery. This period can be lengthy, especially if a court case is involved, and any long-term treatment may need to be delayed until any hearing is over.

The support worker will need to be alert for signs of delayed reactions emerging some time after the event. This role may well fall to the learning disability professional who will need to work with a range of other professionals providing treatment and support to the victim. Either way, the secret to success in this role lies not in

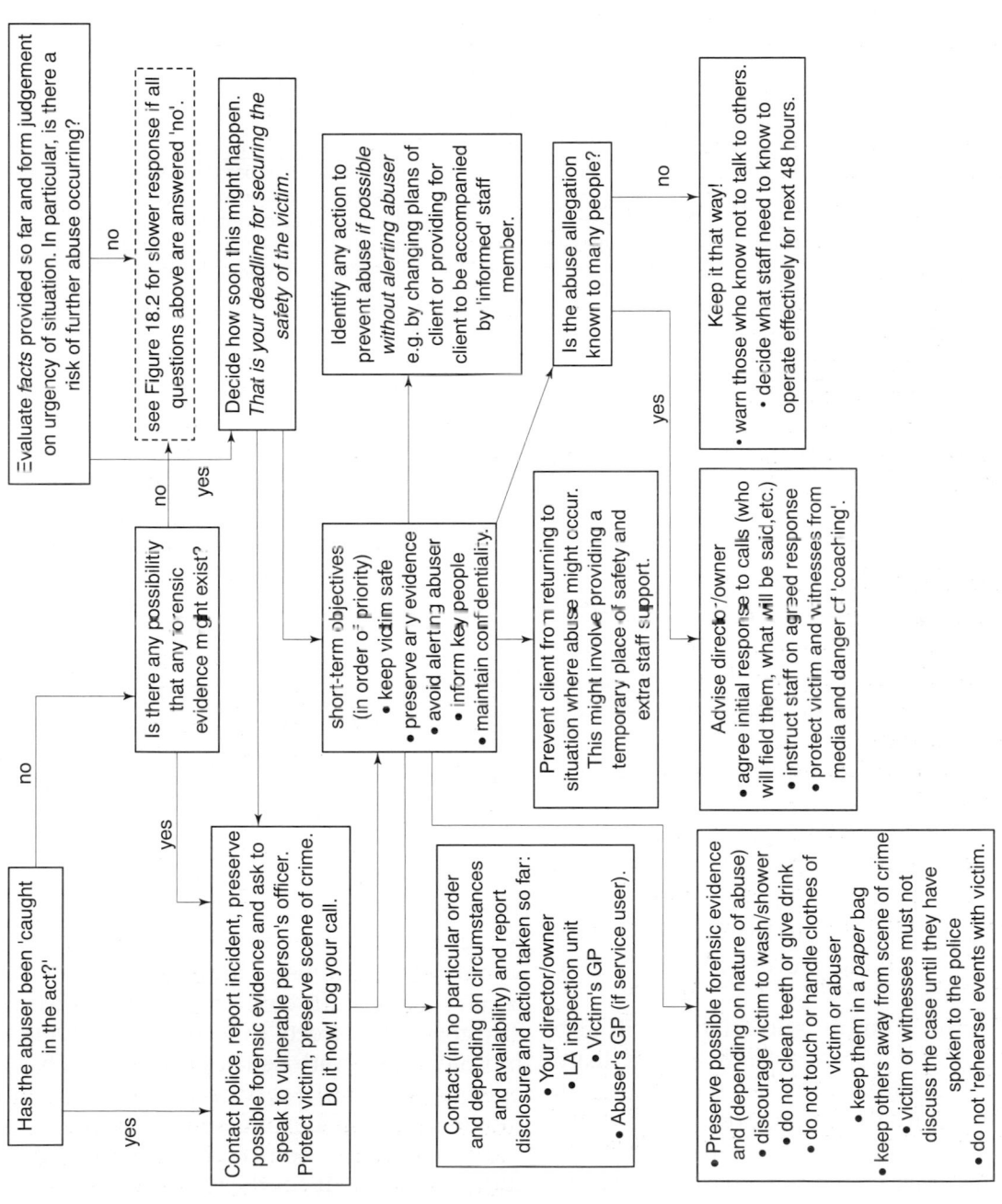

Figure 18.1 Quick response. All this may need to happen within half a day – or less! LA, local authority

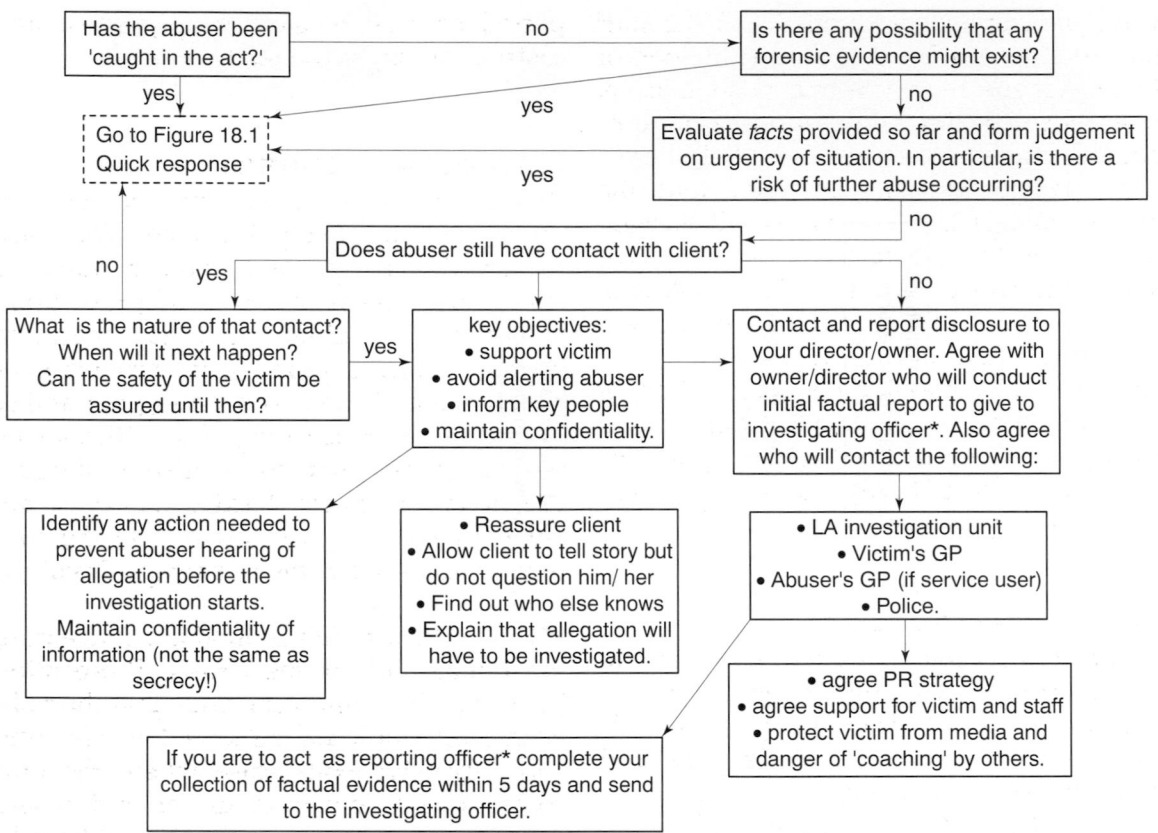

Figure 18.2 Slower response. LA, local authority. *For a fuller explanation of the terms Reporting Officer and Investigating Officer see Churchill et al., 1996

attempting the impossible task of under-standing every aspect of the various technical interventions possible, but rather in seeing the whole picture, knowing where to turn to for help and, with others involved, contributing to the multidisciplinary decision-making process concerning the victim's future.

The victim's family and friends will also need help and support from a staff team who understand what is happening in terms of the investigation, possible prosecution and future planning for the victim. In situations where the agency is held responsible in some way by the family, this is difficult to achieve. Particular difficulties arise in maintaining good relations and

communication when the alleged abuser is a staff or family member.

Supporting the staff

In a contested case involving a staff member as an alleged abuser the effects upon the service and staff team can be disastrous. The corrosive effects in terms of confidence, mutual trust and self-respect of such an episode on staff, service users and their families cannot be overstated. Apart from the inevitable self-recrimination ('Why didn't I spot it earlier?') and pressures arising from the investigation, withdrawals from the service or home may threaten its viability and lead to closure, with all the consequent upheaval entailed. All the staff may feel tainted by the alleged actions of their colleague and some may wish to leave. External counselling and support from outside the immediate service may help here.

It is important to remember that the alleged abuser is innocent until proven guilty, even though he or she should have been automatically suspended following the allegation. They should seek help from their union and/or a lawyer and are entitled to a dispassionate examination of the allegations made against them. Malicious or unfounded allegations of this nature are not unknown and can fatally damage someone's career.

Others need support

The need to continue the service in safety to others during an investigation is paramount and all learning disability professionals need to work with their colleagues and those in other agencies to reduce the adverse effects of an abuse episode.

Support will be needed and *realistic* reassurances given to others (e.g. say 'we will do our best to see it never happens again', don't say 'It will never happen again!' because it cannot be guaranteed). Indeed, past experience suggests that multiple abuse by an abuser is quite common, so uncovering one victim might well lead to others coming forward or other abuse being noticed when people stop to look and think about patterns of behaviour, etc.

Under such circumstances the management of the home or other service will be severely tested. Workplace practices, records and procedures will all need to be scrutinized as well as the actual 'event' itself in order to see how such a thing might in future be avoided and how others might learn from the mistakes made here. In short, both for care staff and management, an abuse disclosure may lead to a prolonged period of high tension, deep distress and distrust amongst the staff team.

Uncertain outcomes

Worst of all, the outcome may be very unsatisfactory for many involved. The track record of the legal profession in pursuing such abuse cases to a successful prosecution is not good – although it has begun to improve of late. Many legal professionals have outdated ideas concerning the ability of people with learning disabilities to be reliable witnesses in court. Also, in the nature of these crimes, hard evidence is not always available, with often only the conflicting accounts of the two people involved to choose from.

When the accused is another service user, the police and/or the Crown Prosecution Service (CPS)[14] often conclude that the public interest would not be served by a lengthy and expensive court case where the outcome is very much in doubt and where the accused, even if found guilty, will probably stay where they now are because there is nowhere else for them to go and prison is not appropriate.[15]

Equally difficult is where the accused (either a service user or staff member) is taken to court and found *not* guilty. A number of issues arise which need consideration:

- Can they have their place (or job) back in the same unit?
- Does this mean that their 'victim' must see them every day?
- Does the accused, the victim and everyone else really understand that a 'not guilty' verdict does *not* mean that the court disbelieved the victim, nor that it was certain that the accused didn't really do it, but only that the court had concluded that there was no proof *beyond reasonable doubt* that they did do it?

- If the accused is a service user who has been found not guilty, do they now think that their behaviour was acceptable and has been 'condoned' by the court so they can repeat it?
- How will they be treated in future by other staff and clients? Can/should they be left alone with others again? Is this really sustainable over a long period of time?
- If there is no proof *beyond reasonable doubt* (e.g. say 80–20%) of their guilt, but the evidence might well *on the balance of probabilities* (e.g. 51–49%) suggest that he did do it, will there be a civil (as opposed to a criminal) prosecution on behalf of the victim? What will this mean for those involved and the service as a whole?
- What needs to be done to put it all back together again for the users, the staff and the service as a whole and to learn from the experience?

Service Users as Abusers

There are particular difficulties for the learning disability professional if the alleged abuser is another service user. Reference has already been made above to the legal issues which can constrain the circumstances under which certain female service users may legally have sexual intercourse. The position of staff monitoring the behaviour of service users in their care and, in particular, of any intimate relationships which may occur, is not an easy one.

Even assuming that they have the support of a clear agency Code of Practice on sexuality and personal relationships, there is always the need to make difficult day-to-day judgements about when a relationship is (becoming) abusive as opposed to being 'merely' exploitative and what interventions (if any) should be made and by whom. Clare and Carson[16] suggest the fol-

lowing issues need to be considered in deciding whether an act or relationship is abusive or not:

- the views of both parties, but particularly those of the person who appears to be the victim, about the sexual and emotional aspects of the relationship;
- whether, and the degree to which, the acts seem to be rewarding to both partners;
- whether other sexual assaults, particularly if of a similar kind, have been committed by one partner (whether proved in a court or not) in the past;
- if similar acts are being repeated, then whether the seriousness or frequency of the assaults is escalating;
- whether the acts are dangerous (i.e. whether they are causing fear, whether they have or could cause physical or emotional harm);
- the extent to which the partners understand the nature and likely effects of their acts;
- the extent to which the partners have control over their behaviour, and can stop it if need be;
- Whether the acts involve threats, coercion or exploitation, for example whether they involve one taking advantge of superior strength, power, ability, or offering inducements which are very difficult for the other person to refuse;
- the implications, directly and indirectly, explicitly and symbolically, of not treating the acts as abuse;
- the possibility that inappropriate stereotyping may be taking place, for example jumping to conclusions about the size, gender or ethnic origin of one party or being influenced inappropriately by someone's past history or reputation.

Where there is any doubt, it is wiser to treat an act as possibly abusive so that further consideration may be given to it.

This is particularly so when there is a continuing relationship between two people with learning disabilities. Under such circumstances care staff often may not consider the potential of one partner to abuse the other.

Remember also that many exploitative relationships, though frequently unpleasant and frustrating to observe in others, are not illegal and there are many instances where people (with or without learning disabilities!) appear to choose to perpetuate an apparently unequal and exploitative relationship. Any interventions by staff should always be carefully considered at a senior level, with outside help if need be, appropriately reinforced by other staff and, crucially, the reasons for any such action recorded.

In such emotionally charged circumstances it is all the more important for staff (who may well have strong personal views about the propriety of such relationships between clients) to be guided by the Code of Practice, to keep in step with other colleagues in handling such matters and to have standard procedures to raise matters of concern which they may have noticed. As has been said before, individual 'freelance' action by staff is potentially damaging and should be avoided. Consistency of approach and treatment is essential for any hope of progress to be achieved.

Assessment and Treatment

Equally important is that agencies should not assume that they have all the necessary expertise in-house to resolve such complex and difficult issues. It should be standard practice for managers to recognize that they may need to access a wide range of specialist assistance in coming to a decision as to whether or not abuse is occurring. Such a decision (as with many others in this difficult area) should never be left to one person alone, but may involve not only those who know the client(s) concerned well from everyday workplace contact but also specialists from outside the agency/workplace who can bring their own expertise and detachment to such deliberations.

Following an alleged incident of abuse involving a service user as a potential abuser, it may be that the police or the CPS decide for any one of a number of reasons not to proceed further with an investigation or prosecution in this case. Learning disability professionals need to understand the overall process here and to appreciate that such a decision does not mean that a crime has not been committed, and also that pursuing a solution to the case by using the criminal justice system is not a risk-free option as Table 18.1[17] shows.

All this should not mean that the incident will not have been properly investigated by the police and there will need to be an additional investigation by the relevant investigating officer of the Local Authority or the agency.[18] This investigation should be conducted in tandem with any police investigation and may need to be continued after any police decision to withdraw and take no further action. It is important both for victim and alleged perpetrator that the allegation is properly investigated and the outcome fully recorded. To do less than this is to add injustice upon injustice (at least for victim or alleged abuser) and to store up additional trouble for the future.

One or two staff will need to be allocated to act as 'supporters' to the alleged service user abuser. This is a difficult task and may well fall to a qualified learning disability specialist on a staff team. It is important that the supporters do not attempt to give legal advice to the alleged abuser, nor that they allow themselves to be seen by the client (or others) as believing or disbelieving the alleged abuser's version of events. This

Table 18.1 Pros and cons of using the Criminal Justice System (CJS)

Advantages of a prosecution	Disadvantages of a prosecution
A clear and final decision will eventually be made	Even if there is a prosecution, the case may never get to court. It may be diverted back to the health care service or no action taken
Involvement of disinterested, official, high status, 'objective' bodies	It all takes time . . . The delay may be stressful and get in the way of assessment and treatment
The suspect is respected as an adult responsible for his or her own actions	Prosecution involves blaming the suspect, rather than the services he or she was, or was not, provided with. The service may be let off the hook
The facts of what happened will be thoroughly tested	Evidence has to be in an 'acceptable' form for the court; otherwise allegations can remain unresolved
Prosecution demonstrates that the service takes abuse seriously	A 'not guilty' result does not prove the perpetrator's innocence or absence of problem
Prosecution indicates the victim is believed	A 'not guilty' result may lead the suspected perpetrator to be reluctant to work with services in future
Suspect's interests can (and should) be protected by a competent lawyer	The victim and other witnesses with learning disabilities could have a very difficult time in court
Decisions are made outside services	Expensive – the resources used in the further involvement of the CJS route might be better spent in providing services
Perpetrator receives clear message about the abusive behaviour	Courts do little to help perpetrators learn about what constitutes appropriate and inappropriate behaviour
Involves recognizing that the victim *was* a victim, not just unfortunate	A 'not guilty' verdict is liable to lead to the victim thinking that he or she was not believed

is a difficult but important role requiring professional detachment and understanding from all concerned.

Additionally, these supporters will be key contacts and sources of information and support for the specialist assessment staff who will need to be brought in to conduct a full assessment of the alleged abuser.[19] These should cover health *and* social care needs as well as his understanding of the abusive nature of his actions. A risk manager will need to be appointed and will convene a case conference to review past actions, the present situation, and future options for the abuser. In all outcomes (bar, perhaps, imprisonment) the learning disability professional is likely to be actively involved in some aspect of care, support and/or treatment of the abusive service user.

Important Role of Care Staff

The provision of continuing care and support to a known service user perpetrator is not without its problems. Learning disability specialists can expect to be asked to supply a lead to others in adopting a positive professional approach to a (probably) highly unpopular and unappealing character whose potential for further abusive behaviour may lead to unfair 'demonizing' of them by others. The staff have an important role to play in leading them towards a normal lifestyle and in demonstrating appropriate behaviour within relationships. Equally important is that the cultural background and the sexual orientation of the perpetrator is respected and not denigrated.

There will also need to be a continuing and constructive exchange between the staff team and any of the specialists providing treatment to the perpetrator. In particular, staff will need to be alert to any signs that a new abusive episode may be imminent and what they must do if this seems possible. Of equal importance is the understanding and monitoring of the perpetrator's compliance with the treatment from such specialists, together with any reporting back on this. Implicit in all this is an understanding by all the staff of the practical, specific requirements of this individual's care plan. These conditions or restrictions may appear very strict (e.g. not to be allowed out alone, not to be left unsupervised with a particular (or even any) client, not be allowed access to alcohol, etc.) but they are doubtless essential to the continued successful placement of that client in a setting which would otherwise be too risky for him to stay in. Behind all this is the constant need to maintain continual vigilance and a full care record on the individual, which may prove invaluable for future care planning or if he or she does (try to) abuse again.

In all this there is ample scope for the learning disability specialist to develop further a number of areas of particular expertise, with the necessary preparation. These could include, for example:

- the delivery of sex education training programmes (these may need to be defined by a specialist) in a manner appropriate to a client's level of understanding;
- observation and assessment of the nature of a relationship between two clients;
- support and monitoring of specialist treatment programmes, with appropriate feedback to the specialist concerned;
- acting as a 'supporter' to an alleged abuser or victim (but not to both!);
- taking the lead in developing an in-house programme of staff training on sexuality, personal relationships and abuse;

- articulating legitimate staff concerns about policy or practice deficits on these matters in a workplace.

Implications for the Future Learning Disability Professional

It can be seen from the above that the learning disability professional cannot afford to ignore the issue of sexual abuse. Perhaps more than any one other single instance in this book, this issue challenges the professional on every front.

- There is a personal challenge which a possible disclosure or suspicion makes on an individual. It is infinitely easier to stifle a nagging doubt over a relationship or ambiguous incident rather than respond in the full knowledge of the future heartache which any action may cause.
- There is a professional challenge in that an allegation of a repugnant act against a vulnerable victim requires a degree of stability and detachment in supporting the victim (or perhaps also the accused) without revealing any personal distaste for what happened, or corrupting the evidence by rehearsing the victim's story.
- Any investigation will require collaboration with a host of other professionals, under difficult circumstances, in pursuit of the best possible outcome. This will not be easy and will require an understanding of the contribution each of those involved may be able to make. Other agencies may, of course, have different priorities and concerns, whilst having the same overall objective of seeing justice is done.
- There is a need to take the long-term view and eschew the mistaken immedi-

ate pursuit of a so-called 'guilty' party. He or she may well return to your team or care having been found not guilty. Any service user has the right to expect a competent professional approach from their care staff and, even if found guilty, they still need care, support and treatment from a professional team.

■ In any abuse incident there is a need to maintain confidentiality of information. This will require discipline from those 'in the know' and understanding from those others who are only told what they need to know in order to operate effectively in their role.

■ The learning disability professional must take an active part in fostering an appropriate workplace ethos on this issue. This may mean having the courage to challenge longstanding attitudes to sexuality or inappropriate workplace practices which undermine attempts at 'openness' on this issue. Such action may well provoke hostility (especially if there is the likelihood of past abuse being uncovered) at all levels, including a complacent (or frightened) senior management.

Abuse issues underline the need for clear policies and procedures for professionals to follow, whatever their own personal views on an (alleged) event. If these are not present, or are not adhered to, abuse will not be detected or reported and will not be handled properly even when it is discovered. The result will be a lottery for all concerned, with many more miscarriages of justice to be heaped upon the victims ill-served by many professions, but most notably by those closest to them who should, above all, know better.

The true learning disability professional cannot afford to retreat in the face of so many likely service and procedural difficulties. Things are changing in this area of practice, more abusers will be successfully prosecuted, the lawyers and police will become more attuned to the needs of disabled victims, courts will adjust their procedures. The question remains as to whether or not the staff involved will pass the litmus test of competence. The learning disability professional has a great deal to offer in this area, both to clients and to colleagues. It isn't easy, but, for the true professional it isn't optional either. Remember that the figures show that in all too many places it *does* happen here, if only people would notice!

Discussion Questions

■ Do you have a clear understanding of what behaviour constitutes sexual abuse?

■ Do you know what you would do if you discovered abuse was happening?

■ Do you know what you would do if you had vague suspicions that abuse was happening but no proof?

■ Does your agency have a policy or Code of Practice which covers *both* sexuality and personal relationships for people with learning disability *and* the issue of sexual abuse? Do you and other staff members have time to discuss these policies and agree on how they will work in practice?

■ Do you know the names and contact numbers of relevant people outside your agency you could approach to report your concerns if you were unable to do so at your workplace?

■ How would you go about supporting a service user who was accused of sexually abusing another client?

■ What support mechanisms exist at

your workplace for staff who are accused of abuse?

- Do you know what is involved in bringing a case to court? How long does it take?

- How 'open' do you think your workplace is to fostering adequate discussion by staff and users on sexuality issues in general and on responding to concerns about abuse in particular? What more could you do to improve the workplace culture in this respect?

- How confident are you that you could work with the other professions involved in abuse cases? Do you know who they are and what they can contribute?

Useful Addresses

The following organizations specialize in matters relating to the sexual abuse of adults with learning disabilities and offer a range of services.

NAPSAC (National Association for the Protection from Sexual Abuse of Adults & Children with Learning Disabilities), Department of Learning Disabilities, University Hospital, Nottingham NG7 2UH (Tel 0115 970 9987)

NAPSAC offers a national network of support and information exchange together with training for care staff and managers. It has an excellent annotated bibliography service to members, publishes a quarterly Bulletin and can help with policy development.

NOTA (The National Association for the Development of Work with Sex Offenders), 50, Hayburn Avenue, Hull HU5 4NA (Tel 01482 343625)

NOTA is a multidisciplinary association whose aim is to support and promote work with sex offenders. It provides a network for professionals, training

events, a national conference and a quarterly newsletter.

RESPOND, Third Floor, 24–32 Stephenson Way, London NW1 2HD (Tel 0171 383 0700)

RESPOND offers a psycho-therapeutic service to people with a learning disability who have been sexually abused and to those who sexually abuse. It can also offer advice, support, training and consultancy to staff and carers on sexual abuse.

VOICE (UK), PO Box 238, Derby DE1 9JN (Tel 01332 519872)

VOICE provides help to those with a learning disability who have been sexually abused. It also assists the families and friends of victims and campaigns for changes in the law and professional practices to help victims obtain justice in the courts.

The following organizations have an interest and expertise in this area, but they also cover a wider field:

ARC (The Association for Residential Care), ARC House, Marsden Street, Chesterfield S40 1JY (Tel 01246 555043)

A national umbrella charity for service providers offering training and advice. Provides open learning material for staff and managers of homes on sexual abuse. Monthly information exchange and computerized residential placement service, Caresearch.

BILD (British Institute of Learning Disabilities), Wolverhampton Road, Kidderminster DY10 3PP (formerly BIMH) (Tel 01562 850251)

Offers both general staff training courses and courses on sexuality and learning disabilities. Resources centre and academic journal.

Family Planning Association, 27–35 Mortimer Street, London W1N 7LJ (Tel 0171 636 7866)

FPA runs courses for direct care staff and have produced some excellent specialist literature in the area of sexuality and learning disability.

Law Society, 50 Chancery Lane, London WC2A 1SX (Tel 0171 404 1124)

The Law Society has a Mental Health and Disability Sub Committee. Contact the Secretary, Penny Letts, at the address above.

Lawyers for people with learning disabilities, c/o Mischon de Reya, 21 Southampton Row, London WC1B 5HS

An unofficial group of lawyers with an interest in this area affiliated to the Law Society. Contact the Chair at the above address.

People First, Instrument House, 207–215 Kings Cross

Road, London WC1X 9DB (Tel 0171 173 6400)
People First is run by people with learning difficulties. Offers a range of training courses on Community Care, sexuality, advocacy and self-advocacy, accessible information and legal legislation to staff and people with learning difficulties.

Public Concern at Work, 42 Kingsway, London WC20 6EN (Tel 0171 404 6609)
Trying to help whistleblowers in the workplace. Welcomes contacts from those individuals who are concerned about bad practice and management's refusal to respond appropriately.

The Tizard Centre, Beverely Farm, University of Kent, Canterbury CT2 7LZ (Tel 01227 764000)
Broad-based academic department offering organizational and management consultancy across a wide range of issues as well as staff training and policy development on sexuality and learning disability, including sexual abuse. Has produced some seminal research on the incidence of abuse.

Further Reading

Government publications

Department of Health and the Home Office (1992). *Review of Health and Social Services for Mentally Disordered and Others Requiring Similar Services.* (The Reed Report.) Cmnd 2088. HMSO, London. Provides the basis for the most recent Government thinking on this subject.

Department of Health and Welsh Office (1990). *Mental Health Act 1983 Code of Practice.* HMSO, London. General guidance on the workings of the Act which may be highly relevant since it covers people with a learning disability, by using backward-looking definitions.

Home Office (1990). *Circular 66/90: Provisions for Mentally Disordered Offenders.* HMSO, London. Suggests to the courts the circumstances under which it may be more appropriate for mentally disordered offenders to be sent for treatment rather than to court and/or prison.

Home Office (1995). *Circular 12/95: Mentally Disordered Offenders: Inter-Agency Working.* HMSO, London. Reinforces the need for agencies to work collaboratively, if mentally disordered offenders are to be identified and successfully diverted for treatment.

Law Commission (1995). *Mental Incapacity.* Law Commission Report No. 231. HMSO, London.

Wide-ranging review of the law as at present. It contains a draft Bill incorporating its proposals and will be highly influential in framing future legislation. It contains some rather controversial proposals on consent to treatment issues.

Other publications

ADSS/NAPSAC (1996). *Advice for Social Services Departments on Abuse of People with Learning Disabilities in Residential Care.* ADSS/NAPSAC, Northallerton & Nottingham. Guidance to SSDs on what sort of services they should be purchasing and the questions they need to ask about abuse issues with providers.

Bean, P. and Nemitz, T. (1995). *Out of Depth and Out of Sight.* Midlands Centre for Criminology. Mencap, London. A review of the working of the Appropriate Adults provisions in the 1984 Police and Criminal Evidence Act, highlighting the fact that these provisions are not invoked by local police stations as often as they should be and that the role of the Appropriate Adult is not well understood nor often adequately fulfilled.

Brown, H. (1996). *Towards Safer Commissioning: A Handbook for Purchasers and Commissioners on the Sexual Abuse of Adults with Learning Disabilities.* NAPSAC 'Need to Know' Series. NAPSAC, Nottingham. Services for learning disabled victims and abusers will only improve when the purchasers become aware of their full responsibilities and begin to commission the right sort of services from competent and informed providers supported by local ancillary services. This book begins to show how that can be achieved.

Brown, H. and Craft, A. (1989). *Thinking the Unthinkable: Papers on Sexual Abuse and People with Learning Difficulties.* FPA Education Unit, London. Based on the proceedings of a 1988 conference on sexual abuse and people with learning difficulties which led to much later work. The book contains five chapters and an introduction and postscript. Useful chapters on the need for safeguards; issues in the sexual abuse of children with mental handicap; sex education and abuse prevention programmes for children with special needs; some detailed clinical material of psychotherapeutic interventions in uncovering and responding to sexual abuse. Of particular interest is the final chapter which outlines the legal position – how the law can help and problems that may arise (by M. Gunn).

Brown, H. and Craft, A. (1992). *Working with the Unthinkable: a Trainer's Manual on the Sexual Abuse of Adults with Learning Disabilities*. FPA Education Unit, London. Recognizing sexual abuse and knowing how to deal with it is a major concern for staff. This manual helps staff to explore this difficult area. Written for trainers running courses for whole staff teams or for individuals from different agencies.

Brown, H. and Egan-Sage, E. with Barry, G. (1995). *Towards Better Interviewing: A Handbook on the Sexual Abuse of Adults with Learning Disabilities for Police Officers and Social Workers*. NAPSAC 'Need to Know' Series. NAPSAC, Nottingham. Interviewing learning disabled victims, witnesses and abusers is not easy, nor something which many people do often enough to become skilled at it. This book provides practical guidance on how to do this difficult task well within the current law.

Brown, H., Brammer, A., Craft, A. and McKay, C. (1996). *Towards Better Safeguards: A Handbook for Inspectors and Registration Officers on the Sexual Abuse of Adults with Learning Disabilities*. NAPSAC 'Need to Know' Series. NAPSAC, Nottingham. Guidance to those officers who are often involved in monitoring and reviewing services, especially when abuse has occurred.

Carson, D. (1992). Legality of responding to the sexuality of a client with profound learning disabilities. *Mental Handicap*, **20** (2), 85–7. Highlights the problems which the law on this subject can cause and begins to explore what is possible, practical and legal.

Churchill, J. (ed.) (1996). *Managers in the Middle*. ARC, Chesterfield. An open learning pack to help managers of services for people with a learning disability deal with issues relating to sexual abuse.

Churchill, J., Craft, A., Holding, A. and Horrocks, C.H. (eds) (1996). *It Could Never Happen Here!* (revised edition). ARC and NAPSAC, Chesterfield and Nottingham. A framework document on the prevention and treatment of sexual abuse of adults with learning disabilities in residential settings.

Churchill, J., Brown, H., Craft, A. and Horrocks, C.H. (eds) (1997). *There Are No Easy Answers*. ARC and NAPSAC, Chesterfield and Nottingham. A series of contributions from a range of authors on aspects of providing treatment, care and support to people with learning disabilities who themselves abuse others.

Clare, I.C.H. (1994). Treatment for men with learning disabilites who are perpetrators of sexual abuse: motivation difficulties and effects on practitioners. *NAPSAC Bulletin*, **8**, 3–6.

Craft, A. (ed.) (1994). *Practice Issues in Sexuality and Lernign Disabilities*. Routledge, London. Three chapters address specific issues relating to sexual abuse: (i) Sobsey, D. Sexual Abuse of Individuals with Intellectual Disability; (ii) Millard, L. Between Ourselves: Experiences of a women's group on sexuality and sexual abuse; (iii) Sinason, V. Working with Sexually Abused Individuals who have a Learning Disability.

Gunn, M.J. (1994). Competency and consent: the importance of decision making. In *Practice Issues in Sexuality and Learning Disabilities* (ed. A. Craft). Routledge, London. Given importance of consent, no-one can afford to ignore this issue which is well treated here.

Gunn, M.J. (1996). *Sex and the Law – A Brief Guide for Staff Working with People with Learning Difficulties* (4th ed). Family Planning Association, London. Essential reading for anyone requiring a concise coverage of the legal issues involved.

Harris, J. and Craft, A. (eds), (1994). *People with Learning Disabilities at Risk of Physical or Sexual Abuse*. BILD Seminar Papers No. 4. BILD, Kidderminster. A useful range of papers from a conference and two workshops held in 1992.

Hollins, S. and Sinason, V. (1993). *Jenny Speaks Out* and *Bob Tells All*. Sovereign Series, St George's Hospital Medical School, London. Two booklets, illustrated line drawings in colour, designed to enable a person with learning disabilities to tell about their experience of sexual abuse.

Hollins, S., Sinason, V. and Boniface, J. (1995). *Going to Court*. St George's Mental Health Library: The Sovereign Series, London. This useful book illustrated by Beth Webb, outlines in pictures a young woman with learning disabilities going through the court process from the point of disclosure to the day in court.

Hollins, S., Sinason, V. and Boniface, J. (1995). *Going to Court*. Illustrated by B. Webb. The Sovereign Series. St George's Mental Health Library, London, in association with VOICE (UK). NB: More books are planned in this useful series including one about police and legal procedures (e.g. *You're Under Arrest!*).

Livingstone, J. with Kitson, D. and Supple, C. (1997). *Equipped to Cope? A resource to help support workers deal with issues relating to the sexual abuse of adults with learning disabilities*. ARC/NAPSAC, Chesterfield and Nottingham. A resource manual for direct care staff which reflects the same approach to issues of abuse as *Managers in the Middle*, but aimed at individual or groups of frontline care staff.

McCarthy, M. and Thompson, D. (1993). *Sex and the 3 R's, Rights, Responsibilities & Risks. A Sex Education Package for Working with People with Learning Difficulties.* Pavilion Publishing, Brighton. A well-received general sex education package for staff working with clients in this area.

McCarthy, M. and Thompson, D. (1995). *Sex and Staff Training.* Pavilion Publishing, Brighton. Generally regarded as setting a benchmark for other staff training packages in the wider area of sexuality and learning disability.

NB: There is a useful source of information in *Sexual Abuse and People with Learning Difficulties: Annotated Bibliography* by Vicky Turk and Hilary Brown (updated January 1992), and NAPSAC publishes a regularly updated bibliography for members.

Notes and References

1 This whole area of the law is currently under review. Detailed recommendations have been made by the Law Commission in 1995 (see *Mental Incapacity,* Report of the Law Commission No. 231. HMSO, London) which, if implemented would bring about considerable changes.

2 Brown, H. and Turk, V (1992). Defining sexual abuse as it affects adults with learning disabilities. *Mental Handicap,* **20**(2), 44–55.

3 There were two, 2-year surveys into the incidence of abuse undertaken in the South East Thames Regional Health Authority area in a research programme based at the Universtiy of Kent and funded by the Joseph Rowntree Foundation. Preliminary findings from the first survey were published in Turk, V. and Brown, H. (1992). Sexual abuse and adults with learning disabilities. *Mental Handicap,* **20**(2), 56–8. The full results can be found in *Mental Handicap Research* in June 1993. Details of the second survey can be found in Brown, H., Turk, V. and Stein, J. (1995). The sexual abuse of adults with learning disabilities: Results of a second two year incidence survey. *Mental Handicap Research* **8**(1), 1–22.

4 The figures quoted here are from the first survey which were, with some minor exceptions (e.g. see below) confirmed by the second survey.

5 In the second 2-year study undertaken the number of male victims identified was significantly higher (at 48%) than in the first study (27%). See Brown, H., Turk, V. and Stein, J. (1995).

6 For a detailed summary of the law on this subject see Gunn, M. (1996). *Sex and the Law a Brief Guide for Staff Working with People with Learning Difficulties,* 4th edn. Family Planning Association, London.

7 The law uses such offensive and outdated terminology because it is constantly referring back to earlier definitions enshrined in law and acts of Parliament. Terms such as 'learning disability' and even 'mental handicap' have no standing in law. Consequently most definitions of learning disability are in fact broader catch-all terms (such as 'defective') which cover both learning disability and mental illness.

8 See the subsequent redefinition of the term in Section 3 of the Mental Health (Amendment) Act 1982.

9 See Section 9(1) of the 1956 Sexual Offences Act.

10 See for example, the Sexual Offences Act of 1967 which makes it an offence for a male member of staff to commit acts of gross indecency on male patients: Section 27 of the 1956 Sexual Offences Act makes it an offence for an owner or occupier of premises to induce or allow a female defective to be there for the purpose of having unlawful sexual intercourse with one or more men. For full details and more on these see Gunn (1996) above (note 6).

11 See the list by Brown and Turk (1992) reproduced in Churchill, J. (1996). *It Could Never Happen Here!,* p. 13. ARC/NASPAC, Chesterfield and Nottingham.

12 For a full explanation of and limitations to the use of these diagrams see Churchill, J. (ed.) (1996). *Managers in the Middle,* Section 7. ARC, Chesterfield.

13 For more on these functions see Churchill, J. (1996). *It Could Never Happen Here!,* p. 53 ff. ARC/NASPAC, Chesterfield and Nottingham.

14 The CPS is an independent body from the police which receives any police report on a possible prosecution and then decides whether or not to proceed. Prior to that the police may, on their own initiative, decide not to pursue further with an investigation.

15 For more on this see Clare, I. and Carson, D. (1997). Practice: wise and defensible decisions. In *There Are No Easy Answers* (eds J. Churchill, H.

Brown, A. Craft and C. Horrocks, pp. 69–88. ARC/NAPSAC, Chesterfield and Nottingham.

16 For more on this see Clare and Carson (1997). *ibid*, p. 70.

17 See Clare and Carson (1997). *ibid* p. 85.

18 Exactly who this person will be will depend upon arrangements which should have been worked out *in advance* between the Local Authority and the provider agency. In any event his report will be lodged with the Local Authority lead officer who has responsibility for monitoring abuse incidents in the area and reporting annually to Local Authorities and to provider agencies. See *It Could Never Happen Here!*, p. 57. This report will also be required by the risk manager who will need to manage the future care of the alleged abuser and advise commissioners/purchasers accordingly (see Murphy, G. (1997). Treatment and risk management. In *There Are No Easy Answers* (eds J. Churchill *et al.*), pp. 120–124. ARC/NAPSAC, Chesterfield and Nottingham.

19 See Murphy, G. (1997). Assessment: establishing the clearest possible understanding of an offender. In *There Are No Easy Answers* (eds. J. Churchill *et al.*), pp. 89–101. ARC/NAPSC, Chesterfield and Nottingham.

Chapter 19

Responding to the Health Needs of People with Learning Disabilities

Owen Barr

Key Issues

- Outline a definition of health
- Summarize the changing morbidity and mortality patterns among people with learning disabilities
- Consider the difficulties people with learning disabilities may encounter when using mainstream health-promotion services
- Review some of the developments in the provision of health promotion for people with learning disabilities
- Provide suggestions for steps towards improving health-promotion services for people with learning disabilities

Health – an Elusive Definition

The word 'health' is used frequently in everyday language; however, definitions exist at differing levels of complexity. These include lay definitions which describe being healthy as an absence of ill health, and a soundness of body and mind. Within such a definition it is difficult to see how people with learning disabilities would be regarded as healthy by members of the general population.

The World Health Organization (1984) defines health as

the extent to which an individual or group is able to, on the one hand realize aspirations and satisfy needs; and on the other hand, to change or cope with the environment. Health is therefore seen as a resource for everyday life, not an object of living: it is a positive concept emphasizing social and personal resources, as well as physical capacities.

(Naidoo and Wills, 1994, p. 21)

This definition provides more scope to view people with learning disabilities as potentially healthy, in that many people with learning disabilities do have aspirations, can cope with varying degrees of change, and have social and personal resources. Therefore under such a definition people with learning disabilities could achieve a healthy state.

Great difficulty exists in producing a defintion of health which will be totally acceptable to all people, but as can be seen from the definitions outlined overleaf, various factors may influence (to differing degrees) an individual's perception of their state of health.

The appraisal of one's state of health is influenced by objective information such as the ability to complete activities, test results and confirmed diagnosis of illness. Personal characteristics (e.g. age, gender, genetic influences) will also contribute to a person's state of health.

Subjective information such as how a person 'feels' is often more significant than objective data when a person is contemplating their health. Despite having no concrete objective data to indicate ill health a person may feel unwell; equally, in the absence of objective data to confirm an improvement in health an individual may feel they are getting better. Therefore, any attempts to establish how an individual views their state of health must incorporate objective and subjective aspects.

Health is also bound by time and culture (Helman, 1994). Many things considered healthy 40 years ago are unlikely to be accepted as such today. Some of the changes witnessed over the past 20 years include altering patterns of diet, exercise, sexual behaviour, overall lifestyle and life expectancy.

Social class has been identified as a major factor to be considered when looking at health services and overall state of health. While it has been shown to be a variable in access to health services, various explanations exist as to how, and to what degree, it exerts an influence (Helman, 1994).

Personal expectations, as well as the expectations of those we come in contact with, be they family, friends or professionals, are incorporated into our personal assessment of our own health state. If carers, family members or the people whom you come in contact with, or who provide service, have low expectations of the acceptable state of health of people with learning disabilities, this could be detrimental to people's state of health.

Negative expectations may influence behaviours of the individual or service providers and can result in self-fulfilling prophecies in which low or negative expectations of an individual's health may lead to the acceptance of a lower state of health as 'normal' by that person or group of people. This is particularly important when considering how a low state of health may become accepted as normal for people with learning disabilities (Figure 19.1a).

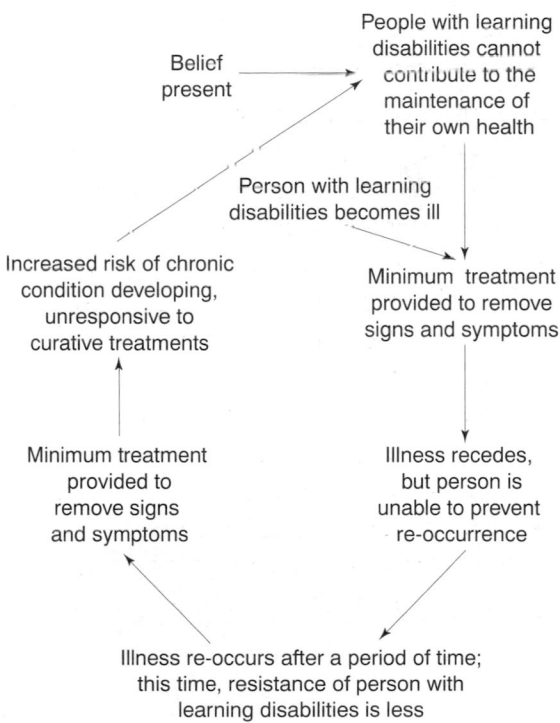

Figure 19.1a Negative self-fulfilling prophecy arising from assumption that people with learning disabilities are unable to contribute to the maintenance of their own health

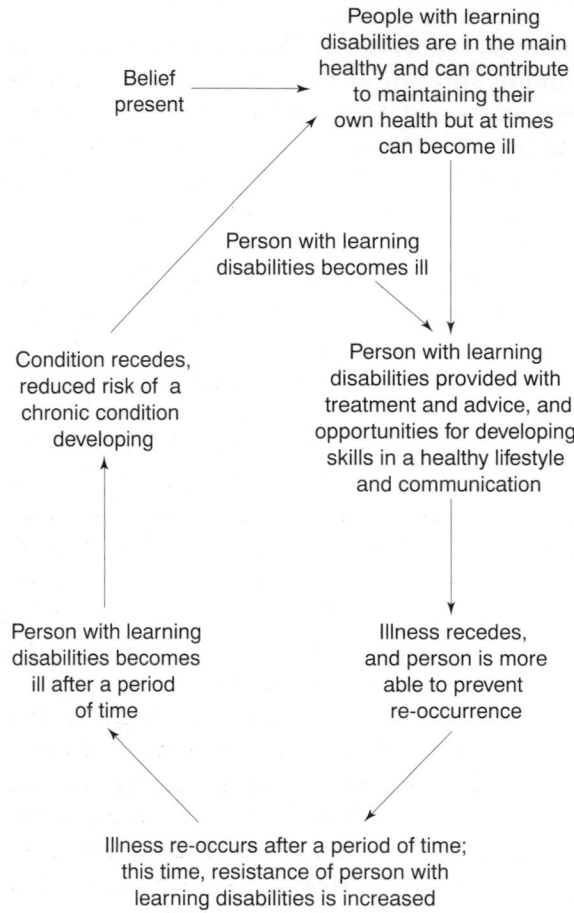

Belief present → People with learning disabilities are in the main healthy and can contribute to maintaining their own health but at times can become ill

Person with learning disabilities becomes ill

Condition recedes, reduced risk of a chronic condition developing

Person with learning disabilities provided with treatment and advice, and opportunities for developing skills in a healthy lifestyle and communication

Person with learning disabilities becomes ill after a period of time

Illness recedes, and person is more able to prevent re-occurrence

Illness re-occurs after a period of time; this time, resistance of person with learning disabilities is increased

Figure 19.1b Positive self-fulfilling prophecy arising from assumption that people with learning disabilities are able to contribute to the maintenance of their own health

Alternatively, self-fulfilling prophecies may be positive, and have a health-enhancing impact on the life of people with learning disabilities (Figure 19.1b). This highlights the importance of reflecting seriously upon the expectations of people providing services to people with learning disabilities. Strenuous efforts must be made to promote positive expectations of health, and reduce the impact of negative expectations and

images that portray people with learning disabilities as ill and unhealthy.

In an attempt to bring together varying theoretical perspectives on what health is, Seedhouse defined health as

a person's optimum state of health is equivalent to the state of the set of conditions which fulfil or enable a person to work to fulfil his or her realistic chosen and biological potentials. Some of these conditions are of highest importance for all people. Others are variable dependent upon individual abilities and circumstances.
(Seedhouse, 1986, p. 61)

The definition has similarities with the philosophy of services for people with learning disabilities; in particular, the emphasis on choice and individuality in priorities, both aspects that are key components of inclusive services (DHSS NI, 1995). Within the parameters of this definition people with learning disabilities, including people with multiple disabilities, may attain a 'healthy state' despite the presence of some physical and psychological disabilities.

Changing Patterns of Mortality and Morbidity Among People with a Learning Disability

Over the past decade a more comprehensive picture of the physical and mental health status of people with learning disabilities has been emerging. Research reports on the abilities and needs of people with a learning disability in relation to their health status have become more frequent. Key findings include evidence of changes in life expectancy; the presence of health risk factors; altering patterns of physical morbidity and mortality; and an increased recognition of the presence of mental illness among people with learning disabilities.

Changes in life expectancy

The life expectancy of people with a learning disability has increased by 40 years over the past 50 years (Jancar, 1988). Women with learning disabilities have a slightly higher life expectancy than men; this is also the situation in the general population. Evenhuis (1995a) in her study includes a person with learning disabilities who is 92 year old, while the oldest person in a study by Kearney *et al.* (1993) is 81 years old.

Although the life expectancy of people with Down's syndrome remains between 5 and 10 years lower than the overall population of people with learning disabilities, this still represents a considerable shift in life expectancy for people with Down's syndrome (Stratford and Gunn, 1996). It has been predicted that 44% of people with Down's syndrome will live to be 60 years old (Carr, 1994), and 1 in 10 will reach 70 years old (Brown, 1996).

The trend in life expectancy is definitely upwards and an increasing number of people with a learning disability are surviving well into old age. However, the mortality rates for people with a learning disability compared to the general population remain considerably higher. People with mild learning disabilities have a rate 1.7 times that of the general population, the rate for people with profound learning disabilities is 4.1 times that of the general population (Dupont and Mortenson, 1990 in Kearney *et al.*, 1993).

Physical health

Increased life expectancy has been in part due to altering patterns of mortality and morbidity among people with learning disabilities. Medical and surgical treatments have improved for conditions such as epilepsy, infections, cardiac defects, head injuries, general trauma and some metabolic disorders. As these advances have become more available to people with learning disabilities there has been a reduction in the number of deaths caused by these conditions (Day and Jancar, 1994).

However, increased longevity among people with learning disabilities has resulted in an increased number of deaths as a result of conditions such as myocardial and vascular diseases, cancer and Alzheimer's disease (Jancar, 1988; Bycroft 1994; Day and Jancar, 1994). Considerable evidence exists to support the concerns about the health of people with learning disabilities in respect of cardiovascular disease, strokes, cancer, mental illness, sexual health and accidents (Bouras *et al.*, 1993; DOH, 1995; Turner and Moss, 1996).

There is some evidence to suggest that many potential health problems and associated health risk factors among people with learning disabilities go undetected. Langan and Russell (1993) found that people with learning disabilities were less likely to be offered cervical screening, breast examination, blood pressure monitoring and advice on the dangers of smoking. One health-screening project (Meehan *et al.*, 1995) reported that out of 191 people with learning disabilities assessed, 176 had previously undetected conditions that either increased their risk of developing ill health, caused pain and discomfort, or reduced their opportunities for social integration (Table 19.1). It is important to remember that these impairments are reported as particularly responsive to treatment, especially when detected at a younger age (DOH, 1995; Evenhuis 1995a,b).

It has been suggested that aspects of the lifestyle of people with learning disabilities may contribute to their increased chances of developing ill health. These factors include a reduced level of fitness, increased obesity,

Table 19.1 Findings from health screening of 195 people between 1992 and 1994. From Meehan *et al.* (1995) with kind permission of *Nursing Times*, London.

Health-screening measures	Number of people with conditions previously undetected
Blood pressure	23
Weight	98
Urinalysis	12
Skin	38
Mouth	60
Hair	30
Feet	72
Breasts	7
Testicles	7
Ears	84
Eyes	36
Blood tests	10
Total	477*

* 83% of people screened had more than one condition

reduced self-care abilities and similar cholesterol profiles to people in the general population (Rimmer *et al.*, 1993, 1994; Turner and Moss, 1996). The incidence of risk factors has also been linked to where people live, significantly higher rates of obesity, smoking, coffee intake and reduced exercise levels have been associated with community residential homes ($P < 0.001$) when compared with people living in hospital or at home.

Although family members and carers may be aware of the signs and symptoms of ill health in people with a learning disability, they may fail to recognize the significance of these and seek appropriate treatment. This could in part be due to low expectations of the health of people with a learning disability.

Mental health

An extensive range of mental illnesses has been reported among people with learning disabilities (see annotated bibliography by Sturmey and Sevin, 1993). However, it is difficult to obtain agreed prevalence rates for the presence of 'dual diagnosis'. In the 17 studies reviewed by Szymanski (1994) prevalence rates ranged from 7.3% to 83% of the people studied within 'selected population' (clinics, hospitals) and from 28% to 64% of people in 'unselected populations' (localities, random samples).

These variations highlight several difficulties with research in this area; namely, reported rates may vary greatly depending on the sampling procedure used. Hospital- and clinic-based studies are likely to report increased rates of illness as this is often the reason for admission. Also, the procedures for diagnosis of both learning disabilities and mental illness vary across studies and are not always directly comparable. While some studies use recognized assessment criteria such as DSM III/IV, others work from recorded diagnosis in care records or confirm diagnosis by a current assessment. Also, while some studies include the category of behaviour disorders, others use only specific conditions. These factors should be considered when critiquing and comparing research findings on the prevalence of mental health problems among people with a learning disability (Borthwick-Duffy, 1994; Sturmey, 1995).

Affective disorders (usually anxiety and depression) are the most commonly reported among people with mild learning disabilities, whereas among people with severe learning difficulties the broad classification of 'behaviour disorders' is reported most frequently. This term is often used when differential diagnosis is not possible due to the limited communication ability and difficulty in expressing how one feels (both central to the process of differential diagnosis).

The fact that people with Down's syndrome have an increased risk of developing

Alzheimer's disease has been known for 50 years (Berg *et al.*, 1992). Indeed, the development of this condition was almost considered inevitable for people with Down's syndrome past 40 years old. Care must be taken that it does not lead to a reinforcement of the stereotype of people with Down's syndrome. This is important because any stereotype has the effect of reducing the individuality of care delivered and increasing the generalizations made.

However, more recent findings highlight the importance of eliminating other possible causes of deteriorating cognitive and physical ability before agreeing or deciding on a diagnosis of Alzheimer's disease (Janicki *et al.*, 1995). In particular, it is necessary to exclude impaired vision, hearing and mobility, trauma, all forms of abuse, infections and drug interactions, metabolic and endocrine disorders and depression (Barr and Campbell, 1995).

Some risk factors have been identified as possibly increasing the occurrence of mental illness in people with learning disabilities. These include stigma, labelling, pressure to achieve within inclusive services, loneliness, boredom, over-control, limited opportunities for development, poverty, multiple bereavements, and physical, emotional and sexual abuse (Monaghan and Soni, 1992; Fraser and Nolan, 1994).

Conclusion

Although much of the evidence provided above could give the impression that people with a learning disability are of much poorer health than members of the general public, this is not necessarily the situation. It appears that for most physical and mental illness the incidence rates are similar for people with learning disabilities and the general population (Moss *et al.*, 1993; Moss and Turner, 1995). The significant change appears to be an alteration in the patterns of physical and mental illness among people with a learning disability over the past few decades.

This could in part be due to increased longevity and therefore subsequent development of the reported conditions. Secondly, increased detection of the conditions reported as a result of increased research in this area could be a factor. It has been asserted that many of the conditions resulting in death among people with a learning disability are avoidable and that 'too often, treatable illness is undetected until it has progressed to a stage where treatment is less effective' (DOH, 1995, p. 14). Many causes of death among people with learning disabilities could be reduced considerably with appropriate health-promotion measures (Kastner *et al*, 1993; Evenhuis, 1995a,b). Possible target areas for health promotion are shown in Table 19.2.

Difficulties Experienced in Accessing Health-promotion Services

Unfortunately, many of the strategies for health promotion and health education have focused on the general population with little consideration given to people with additional needs, such as people with learning disabilities. This was emphasized by Greenhalgh (1994, p. 6) who concluded in her study that 'the interrelated problems of difficulty in diagnosis, incorrect attitudes and low expectations have contributed to a situation which is little short of scandalous'.

It is important that all mainstream health services are accessible to people with a learning disability. In addition, it is also necessary to have access to additional services that can recognize and respond to specific physical, psychological and social

Table 19.2 Possible target areas for health promotion. Developed from DOH (1995)

Coronary heart disease and stroke
Healthy eating, diet (dental care), alcohol, physical activity, stress management

Cancer
Diet, self-examination (female/male), smoking, skin care, sunlight, cervical screening, chronic irritation

HIV/AIDS and sexual health
Hepatitis B, personal relationship education, menstruation care, privacy, touch, saying no, choice, preventing and
    reporting abuse, appropriate social behaviour

Safety
- home – kitchen, bathroom, electricity, fire
- road – transport (car, bus, train), pedestrian, bicycle
- water safety – swimming

Effects of medicines (individualized), alcohol and other substances at risk of misuse

First aid
Cuts, bruises, epilepsy, burns, use of the telephone to contact help from family members, doctor, or emergency
    services

Mental illness
Relaxation exercises, stress managment, assertiveness, expressing feelings, bereavement, life events

factors that influence the health of people with learning disabilities.

Even though health promotion is a major part of current health care provision in hospital, and particularly in community settings, it is clear that people with a learning disability have unequal access to services and advice available. People with a learning disability could face a variety of problems in accessing mainstream health-screening and health-promotion services. These difficulties may relate to their personal characteristics of both people with learning disabilities, carers and staff involved. People with learning disabilities may experience difficulties such as fear of unknown places, people and investigations; difficulty in reading and understanding published material or technical terms; or the need for investigations. The presence of challenging behaviour such as hyperactivity, shouting, or self-injurious behaviour will reduce opportunities to utilize mainstream services. Failure to appreciate the intricacy of socially appropriate behaviour, for example

waiting in queues, taking turns, and acceptable responses to fear and confusion may result in a reluctance among carers and family members to avail of mainstream health-promotion services.

Communication is largely accepted as a two-way process, therefore when people with learning disabilities and staff are unable to communicate with each other, all concerned need to work to find a solution. Often a person with learning disabilities is able to communicate their needs and wishes at home, in the social education centre and when with people who know them locally, but not with unfamiliar people. If this is the situation, it is inappropritate to consider that all the difficulties in communication arise from the person with learning disabilities. The staff unfamiliar with the person with learning disabilities also have communication deficits and should take action to reduce these. Such action may involve identifying what communication system is or could be used, speaking with people familiar with the person with learning disabilities, possibly initially communicating through them until further knowledge and skills are developed.

Staff involved may also need to develop refined skills, for example in adapting normal health-screening measures such as blood pressure monitoring, recording body mass index, or physical examination to be suitable for people with severe learning disabilities.

A critical challenge to be overcome is the assumption that changes in behaviour, physical health or mental health are totally due to the presence of learning disabilities. At the very least, this can result in a reduced quality of life for people with learning disabilities due to a failure to note preventable or treatable conditions, such as an ear infection or toothache. Unfortunately, assumptions about learning disabilities being the cause of changes in a person's health status may result in failure to diagnose fatal conditions early enough for curative treatment, such as cancer or cardiovascular disease. Any temptation to superficially explain a change in someone's behaviour or health status as due to learning disabilities must be resisted and should be challenged as an unsupported and possibly professionally incompetent practice.

Nurses for people with a learning disability are particularly well equipped with their knowledge of health and illness to help overcome some of these problems and, in doing so, increase the availability of health-promotion services for people with learning disabilities. However, effective health promotion is an interdisciplinary endeavour, and staff in services for people with learning disabilities must work with the primary health care and mainstream health-promotion services.

Developing Health-Promotion Services for People with a Learning Disability

As with attempts to define health at the start of this chapter, for many people confusion continues to exist about the definition and distinctions between the terms 'health promotion' and 'health education'. Tones *et al* (1990) draws the following distinctions: health promotion is viewed as incorporating 'all measures deliberately designed to promote health. A major feature of health promotion is undoubtedly the importance of healthy public policy'; whereas health education 'is any planned activity which promotes health or illness related learning, that is, some relatively permanent change in an individual's competence or disposition' (Tones *et al.*, 1990). As can be seen from the definitions, health education is part of the larger process of health promotion. Health promotion is an enabling process and ultimately wishes to enable people to improve their own health.

The response to the health-promotion and health-education needs of people with a learning disability must aim to overcome the challenges already noted in using mainstream services. Strategies utilized should be consistent with the philosophy of normalization, which seeks to increase the social value and the social role of people with a learning disability (Brown and Smith, 1992).

Health promotion may occur at three levels: primary, secondary and tertiary. Each level has specific aims and objectives, and occurs at different times in relation to the progress of the ill health. Primary health promotion occurs prior to the onset of ill health and is aimed at the promotion of health, and the prevention of ill health. The secondary level occurs at times before a person recognizes they are developing ill health and is aimed at the early detection and prompt treatment of ill health. Finally, tertiary health promotion occurs when a condition is established and is aimed at the treatment of the established condition and action to prevent any further disabilities as a result of the condition (Niadoo and Wills, 1994).

Five differing approaches may be utilized when delivering health promotion: these are medical, behavioural, educational, empowerment and social change (Ewles and Simnett, 1992). Each approach involves differing roles for both the health promoter and the recipient of the information. Health promotion in services for people with learning disabilities could utilize all approaches depending on the abilities and needs of the person with a learning disability and the other people involved.

Putting it into Practice

As noted earlier, factors such as the age, experience and ability of all people involved including staff, together with the urgency of need, will influence the selection of the most appropriate strategy. It is necessary to carefully assess the level of ability and needs of each person involved, as this will facilitate careful preparation and presentation of material and activities which are appropriate for the individuals or group members concerned.

Medically focused activities

This involves the regular screening of people for the indicators or risk factors, such as obesity, hypertension and serum cholesterol levels. It tends to focus on people at increased risk of ill health, for example people with Down's syndrome and older people with learning disabilities. In such situations it may involve screening to eliminate specifically associated illness, such as hypothyroidism, cataracts and Alzheimer disease.

An agreed list of screening measures should be developed and should reflect the research findings related to the health of people with learning disabilities. The use of an agreed list also assists increased continuity in health screening, particularly if several members of the health care team are involved in the process at different times. Agreed tests should be related to what is known about people with specific conditions, and can be individualized depending on an individual's previous medical and family history.

The preparation of people for tests and examinations needs to begin in sufficient time prior to the screening to enable family and carers to provide people with learning disabilities with adequate information about what to expect. The use of videos, written or pictorial information, and group or individual activities that are appropriate for the age, cognitive ability and concentration span may be useful in the preparation process. A rehearsal for the assessment may help reassure the person with learning disabilities, family members and staff involved. A gradual introduction to the screening/examinations and opportunities to discuss concerns prior to undergoing screening can also reduce fears. In addition, the presence of staff with whom the person has a trusting relationship can be valuable. It is important to remain aware of the feelings of people with learning disabilities during medical assessment, and adjust the schedule accordingly to increase the likelihood of the successful completion of the assessment.

The medical model has a focus on prompt treatment, and therefore it is necessary to ensure that measures similar to those outlined above are taken in order to increase the prospects of an informed compliance with recommended treatment.

Behavioural-focused activities

Within this approach the emphasis is on bringing about a change in health-related behaviour. Possible target behaviours could be altering one's diet, stopping smoking or increasing the amount of exercise taken (Pitetti *et al.*, 1993). This principally involves teaching new skills that assist a person with learning disabilities replace unhealthy behaviours with healthy behaviours. Role play activities and training exercises in real life situations such as shopping for groceries can provide valuable opportunities to practice new skills and monitor progress (Perry, 1996). It is important that objectives for the health-based training are agreed with the person with learning disability or someone who can represent their interests. As with all behavioural-based teaching programmes, staff must take account of the associated ethical issues, and be able to demonstrate that all interventions should improve the quality of life of people with learning disabilities. The interests of the client must be paramount, clear attempts should be made to provide informed choices, independent representation should be easily accessible, and positive reinforcement strategies should be utilized. No assumptions should be made about the reinforcing properties of stars, charts, tokens or money for all people with learning disabilities. To increase the prospects of success, careful attention should be given to the selection of individual reinforcers for the people involved. Those selected should be health promoting; for example it is misplaced and, it could be argued, unethical to use cigarettes or other potential health-damaging substances as reinforcers.

The success of behavioural approaches relies heavily on careful assessment, planning and implementation. It is necessary to ensure that all necessary resources are in place prior to any programme commencing, and that continuity is maintained throughout the programme. Role models are important and care should be taken to model the desired healthy behaviour (e.g. staff and family members should not be smoking and failing to take exercise while at the same time making these target behaviours for people with learning disabilities). Once a healthy behaviour has been established it is necessary to maintain adequate reinforcement to maintain and generalize the behaviour. This will often involve liaison with family members, day care staff, school teachers and other members of the interdisciplinary team.

Educational-focused activities

This moves beyond the identification of new behaviours to be learnt and focuses on the provision of information as well as on developing new skills. Although this requires a higher degree of cognitive ability than behavioural approaches to be successful, it has clear applications to the majority of people with learning disabilities. The aim is to assist people with learning disabilities understand more about health and illness. This may be targeted at a group of people, or focused on individually identified concerns, such as increasing exercise, menstruation or epilepsy.

Owing to an over-reliance on written communication, and at times abstract images, much of the mainstream health education information is of little use to people with learning disabilities (Nightingale, 1992). Therefore, it is often necessary to prepare specific information leaflets, posters, scrapbooks, line drawings, local photographs, or audio and videotapes. To assist the development of connections between relevant points, information should start with broad general points about health and then gradually move to specific and more detailed points.

The active involvement of people with learning disabilities in the preparation of this material can provide valuable opportunities to discuss the information and may lead to a greater understanding of health. The lack of time taken to explain health information has been highlighted as a major failing of health professions working with people with learning disabilities (Mental Health Foundation, 1996). Images used should have meaning for the people concerned and relate to concrete, easily recognizable (as opposed to abstract) health messages. Fortunately, an increasing amount of specifically designed health education information has become available over the past few years (Table 19.3). Individual and small group work can present opportunities for people to consider what health means to them, develop skills in communication and increase self-

Table 19.3 Broad areas for which commercially produced health education information is now available for people with learning disabilities. From Health Education Authority (1995)

Abuse
Advocacy
Arts and leisure
Bereavement
Communication skills
Consultation and involvement in service planning
Everyday care and personal hygiene
Food and nutrition
Growth and development
Living in the community
Mental health
Parenting
Physical activity
Play
Safety
Sexuality
Substance misuse

awareness. The educational approach should utilize naturally occurring opportunities for health education that arise in daily activities as well as purposeful designed activities.

The educational approach is more than providing information. It is also necessary to evaluate the impact on knowledge and behaviour of the information provided. Simply providing information is no guarantee of achieving any health-related learning. Therefore all health education initiatives should have identified objectives against which their effectiveness can be measured. Failure to evaluate interventions can seriously limit opportunities to support their effectiveness.

Empowerment-focused activities

The primary aim in this approach is to provide people with learning disabilities with the necessary knowledge, skills and opportunities to be involved in the decision-making process about issues that affect their health. This may occur as individuals or as groups. Staff should work to increase the utilization of valued mainstream health-promotion services. This may involve providing information, short courses, and gradually introducing people with learning disabilities to services in a supported manner. General practitioners, practice nurses, other members of the primary health care team and family members may need some encouragement and support to accept that health promotion for people with learning disabilities is a worthwhile venture and any short-term difficulties will be outweighed by longer term advantages.

Self-help groups and advocacy groups could be a key focus for this approach. It is necessary to ensure that, when groups are involved in the decision-making process, representation is adequate to enable the views of all people to be heard. Initially, decisions made may be small, but will gradually progress to larger decisions as knowledge, skills and confidence increases.

It may be possible to develop alliances with other groups that may or may not include other people with learning disabilities to campaign on issues of mutual concern. Careful attention is needed to the dynamics of small group working, mutual goal setting, co-operation, collaboration and lobbying (Gibson, 1991). These areas may form topics for health education (e.g. assertiveness training, decision-making skills) within the group and provided further opportunities for developing understanding.

Empowerment-focused activities may involve the taking of calculated risks, and providing support for the right to make decisions (even if you disagree with the actual decision made). Empowering people to make decisions will result in a change in roles for people with learning disabilities, staff and family members (Braye and Preston-Shoot, 1995). All people must work towards this and be prepared for possible changes in their role and status. Easy access to independent representation is a crucial aspect of developing empowerment-based initiatives.

Social change focused activities

This approach requires collective action on a wider scale and often over a longer period of time than empowerment-based approaches. It involves aspects such as implementing an overall screening policy, providing an adequate budget for health promotion, auditing of services available and taking positive action to overcome limitations identified. The allocation of specific responsibilities for health promotion for people with learning disabilities would involve social change actions, as would developing working alliances between people with learning disabilities, family

members, as well as statutory and independent service providers (Anderson, 1993). It also involves addressing wider issues that impinge on the health of people with learning disabilities, such as poverty, poor housing and limited assistance with transport. Recent community care policies that encourage (and at times appear to put pressure on) people to remain at home, and in doing so may reduce opportunities for them to develop a personal identity or increased independence, need to be examined.

Although a smaller number of people with learning disabilities may be involved at this level, it is important to ensure that their interests are represented accurately. Social change strategies operate over a longer term than the preceding approaches and require the setting of realistic targets within a longer term vision (3–5 years).

Conclusions

Health promotion is necessary for all people with a learning disability and is not solely the domain of people who have a mild-to-moderate degree of learning disability. Indeed, it could be argued that less able people require particular attention in health-promotion activities. Although active involvement and collaboration to increase health may be more difficult to obtain, these remain the aims of health promotion.

Interdisciplinary team members and family members need to have the opportunity to be actively involved in the health-promotion activities, or at the very least be aware of the aims, objectives and content of the programme. Without appropriate role models, the best laid plans in health promotion can easily fail.

Little dispute exists that urgent attention is needed to the health promotion needs of all people with a learning disability. What is now needed is a determined and co-ordinated approach in respect of a health-promotion service which incorporates the abilities and needs of people with a learning disability (Thornton, 1994). This service must target key areas of health which have been identified in the literature as needing attention. There is also an urgent need to research the effectiveness of health-promotion approaches used with people with learning disabilities, in order to establish a body of knowledge to guide and co-ordinate practice, reduce duplication and re-invention of the wheel, and identify those areas that have been effective and ineffective. This research needs to be methodologically sound, completed with rigour and needs to overcome the present deficits identified (Moss and Turner, 1995).

The development and implementation of a health-promotion strategy for all people with learning disabilities will require effective interdisciplinary work, resources and a commitment to provide high-quality services for people with learning disabilities. It is essential that effective liaison is established between specialist learning disabilities services, primary health care services and health-promotion departments. All people working with people with learning disabilities and their families have a responsibility to take action to increase and maintain a better state of health for people with learning disabilities. This should not be viewed as providing an extra service to people with learning disabilities, but instead it is the provision of services they and their families are entitled to as citizens.

Discussion Questions

- What does it mean to you personally to be healthy? Discuss your answer with some colleagues and develop a list of criteria for being healthy in hierarchical order.
- Outline the factors that influence the health status of people with learning disabilities and identify what contribution you can make to improving this. List the knowledge, skills and resources that would assist you to achieve this.
- People with learning disabilities do not require specialist health-promotion services, and should use mainstream health-promotion services in keeping with the philosophy of inclusion. Discuss.
- In discussion with people with learning disabilities identify what their major health concerns are.
- Redesign the information obtained in relation to exercise above; taking care to retain the positive aspects identify and overcome the limitations identified. Evaluate the usefulness of the new information by using it to provide information to people with learning disabilities and obtaining their feedback on it.
- Obtain the available information from your local health promotion on one aspect of a healthy lifestyle (e.g. diet, exercise, stress management). Review the usefulness of this information for the people with learning disabilities you work with, highlighting both positive and negative aspects of the information.

References

Anderson, R.C. (1993). The need to modify health education programs for the mentally retarded and developmentally disabled. *Journal of Developmental and Physical Disabilities* **5**(2), 95–108.

Barr, O. and Campbell, A. (1995). The link between Down's Syndrome and Alzheimer's Disease. *Journal of Dementia Care*, **3**(2), 24–6.

Berg, J.M., Karlinsky, H. and Holland, J. (1992). *Alzheimer Disease, Down's Syndrome: Their Relationship*. Oxford Medical Press, Oxford.

Borthwick-Duffy, S.A. (1994). Epidemiology and prevalence of psychopathology in people with mental retardation. *Journal of Consulting and Clinical Psychology*, **62**(1), 17–27.

Bouras, N., Kon, Y. and Drummond, C. (1993). Medical and psychiatric needs of adults with a mental handicap. *Journal of Intellectual Disabilities Research*, **37**(2), 177–82.

Braye, S. and Preston-Shoot, M. (1995). *Empowering Practice in Social Care*. Open University Press, Buckingham.

Brown, H. and Smith, H. (eds) (1992). *Normalisation. A Reader for the Nineties*. Routledge, London.

Brown, R.I. (1996). Growing older: challenges and opportunities. In *New Approaches to Down Syndrome*, (eds B. Stratford and P. Gunn), pp. 436–50. Cassell, London.

Bycroft, L. (1994). Care of a handicapped woman with metastatic breast cancer. *British Journal of Nursing*, **3**(3), 126–33.

Carr, J. (1994). Long term outcome for people with Down's syndrome. *Journal of Child Psychology and Psychiatry*, **96**(5), 502–11.

Day, K. and Jancar, J. (1994). Mental and physical health and ageing in mental handicap: a review. *Journal of Intellectual Disability Research*, **38**(3), 241–56.

Dept of Health Social Services, Northern Ireland (1995). *Review of Policy for People with a Learning Disability*. DHSS, Belfast.

Dept of Health (1995). *The Health of the Nation. A Strategy for People with Learning Disabilities*. HMSO, London.

Evenhuis, H. (1995a). Medical aspects of ageing in a populaton with intellectual disability: 1. Visual impairment. *Journal of Intellectual Disability Research*, **39**(1), 19–26.

Evenhuis, H. (1995b). Medical aspects of ageing in a population with intellectual disability: 2. Hearing impairment. *Journal of Intellectual Disability Research*, **39**(1), 27–34.

Ewles, L. and Simnett, I. (1992). *Promoting Health: A Practical Guide to Health Education*. Wiley, Chichester.

Fraser, W. and Nolan, M. (1994). Psychiatric disorders in mental retardation. In *Mental Health in Mental Retardation. Recent Advances and Practices* (ed. N. Bouras), pp. 79–92. Cambridge University Press, Cambridge.

Greenhalgh, L. (1994). *Well Aware. Improving access to health information for people with learning difficulties*. Milton Keynes General NHS Trust, Milton Keynes.

Gibson, C. (1991). A concept analysis of empowerment. *Journal of Advanced Nursing*, **16**(3), 354–61.

Health Education Authority (1995). *Health-related Resources for People with Learning Disabilities*. Health Education Authority, London.

Helman, C. (1994). *Culture, Health and Illness*, 3rd edn. Butterworth Heinemann, Oxford.

Jancar, J. (1988). Consequences of longer life for the mentally handicapped. *Geriatric Medicine*, **5**, 81–7.

Janicki, M.P., Heller, T., Seltzer, G. and Hogg, J. (1995). *Practice Guidelines for the Clinical Assessment and Care Management of Alzheimer and other Dementias Among Adults with Mental Retardation*. American Association on Mental Retardation, Washington.

Kastner, T., Nathanson, R. and Friedman, D.L. (1993). Mortality among individuals with mental retardation living in the community. *American Journal of Mental Reatardation*, **98**(2), 285–92.

Kearney, G.M., Krishnan, V. and Londhe, J. (1993). Characteristics of elderly people with a mental handicap living in a mental handicap hospital: a descriptive study. *The British Journal of Developmental Disabilities*, **XXXIX**(1), 31–50.

Langan, J. and Russell, O. (1993). *Community Care and the General Practitioner. Primary Health Care for People with Learning Disabilities*. (Summary of final report to the Department of Health). Norah Fry Research Centre, Bristol.

Meehan, S., Moore, G. and Barr, O. (1995). Specialist services for people with learning disabilities. *Nursing Times*, **91**(13), 33–5.

Mental Health Foundation (1996). *Building Expectations: Opportunities and Services for People with a Learning Disability*. Mental Health Foundation, London.

Monaghan, M.T. and Soni, S. (1992). Effects of significant life events on the behaviour of mentally retarded people in the community. *The British Journal of Mental Subnormality*, **XXXVIII**(2), 114–21.

Moss, S. and Turner, S. (1995). *The Health of People with Learning Disability.* Hester Adrian Research Centre, Manchester.

Moss, S., Goldberg, D., Patel, P. and Wilkin, D. (1993). Physical morbidity in older people with moderate, severe and profound mental handicap, and its relation to psychiatric morbidity. *Social Psychiatry and Psychiatric Epidemiology*, **28**(1), 32–9.

Naidoo, J. and Wills, J. (1994). *Health Promotion. Foundations for Practice.* Baillière Tindall, London.

Nightingale, C. (1992). Pointing the way ahead. Health education for people with learning disabilities. *Professional Nurse*, 612–15.

Perry, M. (1996). Treating obesity in people with learning disabilities. *Nursing Times*, **92**(35), 37–8.

Pitetti, K.H., Rimmer, J.H. and Fernhall, B. (1993). Physical fitness and adults with mental retardation. An overview of current research and future directions. *Sports Medicine*, **16**(1), 23–56.

Rimmer, J.H., Braddock, D. and Fujiura, G. (1993). Prevalence of obesity in adults with mental retardation: implications for health promotion and disease prevention. *Mental Retardation*, **31**(2), 83–8.

Rimmer, J.H., Braddock, D. and Marks, B. (1994). Health characteristics and behaviours of adults with mental retardation residing in three living arrangements. *Research in Developmental Disabilities*, **16**(6), 489–99.

Seedhouse, D. (1986). *Health: Foundations for Achievement.* Wiley, Bristol.

Stratford, B. and Gunn, P. (eds) (1996). *New Approaches to Down Syndrome.* Cassell, London.

Sturmey, P. (1995). DSM-III-R and persons with dual diagnosis: conceptual issues and strategies for future research. *Journal of Intellectual Disabilities Research*, **39**(5), 357–64.

Sturmey, P. and Sevin, J. (1993). Dual diagnosis: an annotated bibliography of recent research. *Journal of Intellectual Disabilities Research*, **37**(5), 437–48.

Szymanski, L. (1994). Mental retardation and mental health: concepts, aetiology and incidence. In *Mental Health in Mental Retardation. Recent Advances and Practices* (ed. N. Bouras), pp. 19–33. Cambridge University Press, Cambridge.

Tones, K., Tilford, S. and Robinson, Y. (1990). *Health Education: Effectiveness and Efficiency.* Chapman & Hall, London.

Thornton, C. (1994). Primary health care for adults with learning disabilities who live in the community – is a specialist nurse required? *Journal of Psychiatric and Mental Health Nursing*, **1** (2), 125–6.

Turner, S. and Moss, S. (1996). The health needs of adults with learning disabilities and the Health of the Nation strategy. *Journal of Intellectual Disabilities Research*, **40**(5), 238–50.

World Health Organization (1984). In Niadoo and Wills (1994). *Health Promotion. Foundations for Practice.* Baillière Tindall, London.

Part Four

Professional Roles and Their Interrelationships

Chapter 20

The Professions and Their Interrelationships

Jenny Weinstein

Key Issues

- Current systems of service delivery require close collaboration between different health and care professionals to serve the best interests of users.
- Different professionals sometimes hold conflicting views about the best way to serve users and carers and these differences can lead to breakdowns of communication between them.
- Differences between professionals may be minimized if users and carers are enabled to play a stronger role in the planning and decision-making for their care.
- The rapid changes in the roles of professionals, caused in particular by the introduction of the market, are creating problems of work overload, insecurity and loss of identity for many health and care professionals.

This sometimes increases defensiveness and impairs effective working together.
- Nevertheless, the barriers to and success factors for successful interprofessional collaboration have been identified by research.
- All health and care professionals should be prepared at pre- and post-qualifying levels with the competence (in terms of relevant knowledge, values and skills) which they need for interprofessional working.

Introduction

When a group of health and care professionals is asked about the advantages of collaboration or interprofessional working, they will invariably say that it is beneficial to service users. Child abuse inquiry reports (Blom-Cooper, 1985) and recent investigations of mental health scandals (Ritchie *et al.*, 1994) point to breakdowns in interprofessional communication as contributory factors. Those that hit the headlines are serious tragedies, involving loss of life or serious injury, but there are also numerous day-to-day examples of situations where service users have found themselves confused, or subject to conflicting advice or fragmented services because of inadequate co-ordination between services (Hornby, 1993).

Better collaboration sounds simple enough, but experience shows that it is in fact extremely complex. The stresses and strains of achieving inter-agency co-ordination, with all its bureaucracy, procedural difficulties, culture clashes and so on can become such an all-consuming activity in its own right that the users and carers are in danger of being excluded altogether (Biggs, 1993).

The position is exacerbated by the fact that health and care professionals are themselves ideologically under attack from both Left and Right. The Left have campaigned for the demystification of professional knowledge and the sharing of professional power with the consumer (Johnson, 1972; Illich, 1977) while the Right want the professionals to become less autonomous and more accountable to cost-conscious managers (King, 1987). The Right has questioned the need for so many professionals to undertake expensive training and argued that vocationally trained individuals (e.g. 'streetwise grandmas') could undertake many of the tasks currently undertaken by professionals (Weinstein, 1994). These threats have divided the professionals further in that some, concerned about lowering standards and losing specialist expertise, have taken refuge in defensiveness and a determined resistance to change; while others, enthusiasts for the market and the notion of 'consumer choice' are wholeheartedly implementing the new approaches (Bottery, 1995).

These issues are affecting all the professionals who work with people with learning disabilities – doctors, psychologists, community nurses, occupational therapists, housing officers, teachers, social workers, speech and language therapists, and many others. All these groups are under considerable pressure owing to worries about job insecurity, enormously increased workloads, especially paperwork, and concerns about cuts and reduced services to clients.

Government policy and guidance papers are full of exhortations to professionals and agencies to co-ordinate and work more closely together. New funding is often dependent on evidence of joint planning. However, on a macro-level, the structures, procedures and financing of the key agencies are so separate and complex that co-ordination involves cumbersome, time-consuming processes which are understandably abandoned under the strain of day-to-day pressures. At grass roots level, uni-professional training is still very insular and people are not prepared, at qualifying and pre-registration level, with the skills necessary for effective interprofessional working.

This chapter examines in more depth some of the problems which can impede interprofessional collaboration: differences in values and attitudes towards service users; insecurity and competition caused by the rapidly changing roles and status of professions; and the barriers to co-operation which exist at national, organizational and interpersonal levels. It suggests that the most important way of overcoming these is by ensuring that interprofessional work is user-driven and user-led (see also Chapter 13) so that decisions are based on stated user preferences rather than on the views, attitudes or outcome of power struggles between professionals. In addition, it recommends that people from all the professions should develop, as part of their basic training, the relevant knowledge, values and skills to facilitate successful interprofessional working. To this end, a list of competences for interprofessional working is suggested and recommendations are made as to how these might be acquired.

Conflicting Attitudes of Different Professionals Towards Users

Problems of collaboration between professionals have sometimes been attributed to differences in their 'values' or their approaches to 'ethics'. In practice, the values or ethics of a professional often mean the ideological or philosophical ideas that motivate their practice and influence their attitudes and beliefs about 'what is best' for the service user. Marx (1969) describes professional ideology as 'shared belief systems which guide and justify purposeful therapeutic actions'. While all professionals would be likely to agree that the users and their needs must come first, they may have conflicting views about how this can be achieved.

This is illustrated by a case study of community care undertaken by Dalley (1991) who found that 'In relation to a number of issues, doctors . . . were located at one end of an ideological continuum with field level social workers at the other. Nurses . . . were ranged between them'. Doctors were more likely to favour residential care, where, as they saw it, people were adequately cared for and risk was minimized, while social workers were much more in favour of community care because they believed that people's rights to make choices were more important than protecting them from possible harm. These differences may be linked to the fact that some professionals are more likely to iden-

tify with the users; others with the carers – another potential source of conflict.

Values and attitudes also influence the different theories and approaches to practice that professionals adopt. Normalization theory (Wolfensberger and Thomas, 1983) challenged the institutionalization of people with learning disabilities which led to the generally welcomed closure of the large mental handicap hospitals in the 1980s. However, this approach has since been criticized by the disability movement and by writers such as Chappell (1992), because it still leaves the power and decision-making about services in the hands of the professionals. Some professionals, nurses and social workers, for example, who work with people with learning disabilities may be far more radical than others, such as doctors and psychologists, in espousing the social, rather than the medical model of disability and in their interpretation of the notion of 'empowerment' (Means and Smith, 1994, p. 74).

The degree to which professionals consider and discuss their clients in a political and sociological context rather than simply as 'individuals with problems' can be another subject of conflict and misunderstanding. For example, the value base of social work teaches explicitly the importance of actively countering racism and discrimination. It also emphasizes the importance of valuing and respecting diversity between clients – such as differences in their language, culture, religion or sexual orientation. While many health professionals have adopted similar attitudes, others find this approach hard to understand because, they argue 'we treat all our patients the same'. A major problem for some service users is that many professionals do assume that everyone's needs are 'the same'. Hospital, field, residential and day care services therefore fail to cater for people's differences (e.g. alternative diets, wheelchair access, interpreters/ signers or other particular services).

Another debating point for different professions may be the 'voice' and 'exit' models of user empowerment which are helpfully elaborated by Means and Smith (1994, p. 82): they differentiate 'the *market* approach' which 'seeks to empower consumers by giving them choice between alternatives and the option of "exit" . . . (i.e. finding another service . . .)' from 'the *democratic* approach' which 'would keep more services in the public sector but seeks to empower users by giving them a "voice" in services and thereby the chance to change (i.e. transform) their existing service . . . '.

The responsibility of the professional is to minimize risk of harm to the patient and provide maximum care.	The responsibility of the professional is to ensure that the user chooses own preferred lifestyle, even if this involves a degree of risk to user's health/welfare.
'Normalization' People with learning disabilities and physical disabilities should be enabled as far as possible to live 'normal' lives.	*'Social model of disability'* The problem for people with disabilities is not their disability but the way in which society is organized to exclude them.
The job of the professional is to assist people who have individual problems such as illness, disability or social difficulties. They should not be involved with politics.	Many of the problems people have are caused by poverty, poor housing, discrimination and other political and social phenomena. Professionals should concern themselves with the causes of problems, as well as the problems themselves.
Professionals and public services are not discriminatory because they treat everyone the same.	Professionals and public services are discriminatory because they do not cater for people whose race, culture, religion or disability make it difficult or even impossible for them to access services which will meet their particular needs.
The professional should concern her/himself as much with the carers as with the users of services.	While the carer is important, and should be involved and consulted, the service user must be the prime client and the user's views should ultimately determine the nature of the service given.
The introduction of the 'market' is a good thing for service users. It means that they have choice. Competition will lead to improvement in services.	The introduction of the 'market' is not good for users. They are not the direct purchasers of services. 'Value for money' often means 'cheapest' and the most vulnerable groups in the community have neither the 'voice' nor the money to buy the services they need.

Box 1 Examples of ideological/value/ethical differences between professionals

Some professionals, especially those who have become managers, may welcome the market as a means of offering 'consumer choice'. On the other hand, those at the coal face are concerned that the market approach will undermine the welfare state and thus disadvantage people who, whether because of age, mental health or learning disability, are far too poor to be in a position to 'exit' from existing services or to seek and purchase alternatives.

Strongly held differing beliefs on these kinds of issues have been found in many studies to constitute an important barrier to collaboration. One way of dealing with this would be for the professionals to train together at an earlier stage, before attitudes and stereotypes become established. Another would be for them to confront their differences more openly and to debate the issues, not so much in general terms but in relation to individual service users with whom they are working. Some examples of conflicting views are provided in Box 1.

However, far the most effective solution would be for the user her or himself to have a much stronger say in the decision about 'what is best'. So, for example, where the doctor feels that Mrs Hussein would be much better off in a nice Sheltered Home where she would be properly looked after and the social worker thinks she would be happier living independently, the key question is – what does Mrs Hussein think? How far is she being provided with adequate jargon-free information, translated into her own language, if necessary, and helped, without being patronized, to consider the options so that she can make the decision herself? Does she have any particular religious, language, dietry or other needs which must be taken into account?

The only way to ensure that collaboration will benefit users and carers is to involve them directly in any initiative from the outset. The temptation to bring the profes-sionals together first, and consult the users later, must be avoided. It is tokenistic and likely to bring about an 'us' and 'them' situation with angry users and defensive professionals each trying to protect their own ground.

It is easy to make the mistake of bracket-ing 'users and carers' together as though their interests were the same. For example, some people with learning disabilities may feel that their carers are over-protective and want more intervention from the profes-sionals than is comfortable for the user. Professionals may think that a user group such as people with learning disabilities 'do not know what they want'. Self-advocacy groups such as People First have shown very clearly that this is far from the case (see example in Box 2).

The list in Box 3 provides some key poin-ters for good practice in working closely with users which, if followed, would also improve interprofessional collaboration.

The next section suggests that the bom-bardment of change being experienced by professionals may divert them from focus-ing on the users because of the threats and insecurities they themselves are facing.

The Evolving Roles of Professionals

The roles of health and care professionals have <u>changed</u> beyond recognition in the last decade, mainly as a result of the intro-duction of the market and the mixed econ-omy of welfare. Professionals have resisted the changes for a number of reasons. The market requires quantification and measure-ment of outcomes which some professionals claim as an inappropriate means of evaluat-ing their performance because it misunder-stands the concept of care. In other words: 'the introduction of the cash nexus into the

Croydon Social Services Department organized a large conference for local professionals and users when the Griffiths Report was first published to consult about expectations in relation to community care. People with learning disabilities, people with mental health problems, people with physical disabilities and older people were all represented. The people with learning disabilities were the most vocal. Their demands included:

- not having to go to the day centre if they feel like having a day at home;
- not being taken out in a large obvious group but going in ones and twos;
- having the opportunity of a holiday abroad;
- having the opportunity to participate in sports for disabled people;
- going to evening classes;
- being consulted and given choices about small domestic day-to-day issues.

Box 2 Case example

- Involve users and carers but recognize and allow space for their different views.
- Involve users and carers at all levels: planning, care management and service delivery.
- Ensure that users are part of the interprofessional team from the outset.
- Do not use professional jargon which excludes participation by users.
- Give users real choices by providing sufficient information, time and support for them to come to decisions.
- Acknowledge and be prepared to counter the discrimination which users experience by virtue of their disability and/or because of other disadvantages such as race, gender or poverty.
- Do not sacrifice the users' interests through interprofessional power play or point scoring.
- Be led by the user, in your interprofessional interaction, planning, care management and service delivery.

Box 3 User involvement in interprofessional collaboration – key pointers for good practice

relationship between purchaser and provider can lead to a slippery slope in which professional judgements can be "bought and negotiated" rather than accepted as of right' (Carrier and Kendall, 1995). Other concerns are that 'skill mix' will lead to deprofessionalization and a lowering of standards and that devolution of decision-making to local Trusts and units will undermine the maintenance of UK standards and lead to wide variations in the quality of service delivery across the country.

Box 4 lists some of the key changes which

are affecting the roles and status of health and care professionals.

While recruitment to medicine and the other therapy professions remains very competitive, retention is becoming a serious problem for many of these groups. As yet, there is only anecdotal evidence as to why this might be but demoralization, declining status and worsening remuneration and working conditions are thought to be contributory factors.

A closer look at the current position in general practice provides a useful illustra-

- The introduction of the mixed economy of welfare.
- Revolutionary discoveries in medical science which mean shorter stays in hospital and more focus on primary care.
- The closure of large institutions and the move to community care.
- More assertive, knowledgeable and critical service users with access to charters and complaints procedures leading to the demystification of 'professional expertise'.
- Increased managerial, administrative and financial responsibilities for professionals which take them away from patients/clients.
- Skill mix – i.e. the changing balance in numbers and roles of professionally qualified staff and support workers.
- Job insecurity, competition and the contract culture introduced into the public sector.
- The increased use of new technology which presents new ethical dilemmas.
- The introduction of quality assurance systems, audit and performance measures.
- A shift in emphasis in professional education from the acquisition of knowledge towards the development of skills and the ability to reflect critically.

Box 4 Examples of changes that have influenced the role and status of professionals

tion of many of the issues. GPs are notorious for failing to collaborate effectively with other professions (Dingwall, 1978; Birchall and Hallett, 1995). Non-medical health and care professionals will happily unite in jokes and criticisms at the doctors' expense. However, a closer look will find the 'arrogant superior and domineering' doctor facing similar struggles to those of other health and care professionals. A report by the RCGP (1994) indicates that GPs are more demoralized than they have ever been. There is a severe shortage of GPs with older doctors wanting to retire much earlier than previously and fewer young doctors wanting to become GPs. Watkins *et al.* (1992, p. 45) cite a survey in which a group of doctors was interviewed approximately 10 years after they had qualified in 1981 and 46% regretted their choice of career. They also point out that in the 1990s complaints against family doctors have increased by more than 50%.

GPs are dissatisfied with their ever-increasing workload, their very long hours

and the vast amounts of administration involved in budgeting and fundholding. The change of orientation towards primary care and community care has meant significant new responsibilities for sicker and more vulnerable people who might previously have been in hospital. Some models advocate the GP as the central or lead professional in community care and primary care with whom all the other professionals will plan and liaise. In large fundholding practices, which employ a range of health and care professionals to work as part of the primary health care team, this model can work well, but it is still more often the ideal than the reality. Stott (1995) describes the shift and its problems as follows:

An increasing need for chronic disease care and health promotion and the shift of acute health care from hospital to community have been associated with a rising emphasis on general practice based teamwork, special interests, consumerism, information support systems and commercial incentives to conform to what Government regards as appropriate clinical activity. . . . The political rhetoric builds on the strengths of a traditional general practice based National Health Service. The reality is a major lurch towards changing the doctor–patient relationship to provide a service to patients by a variable sized primary team.

Social work is another example of a profession radically affected by the introduction of the market. In this case, the impact has, in some ways, been even more fundamental because it has challenged the very heart of the identity of social workers and the very nature of their work. 'What has emerged is a reconstruction of social work and the way in which it operates which is very consistent with the central themes characterising the reconstruction of welfare more generally' (Parton, 1996, p. 10; see Box 5).

Twenty years ago, on their training courses, student social workers were taught a range of therapeutic interventions, based mainly on psychology, with a significant counselling component, collectively known as 'case-work'. This approach concentrated on understanding the individual in the

context of their immediate family and close relationships. In the late 1960s and early 1970s, the emphasis changed on some courses to focus on sociology and politics. Students were encouraged to consider the problems and behaviour of their clients in relation to their wider environment, in particular the poverty and deprivation with which they struggled. In the 1980s and early 1990s this discourse was extended to include the nature of structural and institutional oppression, racism and discrimination and its impact on the life chances and access to services of marginalized groups.

In the 1970s, 'group work' and 'community work' were popular social work interventions, aimed to encourage clients to support each other in demanding improved services such as welfare rights, housing or child care facilities. This was seen as 'empowering' people to fight for their rights to a decent life rather than stigmatizing them as 'problems or misfits'. Considerable energy, enthusiasm and commitment was vested in these kinds of struggles, with and on behalf of clients. During the 1980s, when it was part of the ethos for social workers to identify with campaigns to fight the cuts, defend the unions, prevent the closures of schools, hospitals and nurseries and to oppose racism and discrimination in service delivery, they came under severe attack from the Right who saw them as part of 'the enemy within'.

A newly qualified social worker entering the service in the mid-1990s will have been prepared for an entirely different kind of job. S/he will be expected to make assessments and develop packages of care, to undertake risk assessment and to intervene in accordance with relevant legislation and procedures, to write reports and to use information technology and to work openly and in partnership with service users and their carers who are now called 'consumers' rather than 'clients'. Social workers may

- The purchaser/provider split.
- Services based on need and the assessment of risk, rather than demand.
- Devolvement of budgets.
- The promotion of choice through consumer competition.
- Contractual rather than hierarchical responsibility.
- The introduction of business planning, target setting, performance indicators and outcome measures. (Parton, 1996, p. 10)

Box 5 Main features of changes in the delivery of welfare affecting the social work role refer people for counselling but this will be provided by someone else (often an ex health or care professional who has turned to counselling for a more satisfying job), and political campaigning, where it still occurs, is strictly extra curricular and marginalized. The cartoon in Figure 20.1 illustrates some of the changes over the last three decades.

While social workers have always had to ration resources and police risk, there was a degree of apology and defensiveness about these roles and responsibilities and their preferred image was primarily as the client's counsellor and the client's champion. The ascendancy of the market has forced a significant shift of emphasis from the latter role to the former and has caused a crisis of identity and serious demoralization for many social workers. Some social workers hoped that this would be ameliorated through the creation of a General Social Services Council which would legitimize

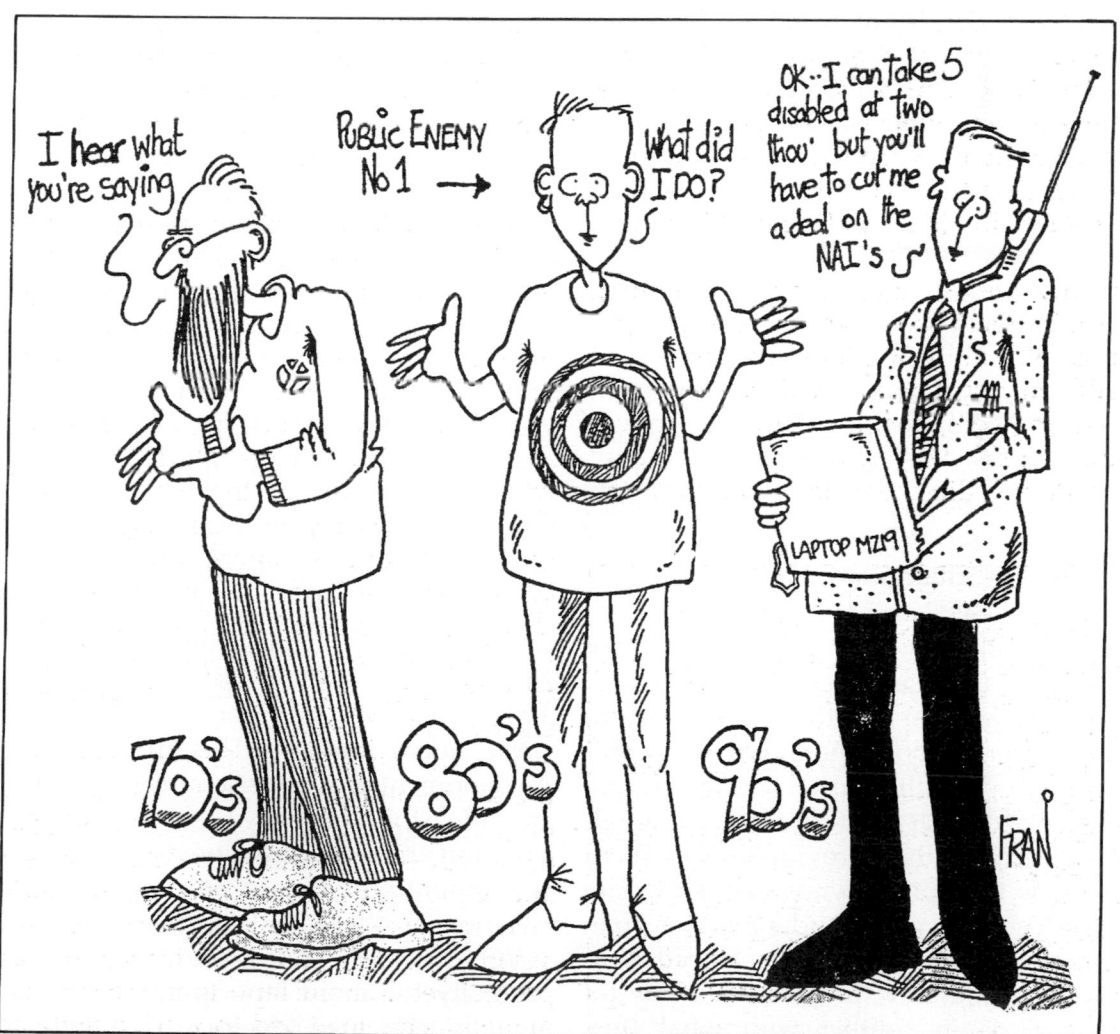

Figure 20.1 The changing face of social work. NAI, non-accidental injury, is social work jargon for child abuse. Reproduced with kind permission of the artist, Fran Orford

- Address the problems associated with single-discipline training and, in particular, the inflexibility for both the trainee and the organization.
- Redesign professional training to deliver the generic professional rather than single occupations.
- Introduce a common core programme for all health care workers, including medical students.
- Recruit trainee therapists, trainee medics and trainee nurses from experienced patient carers instead of from school leavers to ensure suitability for the job and less chance of drop out later on.
- Design jobs around occupational standards with the right to practise subject to assessment of competence.
- Utilize the accreditation of prior learning (AP(E)L) to enable trainees to enter programmes at different stages, depending on their experience.
- Ensure that employers play a leading role in all aspects of education and training.
- Use occupational standards to develop multidisciplinary teams and identify common skills between professions.
- Provide all staff and trainees with a portfolio in which to record achievement for the purposes of further training or career transfer.
- Bring together the different funding systems for health education.

Box 6 Some of the proposals from the report on *The Future of the Health Care Workforce* (Conrane Consulting *et al.*, 1996)

social work as a 'registered profession'. Others see the creation of such a body, which would be part of 'the establishment', as the final betrayal by social workers of their role as champions of the poor and the dispossessed.

Social work may be an extreme example but many of the issues faced by social workers will be familiar to others in the Health Service: occupational therapists and community nurses who are working as care managers; district nurses who supervise assistants rather than provide direct patient care and therapists whose services are rationed according to budget rather than delivered in response to patient need. Professionals frequently find that their day-to-day work is in conflict with what they believe to be their fundamental professional values (Weinstein, 1996).

A report by Conrane Consulting *et al.*

(1996) on behalf of a number of NHS management organizations anticipates further developments along these lines for the NHS workforce of the future. Their recommendations focus on developing an increase in functional flexibility of all NHS staff. The outcome would be the same scenario as that first mooted by the Audit Commission in 1986 which was so vigorously opposed by professional bodies. This proposed the development of a 'generic carer' who would provide the majority of direct hands on care and co-ordination for patients in the community. Non-professional, Scottish /National Vocational Qualification (S/NVQ) qualified staff, would increase incrementally by about 20% in ratio to professionally educated doctors and therapists who would undertake specialist roles only. This revolutionary change would be achieved by radically altering the way health care staff are trained. Box 6 comprises some of the main suggestions of the steering group.

These kinds of proposals are seen by many professionals as a threat to their power and autonomy. It has made them more protective of their territory, more inward looking and less inclined to share and collaborate with other professionals whom they view as potential competitors. However, these 'head in the sand' attitudes will neither assure the maintenance of standards nor curb the excesses of the market.

Carrier and Kendall (1995) suggest a way forward which both acknowledges the necessity for closer collaboration while constructively resisting deprofessionalization and the lowering of standards. They propose a thorough reconsideration of professional ethics and values in the context of current service delivery systems. In this author's view, if such a review was undertaken interprofessionally it could provide an important basis for mutual respect and understanding. It could also ensure a jointly agreed minimum standard held by all professionals as a means of holding at bay the criteria of cost effectiveness, as the only valid measure. Carrier and Kendall (1995) also advocate that professionals should be prepared to review and change practice and to redraw boundaries in line with current needs, without diluting standards. This would be achieved by developing a co-ordinated approach and continuous interprofessional evaluation of the new ways of working.

This section has identified some of the political, ideological and economic factors which are affecting the roles and status of professionals. The next section examines the structures and processes through which collaboration occurs and identifies some of the barriers to success.

Barriers to and Success Factors for Effective Interprofessional Collaboration

Multidisciplinary team work can imply anything on a continuum from the tight-knit team working from its own base to much wider networks across and between different agencies (Øvretveit, 1993). Hunter and Wistow (1987) identify three levels at which collaboration needs to take place: *national or interdepartmental, local or inter agency* and *field or interdisciplinary*. Øvretveit (1993) identifies three processes which correspond with these three levels: the *market* process whereby co-ordination is via exchange of services for money; the *bureaucratic* process where structures and procedures are established to facilitate collaboration between agencies; and *association* whereby collaboration is based on trust and communication between people from different professions at field level.

On a national level the Government has advocated collaboration in all its circulars and guidance documents since the White Paper on community care (DOH, 1989). However, successive ministers have failed to acknowledge the structural, financial and procedural barriers that exist or to provide the necessary resources required to overcome them. While a holistic approach to service users is urged, finance is designated for either 'health care' or 'social care'. Social Services tend to be means tested while Health Services are still expected to be free at the point of delivery. The oft quoted 'health bath' or 'social bath' and the debate about who should pay for nursing home care graphically exemplify these contradictions. Problems of service users being shunted between agencies who each deny budgetary responsibility are frequently due to these arbitrary financial divisions. In an early study of community care, Challis et al. (1989) recommended a joint agency approach with a single budget, while Øvretveit (1993) points out the downside of adopting such a model which would limit flexibility and choice.

On the inter-agency level, Local Authority Social Service Departments are expected to submit annual joint plans with Health Services to meet the community care needs of their locality. While this process has brought some improvement in co-ordination, the reality in practice is that the two agencies operate very differently and quite independently from each other.

Housing has become a key agency in the community care equation, and here too communication and liaison leave much to be desired. Attempts are being made to address this in some localities where Housing and Social Services have been combined into a single department but far more detailed work is needed to provide a 'seamless service'. The Department of the Environment and the Department of Health have drawn up a checklist for assessing closer collaboration between Housing and Social Services (Community Care, 1996, p. 5; see Box 7).

From the perspective of individual practitioners, as already indicated, the emphasis on teamwork and collaboration is occurring in a climate where competition and job insecurity lead to increasing protectionism and distrust. This problem is exacerbated by the continuing tendency to train and socialize health care professionals narrowly within their own discipline (Hilton, 1995), embedding many of the problems at an early stage.

Research which compared team performance amongst primary health care teams with a range of teams from different occupational settings found that the primary health care teams have less clear objectives, lower levels of participation, lower levels of interaction-frequency and poorer task orientation than the others (West and Poulton, 1995).

A number of authors and researchers have indicated a range of success factors for interdisciplinary teams (Pearson and Spencer, 1995; West and Field, 1995a, b). These include, the need for common understanding and common goals and objectives, regular interaction between members, equal participation by and valuing of all members, meaningful and challenging tasks for all participants, and joint evaluation and action planning. It is important to establish clear decision-making processes with a small enough number of people for this to be realistic. Issues of hierarchy, status, race, gender and other structural differences, which either exclude key people or give one or two individuals more say than they deserve, need to be confronted openly. Everyone needs to feel that their special skills are being used to the full and that their unique contribution is recognized

- Effective mechanisms for joint planning.
- Social Services influence in spending Housing resources.
- Housing involvement in developing community care plans, and Social Services participation in the Housing strategy.
- Joint training including secondment or work experience between departments.
- Mechanism to identify and address the needs of people in hospital.
- Policies that are preventive and not just reactive.
- Account taken of users' and carers' views.

Box 7 Checklist for improved co-ordination between Housing and Social Services and valued. When some team members do not pull their weight, it may be because they feel alienated or marginalized; valuing and respecting their contribution will improve the team's effectiveness.

Clear jargon-free communication must be established in a relaxed atmosphere where people feel comfortable enough to ask if they do not understand, or to say if they disagree. A blaming culture should be

- Lack of shared aims or goals.
- Different language/jargon.
- Conflicting values/ethics/attitudes.
- Different cultures.
- Status differences – minority dominate.
- Race and gender issues – lack of involvement and participation by key members.
- Lack of knowledge about each other's roles.
- Lack of clarity about tasks and responsibilities.
- Power struggles – who is the 'key-worker' or who is in charge?
- Unexpressed conflict leading to poor communication and distrust.
- Inability/unwillingness to share.
- Lack of knowledge about group/organizational dynamics.
- Lack of self-awareness.
- Rigid and narrow view of own remit.
- Lack of clarity about inter-agency procedures and decision-making processes.
- Size of team too large for successful interaction.

Box 8 Barriers to interdisciplinary functioning have been identified as:

- Common understanding and common goals and objectives.
- Clear jargon-free communication.
- Effective leadership.
- Regular interaction between members.
- Equal participation by and valuing of all members.
- Meaningful and challenging tasks for all participants.
- Joint evaluation and action planning.
- Clear decision-making processes.
- Small enough number of people to facilitate thorough and regular communication.
- Open acknowledgement of power issues related to hierarchy, status, race, gender and other structural differences.
- Open acknowledgement and resolution of conflict.
- Recognition of the unique contribution of each member of the team.

Box 9 Success factors for working in an interdisciplinary team.

avoided. Instead, the team should work together to evaluate their performance and to identify and rectify problems and ineffectiveness. Leadership is needed in teams as long as it is supportive and facilitative providing vision and motivation. Critical and domineering leadership will lead to demoralization and ineffectiveness.

In an effective team, the issue of professional status differences will not be a problem, neither will confidentiality, the allocation of tasks or the referral process. There will be trust and confidence between members and the advice which patients receive will be consistent. Where these factors cause problems, the use of a facilitator to help the team diagnose and resolve their problems can be very helpful.

Boxes 8 and 9 summarize some of the barriers to and success factors for effective interprofessional collaboration in teams.

This section has identified some of the structural and interpersonal problems that prevent effective collaboration and suggested ways that these may be tackled at local level. The next section suggests ways in which professionals can be prepared to overcome barriers to collaboration and acquire the necessary knowledge values and skills for effective interprofessional working.

Competences for Interprofessional Working

While it is beyond the scope of this chapter to address the many complex structural financial and procedural changes which would be needed to overcome some of the barriers identified above, some proposals are made below about how professionals could be more effectively prepared to work interprofessionally. Success factors for effective interdisciplinary teamwork

have been identified through research and listed in the previous section. It should be possible to facilitate these by preparing health and care professions with the necessary competences for interprofessional working at the qualifying/pre-registration stage.

It is important to note that as the roles and relationships of professionals are changing in practice, their education systems are also in a state of upheaval, causing parallel debates and controversies. In particular, there are strong disagreements surrounding the use of the word 'competences' in relation to professional education. Some critics (Webb, 1992) regard the process of breaking down professional training into observable actions which can be monitored and assessed (Ellis, 1988) as over-simplified and mechanistic. They argue that this methodology cannot be applied to complex roles that require extensive specialist knowledge, the ability to make difficult decisions and continuous 'reflection in action' as described by Schon (1987).

In this chapter, the use of the word 'competence' does not imply a reductionist approach. It means a combination of specialist knowledge, values and skills which enables the professional to perform to a satisfactory standard in the work context. This kind of competence, which some prefer to call 'capability' is essential to interprofessional working. Attention is beginning to be paid both on uniprofessional courses (Whittington, 1992) and on programmes of joint or shared learning (Barr and Shaw, 1995) to preparing new professionals with the competences they will require to undertake effective interprofessional collaboration in the service of users. Building on some of the work that has already been achieved, a more systematic approach to the achievement of competences for interprofessional working is suggested below.

The Care Sector Consortium (CSC), which

2.3. Enable practitioners and agencies to work collaboratively to improve the effectiveness of services, products and activities which contribute to health and social well-being.

6.2. Develop and sustain joint working across different agencies to promote health and social well-being.

8.2. Co-ordinate initiatives and programmes to raise awareness of health and health issues.

9.4. Contribute to the joint planning, implementation, monitoring and review of care interventions for groups of clients.

9.5. Co-ordinate an interdisciplinary team to meet clients' and carers' assessed needs.

Box 10 Units and elements from *Draft National Occupational Standards for Three Groups of Health Care Practitioners* (CSC Consultation Documents: Standards overview July 1996, prepared by Prime Consultants)

is the Occupational Standards Council for health and social care is, at the time of writing, developing National Occupational Standards for three groups of health care practitioners. Box 10 provides examples of some of the units and elements which have been identified in relation to interprofessional collaboration.

The standards in Box 10 are those which would be expected of a practitioner 1–2 years into practice. Rather than breaking these down into elements, range statements and performance criteria in the style of NCVQ, it is suggested that for education and training at professional level it is more useful to think in terms of the relevant knowledge values and skills that students would need to acquire in order to achieve these standards.

Knowledge areas could be taught in interprofessional groups at college where students might work on joint projects or use a problem-based learning approach. Skills and values could be developed and assessed in practice placements working with other professionals from whom they would receive support and feedback. Those professionals who were not prepared in this way on their initial training could acquire

their interprofessional competence as part of continuing professional development.

The knowledge, values and skills listed in Boxes 11–13 have been developed from the author's personal experience of and research into interprofessional work. This was assisted by the work of Engel (Engel, 1994) who suggested some competences for interprofessional work; Kane (1976) who produced a list of knowledge, skills and attitudes for working interprofessionally; and CCETSW (1995) who laid down values requirements for qualifying social workers.

Summary and Recommendations

- Interprofessional collaboration is esential to high quality health and care service delivery. The key to effectiveness is a user-led system whereby the user (and carer) work in equal partnership with the professionals. This approach must be developed at national, organizational and field levels facilitated by appropriate structures and resources.

- The current climate is a very difficult one

Other agencies and professions

- Knowledge of current social policy and its impact on the provision of health and welfare services.
- Knowledge and understanding of the roles of other related professionals, the ways these are changing and the impact this may have on their ways of working.
- Knowledge and understanding of the procedures involved in referral to other agencies.
- Knowledge and understanding of a range of different organizational structures and systems, including finance and budget allocation.
- Knowledge and understanding of interorganizational structures and processes.
- Knowledge and understanding of organizational and interorganizational dynamics.
- Knowledge and understanding of other professions' likely perceptions or misconceptions of own profession and role.

Working as a team or group

- Knowledge and understanding of group dynamics, including group process, stages of group development, leadership styles, decision-making, characteristics of performing and non-performing groups.
- Knowledge and understanding of own role in groups.
- Knowledge and understanding of institutional oppression and discrimination and the way in which this influences the ability of women, black people, service users or people with disabilities to be appropriately represented and influential in group process and decision-making.

Managing change

- Knowledge of the impact of change on staff at all levels in organizations.
- Knowledge of own reaction to change.
- Knowledge of positive strategies for managing change including clear communication; involvement of people in decision-making as far as is appropriate; acknowledging and dealing with loss and conflict; making plans within realistic time scales and keeping to these.
- Knowledge of relevant research methods and systems of audit and evaluation to improve and develop interprofessional effectiveness.

Box 11 Knowledge required for interprofessional working

in which to foster collaboration because professionals themselves feel under so much pressure from the rapid rate of change and the contradictions posed by a market approach to welfare. One response, which must be resisted, is to become rigidly protectionist and to close ranks within a single profession. The other equally dangerous solution is to

be carried away by the logic of the market and forget the real purpose of providing health and welfare services.

- A more effective approach may be to share the problems and to constructively review professional values and ethics collaboratively in the light of the market and the rapid developments in technology. A shared value base between the profes-

- A preparedness to acknowledge and explore own values and prejudices and the impact these may have on relationships with users, carers and fellow professionals.
- A user-centred perspective which fosters active participation of users in all decisions about their lives and their care, which respects their rights to choice, self-determination and confidentiality and which builds on strengths.
- An approach which respects and values difference and recognizes users, carers and fellow professionals as unique individuals with their own needs, culture, beliefs and values systems.
- Respect for the knowledge skills and commitment of people with a different professional training.
- Recognition of the need of all team members for recognition, appreciation and self-esteem.
- A preparedness to counter all forms of discrimination, racism, inequality and injustice and to practice in a manner which does not stigmatize or disadvantage users, carers, care workers or fellow professionals.
- A commitment to improving services to users by continuous reflection and the research and evaluation of outcomes and performance.

Box 12 Values required for interprofessional working

sions may form a more effective barrier against deteriorating standards than uniprofessional 'tribalism'.

- Similarly, the professionals need to work together without being defensive, to acknowledge where boundaries need to be redrawn and practices changed to meet modern service delivery needs. Together, they could argue that professionally trained staff should continue to provide hands on services to users but with improved co-ordination and shared training, this can be achieved without unnecessary overlap or wasting resources.
- All trainee professionals should be prepared with the necessary competences for interprofessional practice on their qualifying preregistration courses. Where possible shared learning in college and in practice should be facilitated.

Discussion Questions

- Look at Box 1 and discuss your own views on each issue. Do you think it would be possible for health and care professionals to develop a common set of values and ethics? If not, what are the barriers to this?
- Do you think services would be improved if a single agency covering all aspects of community care was established to replace separate Housing, Social Services and Health Departments?
- What strategies would you recommend for training and supporting health and care professionals to work together more effectively? For example, would you support:

- Develop trust and confidence in others by carrying out own professional role clearly and competently.
- Be reliable and punctual and keep other professionals closely informed about work with people whom they have referred or with whom they are working.
- Communicate and negotiate clearly and without jargon, orally and in writing, within small groups, larger organizations and between organizations.
- Acknowledge honestly own lack of knowledge or understanding about views or actions of other professionals and listen actively to explanations or opinions.
- Use communication and negotiation skills to explain own professional role, agree goals and priorities, allocate tasks, implement decisions, evaluate outcomes and renegotiate action where necessary.
- Express respect and appreciation for the contribution of all team members and fellow professionals.
- Share tasks and be flexible about the division of roles and responsibilities.
- Recognize and empathize with the complexities of the work of other professionals and the difficulties that they may encounter in undertaking their tasks.
- Encourage and facilitate the active involvement of users, carers, care workers or fellow professionals, who by reason of status, gender, race or other structural disadvantage, may feel less confident about their role and contribution.
- Acknowledge and resolve differences of view or conflict openly and without personal rancour.
- Develop strategies for coping with change, ambiguity and uncertainty and for helping others to do so.
- Seek advice, information and support from others to improve own performance.
- Constructively provide advice, information and support to others when requested.
- Continually reflect on own performance and means of improving this and engage with others on joint evaluation and development of practice.

Box 13 Skills required for interprofessional working

(a) a common foundation year for all health and care professionals as a basis for further uniprofessional training?
(b) more joint training and shared learning throughout qualifying training?
(c) focusing more on 'on the job' development and training at the post-qualifying stage?

REFERENCES

Audit Commission (1986). *Making a Reality of Community Care*. HMSO, London.

Barr, H. and Shaw, I. (1995). *Shared Learning: Selected Examples from the Literature*. CAIPE, London.

Biggs, S. (1993). User participation and interprofessional collaboration in community care. *Journal of Interprofessional Care*, **7**(2), 151–9. Marylebone Centre Trust, London.

Birchall, E. and Hallett, C. (1995). *Working Together in Child Protection*. HMSO, London.

Blom-Cooper, L. (1985). *A Child in Trust*. Kingswood Press, Harrow, Middlesex.

Bottery, M. (1995). *Education Markets, Post-Fordism,*

Chapter 21

Professions in Teams

David Sines and Owen Barr

Key Issues

- Changes influencing teams
- Assumptions about teamwork
- When is a group of people a team?
- Levels of collaboration
- Operational cultures
- Enhancing teamwork
- Indicators for effective teamwork
- Working across boundaries
- Teamwork and crisis intervention
- Challenges

Introduction

In 1992, Brown concluded his chapter on 'Professions in teams' on a positive note. He believed that community mental handicap teams (now referred to as community learning disability teams) would continue to develop and 'show the way forward in multidisciplinary approaches to service provision' (p. 385).

Several major changes, that have implications for community learning disability teams (CLDTs) have occurred in Health and Social Services since then. Some of the changes are developments of previous structures and include aspects such as the increasing focus on mixed economy of care; major developments in the service provision by the independent (private and not for profit) sector; more clients and their families acting as consumers of services with increased opportunities for representation; further reductions in the amount of hospital provision for people with learning disabilities; an increased emphasis on people living at home; and the development of respite care provision.

Other changes have arisen with the implementation of new arrangements for service provision. These include mandatory taking of 'Trust status' for Health Services (combined Health and Social Services Trusts exist in N. Ireland); the national introduction of care management; the national introduction of General Practitioner (GP) fundholding; and plans for Direct Care Payments.

In the professional arena there has been the development of Continuing/Higher Education Framework by the UK National Boards for Nursing, Midwifery and Health

Visiting, the UKCC standards for Post-Registration and Practice Project (PREP), a focus on competence-based training seen most clearly in National Vocational Qualifications (NVQs), and the development of an increased number of interdisciplinary courses, some providing dual nursing and social work qualifications. The ability to work competently as a team member is a key competence in most current undergraduate professional curricula, and is a central theme in the majority of continuing professional education.

As a result of these changes, the expectations of what will be provided have been raised. People with learning disabilities and their families expect more flexible, accessible and individually tailored services. The emphasis on the cost of services has led to many managers expecting greatly increased work output with little or no extra resources.

In the short space of time since 1992, much has changed in the way in which services are planned, funded and delivered. At times members of CLDTs could be forgiven for thinking that they are compromised between the raised expectations of people with learning disabilities, families and managers, and the ever-increasing pressure for cost efficiency.

This chapter considers the changing nature of teamwork within services for people with learning disabilities. In doing so, it considers issues relating to the definition and functioning of teams and how teamwork may be enhanced.

Why Have a Team?

This question often meets with a puzzled expression and a series of vague answers such as, 'because teams are more effective', 'teams are better', or 'it increases the quality of the service'. It appears at times as if

the question has not been seriously considered, and an assumption exists that teams, in particular multidisciplinary teams, are always positive. However, there is no room in services for assumptions about any aspect of services – all decisions should be based on a balanced consideration of the available evidence.

Considerable attention has been given to the value of teamwork over the past few years in relation to areas such as care of people who are elderly; child protection; mental health services; palliative care; and primary health care (Owens et al., 1995). Prior to 1992, several significant studies by McGrath and Humphreys (1988 cited in Hudson, 1995), Brown and Wistow (1990) and McGrath (1991) provided supporting evidence that CLDTs made a valuable contribution to services for people with learning disabilities and their families. These studies also highlighted difficulties to be overcome in relation to the priorities set within the teams; leadership; internal communication; accountability; and strategies for team evaluation. A recent study by Aylott and Todcaram (1996) also confirmed the important contribution that a CLDT had made to the lives of people with learning disabilities and their families. These authors highlighted the need to ask for feedback on services for service users and purchasers of services in an attempt to streamline the service provided to what is required. Among their findings considerable differences were noted in the expectations of people with learning disabilities and their carers; a high desire for greater emergency/on-call access was a priority for people with learning disabilities and families; and people with profound learning disability had less contact with the CLDT than people with mild learning disabilities. Careful attention needs to be given to the last finding, especially in the light of the focus on current services responding to those in the greatest need. Unfortunately, few studies into the work of CLDTs have been published in the past few years. This is surprising in the light of the fact that over the past 5 years CLDTs have probably been under more scrutiny than ever before. It is likely, therefore, that a substantial number of local studies and evaluations have been undertaken, but in many cases this information has not been shared with a wider audience and appears destined to remain at a local level. Unfortunately, this seriously restricts the opportunities to learn from the experience of others. However, the value of CLDTs does not appear to have been widely assessed in the past 5 years. This adds further weight to the argument that an assumption about the usefulness of teamwork exists.

The potential benefits of cohesive teamwork are considerable for people with learning disabilities, their families, team members and the overall service organization (Table 21.1). Benefits may primarily relate to one group of people but in reality, owing to the interrelationships among those involved, improvements or weakness in groups of people will have an impact on everyone else to a greater or lesser extent.

The achievements of CLDTs to date have been summarized by Hudson (1995) and include recognizing that planning must be needs led; involving clients and their carers;

Table 21.1 Some anticipated benefits of teamwork. Developed from Rawson (1994), Hudson (1995) and Pritchard (1995)

People with learning disabilities/families

- Increased co-ordination of services.
- Key-worker system operates more effectively.
- Continuity of care increased.
- Greater speed and accuracy of response to client needs.
- Rare skills used more appropriately.
- Enhances preventive work.
- Holistic approach to individual service planning.

Team members

- More effective communication between professionals.
- Greater appreciation of colleagues' roles.
- Increased learning opportunities for team members to enhance their skills and knowledge.
- Broader perspectives on services.
- Shared values.
- Reduced defensiveness and territorialism.
- Peer support and informal learning between members.
- Increased job satisfaction and better able to cope with stresses and strains of the job.

Service organization

- Increased flexibility in roles.
- Reduced costs due to the sharing of offices and other equipment.
- Breakdown of divisive professional barriers.
- Reduces potential overlaps and gaps in services.
- Contributes to the promotion of positive image of a progressive service.

assisting to clarify professional roles; demonstrating ways of working together; strengthen co-operation between Health and Social Services at client, local and strategic planning levels; and establishing a substantial specialist fieldwork resource and securing 'ringfenced' funding.

The potential benefits provide strong incentives to develop interdisciplinary teams. The temptation should be avoided to set up teams primarily because they will improve the image of the service; it is a 'trendy' thing to do; everybody else is doing it; or amalgamation is a back door to saving money.

Not all voices are in favour of the present form of 'teamwork' and some doubt has been cast on the assumption that teamwork is always positive, or even on balance a positive option. Braye and Preston-Shoot (1995) asserted that the 'track record of multidisciplinary teamwork remains unimpressive' (p. 147).

Difficulties that may arise when attempting to increase the amount of multidisciplinary teamwork include aspects such as development of a culture of conformity; suppression of conflict and innovation; too many people involved in the decision-making process (slowing-down process); increased tiers of management; expensive to maintain; and poor quality of decisions made due to the influence 'group think' (Janis, 1983). Careful attention should be given to the possibility of this deficiency in decision-making within CLDTs. As such, all team members should be vigilant for the antecedent conditions, characteristic symptoms and defects in decision-making (see Table 21.2).

The need to seriously reflect on the desire for teams is clear in the note of caution provided by Hattersley (1995) who states that 'many organisations evolve gradually, without explicit review, and the resulting "monsters" can often establish their own demands for collaboration which exist only because of unnecessary division and barriers which have developed' (p. 261).

The primary reason for setting up a CDLT, or any other team within Health and Social Services should be that the new structure will provide a higher quality service to clients and their families than the previous arrangements.

When is a Group of People a Team?

The word 'team' is used as if everyone has a clear understanding of what it means. However, this clear understanding is not present and teamwork has become a 'catch all' phrase that is more often used than practised. Leathard (1994) provides evidence of the confusion about teamwork when she identifies 52 terms that have been used to describe joint working. This degree of confusion is the first major obstacle to teamwork; without a clear understanding of exactly what is meant by 'teamwork' several people could be using similar language and meaning different things.

The concept of a team is more than a group of individual practitioners who are placed together, renamed and referred to as a team. Although this collection of people may have the potential to become an effective team, if all they have in common is a location or collective name then they are a group and nothing more. Such a collection of people could be designated as a 'pseudo team'. That is

a group of people who are called, or who call themselves, a team . . . but don't actually try to co-ordinate what they are doing or establish collective responsibility . . . in reality they act on a purely individual level and are concerned only with their own departments and responsibilities. (Hayes, 1997, p. 129)

Table 21.2 Components of 'group think' decision-making. Developed from Moorhead *et al.* (1991)

Antecedents	Characteristic symptoms	Defects in decision-making
Cohesive group	Team believe they are invulnerable	Few alternatives considered
Leader preference for a particular decision	Rationalization to discount any warnings against the preferred decision	No re-examination of alternatives
		Rejecting of expert opinions
Insulation from experts who would be able to challenge decision	Team members believe without doubt in the morality of their decision	Rejecting negative information
		No contingency plans
	Stereotyped views held of other people outside the team	
	Pressure on people who dissent from the preferred decision to change their view	
	Self-censorship by group members if they deviate from the preferred decision – group members undervalue their own importance	
	An illusion of the need for and presence of unanimity 'Mindguarding' – key team members withhold information that may result in a challenge of the decision from other team members	

Real teams are characterized by ownership of shared aims and objectives, a defined membership, and a clear structure. To become an effective team, a commitment to working together, which is built on mutual trust and respect, and a strong bond between members are also required.

The majority of teams that provide services to people with learning disabilities are now multidisciplinary in their membership. However, not all teams are multidisciplinary – some single-profession teams remain. These are normally of two varieties.

First, generic teams exist within professional groupings often among the professions allied to medicine, such as occupational therapy, speech therapy and physiotherapy. Members of a locality-based service team may provide services to people with learning disabilities as one of a number of clients' groups they visit. These staff may also be part-time members of a CLDT as well as members of their professional team. CLDTs could have a combination of full-time, part-time, core, contracted or associate team members (Øvretveit, 1993).

Second, single profession teams continue to exist in some nursing and Social Service

Departments. These teams are specific teams of staff who only work with people with learning disabilities and their families. Even though they may work in co-operation with other professional groups, they are managed completely separately. The members of such a team identify with a uniprofessional orientation and not on shared values across a number of professional groups. Indeed, the objectives of single profession teams and multidisciplinary teams may at times be in conflict with each other.

Recently, a distinction has been made between multiprofessional work and interprofessional work. Carrier and Kendall (1995) stated that

multiprofessional work is a co-operative enterprise in which traditional forms and division of professional knowledge are retained. . . . Interprofessional work implies a willingness to share and indeed give up exclusive claims to specialised knowledge and authority, if the needs of the clients can be met more effectively by other professional groups. (Carrier and Kendall, 1995, p. 10)

This distinction challenges staff to consider in more detail the extent to which they work as a team.

No set formula exists for the membership of CLDTs and considerable variation has been shown to be present (McGrath and Humphreys, 1988; Brown, 1990; Jenkins and Johnson, 1991; Aylott and Todcaram, 1996). The size and function of CLDTs often differ from one place to another. This variation is influenced by aspects such as the previous service structures; resources available including money and people; the level of commitment to teamwork; local politics; and a vision of future services.

At present, no concrete and universally accepted definition for a team, be it unidisciplinary, multidisciplinary or interdisciplinary, exists. In summary, the commonly agreed characteristics of effective teams include a defined membership; agreed values, aims, objectives and priorities; a clear structure and team procedures; and a commitment to work together.

Collaboration – a Crucial Factor

Current 'teams' within services for people with learning disabilities could fall into any of the following categories: groups, teams, multidisciplinary teams or interdisciplinary teams. A crucial distinguishing factor is the level of collaboration evidenced. Collaboration requires time and favourable conditions for the team to develop. Thus, the antecedents of collaboration include individual readiness of all (or at least the majority of) team members; understanding and acceptance of one's own role and expertise; confidence in one's own ability; recognition of the boundaries of one's own discipline; effective group dynamics (communication skills, respect and trust); an environment with a team orientation; organizational values of participation; interdependence; and a leader supportive of autonomy (Hennemann *et al.*, 1995).

Three levels of collaboration that reflect differences in the quality of interaction between team members have been outlined by Pritchard and Pritchard (1994). First, teams may have a *nominal* level of collaboration that is characterized by the absence of explicit goals; common stereotypes being held by members; the adherence to provide hierarchical distinctions in status; and a lack of mutual trust and respect between members. Poor-quality communication is present, leading to confusion, frustration and conflicting information being provided to team members, people with learning disabilities and their families.

Collaboration is indeed present in name only.

Despite being considered to be more developed, the *convenient* level of collaboration has several major shortcomings. These include an expectation that team members will follow, without question, the orders of the person perceived as having the most professional status (often the doctor). Limited trust and mutual respect between members, little detailed understanding of other team members' roles, and inconsistent communication resulting in poorly co-ordinated assistance and advice to clients and their families are also present.

The final level of *committed* collaboration involves explicitly shared team goals; an accurate understanding of one's own role and the role of other team members; and the presence of mutual trust and respect for other team members. Each team member is viewed as a valuable contributor to the overall success of the team, and accurate communication and advice to clients and their family members is provided.

Hennemann *et al.* (1995) identified further defining variables of collaboration that can be seen in the structure of the team; in team members' work with clients; among team members; and within the overall service. These were the sharing of power based on knowledge and expertise instead of role or title; and clear procedures for managing conflict within the team. Interaction between team members involves regular open and honest communication between all members; shared planning and decision-making; and co-operative endeavour in which team members are interdependent on each other for the successful achievement of agreed goals.

Establishing and maintaining successful collaboration is not a straightforward process and often obstacles relating to organizational, professional and personal influences have to be overcome (Table 21.3). If teamwork is to become and remain effective, these issues must be addressed and clear action taken to remove or reduce the number and degree of obstacles present (see 'Enhancing team working', p. 351).

Operational Policies and Operational Culture

Well-developed operational policies are essential to the effective functioning of any team. A comprehensive operational policy will cover aspects such as aims; priorities; client group; catchment area; team philosophy; team membership; issues arising in relation to the conduct of team meetings; team leader role; professional advisor roles; team systems and procedures; and information on team accountability and performance reporting (Øvretveit, 1993, pp. 195–6). Operational policies provide team members with a structure and guidelines to be followed in the day-to-day work of the team. Such policies should be developed in collaboration with team members and must reflect the situations and difficulties they face and should be reviewed regularly, possibly annually, or sooner if an issue arises that the operational policy does not cover. For operational policies to be effective, team members must have a working knowledge of them. Operational policies that team members are unfamiliar with, and lay on shelves unopened, may create the illusion of a well-organized team (on paper), but provide no real structure to assist effective teamwork.

Brown (1992) argued that operational culture was at least as important, if not more important, than operational policies to the effectiveness of the team. Even when operational policies are present, the failure to give adequate attention to the influence of operational culture can bring a team to the point

Table 21.3 Obstacles to successful collaboration. Developed from Øvretveit (1993), Hattersley (1995) and Hayes (1997)

Organizational

- Difference in pay and conditions between team members.
- Inadequate time made available for team members to get to know each other.
- High staff turnover and periods of reduced staff numbers.
- Lack of autonomy (actual or perceived).
- Lack of support and commitment.
- Team too large/too small.
- Lack of resources.
- Lack of feedback/recognition.
- Competitive individual appraisal.
- Peer pressure or management pressure to conform.
- Being made to become part of a 'team'.
- Over control by managers/professional advisors outside of team.

Professional

- Differences in values and philosophy.
- Professional (and/or personal) defensiveness due to pressure to expose poor practices in a bid to increase quality of service delivery.
- Development of professional cliques.
- Unnecessarily complicated and exclusive language/jargon.
- Felt need to keep a professional distance.
- Desire to keep professional knowledge and skills.

Personal

- Varying expectations of one's role in relation to degree of client work involved.
- Struggles to assert personal power within the team.
- Sabotage of team effort due to perverse incentives (such as maintaining previous position).
- Previous limited or negative experience.
- Lack of confidence in one's own ability to function as a team member.
- Lack of interpersonal communication skills, in particular – assertiveness.
- Fear of reduced autonomy.

of breakdown. The crucial influence of operational culture has also been highlighted by Mullins (1996) and Hayes (1997).

Operational culture has been defined as

the patterns of relationships and sets of assumptions which team members hold about themselves and their colleagues . . . the routine and often unspoken ways that members define their roles and their professional relationships. (Brown, 1992, pp. 372, 377)

This involves unwritten rules, rituals, customs, slogans, myths, shared beliefs, patterned conduct and the impact of wider organizational systems on team functioning (Hayes, 1997).

Attempts have been made to delineate four types of operational culture (Mullins, 1996). Within a homogenized culture all team members have equal status, but no clear roles or leader exist. Team members fear being singled out and they seek safety in remaining unnoticed; autonomous behaviour and speaking out is not valued. The team fails to achieve the assigned tasks, lacks innovation and creativity and appears to have lost its purpose. Team members develop a sense of helplessness about their situation that may result in reduced effectiveness.

An institutional team culture is recognizable by the presence of a designated leader who controls team members, limiting their autonomy. Team members have assigned roles, a fear of being singled out or punished, and they find safety in following imposed rules. In this culture, team members lose sight of their own individual purpose and feel frustrated because they can see no way to change their situation. Although team tasks may get achieved, there is an absence of innovation and flexibility, in part due to a culture of conformity and obedience.

Autocratic team cultures are in some ways similar to the institutional culture, with the presence of assigned roles, a focus on conformity, a fear of speaking out and the presence of a structural hierarchy. Team members only work under direction of the leader, they feel unsafe, insecure and unsure of the leader. Again, the illusion of an effective team can be brought about by the achievement of team tasks. However, these tasks and team priorities are almost exclusively dictated by the leader and team members lose any sense of individual purpose. Such a culture stifles flexibility and will greatly reduce the ability of the team to work in a client-centred or needs-led manner. Indeed, it may contribute to the development of an 'expert knows best' relationship between team members and service users, as this is the role model team members have been exposed to.

Within an intentional operational culture, roles and status are flexible and reflect the changing needs of the team. All team members feel a responsibility for the successful achievement of agreed team goals and in pursuit of this, autonomous behaviour of team members within limits agreed by each team member is valued. Challenge, conflict, frustration and sharing points are considered part and parcel of teamwork and channelled constructively towards the development of innovative team responses. Team members feel secure and empowered to act. Such a team culture promotes personal and professional growth, and is able to adapt to the frequently changing nature of service.

It is foreseeable that these cultures could exist in full or part within any CLDT, and each will have a crucial influence on the effectiveness of the team. It is therefore important that team members consider the predominant culture within their team and reflect on the implications of this for the effectiveness of the services they provide and what (if any) changes are required to enhance positive aspects of teamwork. The involvement of some people with learning disabilities, families, or some other people outside of the team in these discussions may shed light on functional aspects of the team that team members are not aware of.

Enhancing Teamwork in CLDTs

A combination of roles

The desire for interdisciplinary teamwork must be matched by financial resources, commitment and practical support from managers in Health and Social Services. Effective teams are complex structures and require an investment of time, money, personnel and personal commitment. The establishment and maintenance of high-quality teams is much too important to be an arbitrary assignment of people to new structures or offices and calling them a team.

A major obstacle to effective and efficient teamwork is lack of clarity over individual leadership and overall team roles. Prior to a team being set up it should be clear that a need for this team exists, and what their intended role will be. This will assist in the identification of potential team members and provide interested staff with some information to consider if they are interested in becoming a team member. In particular, it is necessary to be clear about the relationship between existing teams and any new team that is to be developed. Being unclear of these relationships can result in a team being 'adrift in overall services' and has been identified as a major cause of reduced effectiveness and eventual team failure (Øvretveit, 1993).

The leadership style exercised within the team will be influenced by the maturity of the team members as individuals and the team as a functional unit. The higher the ability and motivation of team members, the greater the opportunity to opt for an approach that focuses on shared decision-making within agreed limits, delegation, and a degree of individual autonomy. Key decisions must also be made in respect of the responsibilities, authority and accountability of the team leader and team members. This must clearly identify pathways for both managerial and professional accountability, and the agreed arrangements for clinical supervision.

One of the strategies for reducing conflict over who was the 'boss' in multidisciplinary and interdisciplinary teams has been to elect a chairperson or appoint a co-ordinator instead of having a fully accountable manager. A chairperson is elected by team members normally for a specific period of time and is unpaid for their additional role. They have responsibility for chairing team meetings and may be given additional responsibilities by the team. They are usually accountable to the team meeting and are authorized to ensure the best use of time at team meetings, but are not authorized to take action outside of the team unless this is decided by the team. On the other hand, the co-ordinator is normally appointed, and in turn may hold a reduced client workload to enable them to attend to their new tasks. They are mainly responsible for chairing team meetings, upholding and reviewing team policy and other delegated management tasks. The co-ordinator is accountable to the team or a manager and is authorized to take action to uphold policy. This could involve requesting team members to alter their behaviour, but not to over-rule case decisions (Øvretveit, 1993).

The most effective problem-solving teams have been shown to have team members who undertake a combination of complementary roles (Belbin, 1993). These roles and corresponding characteristics have been given the following names: *plant* (creative, imaginative, unorthodox), *resource investigator* (extrovert, enthusiastic, communicative), *co-ordinator* (mature, confident, good chairperson), *shaper* (challenging, dynamic, thrives on pressure), *monitor–evaluator* (sober, strategic, accurate judge), *teamworker* (co-operative, perceptive, diplomatic), *implementer* (disciplined, reliable, conservative, efficient), *completer* (conscientious, anxious, delivers on time) and, finally, a *specialist* (single-minded, self-sharing, dedicated, skills in rare supply).

One person may fulfil more than one role, therefore all roles may be present in a small team. Particular team members as individuals may lean towards one role more than another; however, to increase team effectiveness it may be necessary for some team members to adopt a team role that is absent from the team in order to increase team effectiveness.

Three essential points are made in relation to the combination of roles: first, a team with a combination of roles is more effective at problem-solving than a team of 'experts'. Second, all team roles have weaknesses as well as strengths; it is necessary to accept both aspects of people's roles. Finally, all team roles are of equal importance, because it is the combination of roles, not the presence of any single role, that brings about team effectiveness.

Developing a team identity

Interdisciplinary teams, by their design, bring together a collection of people from a range of professional, personal and, at times, geographic and cultural backgrounds. The essence of teamwork is to combine the abilities of these people into a cohesive unit. Part of this process involves the development of a team identity.

Identity is a complex issue that involves aspects of self-esteem, self-image and status. In addition, it is closely linked to how a person evaluates their self-worth, confidence and overall ability.

Therefore, any change related to identity needs to be handled sensitively and will best be achieved over time. The process of change can be a frightening experience and people's sensitivities should be considered.

Tensions may well exist and need to be carefully resolved between people's previous professional and personal identity, and their new position in the CDLT. Some team members may feel their status, security, authority, career or professional judgements are being challenged.

Each team should have a distinctive identity that reflects the role of the team, and the team membership. This is important, as some CDLT members may participate in more than one team and it helps clarify their involvement in each team they belong to. Team identity is more than the name of the team and evolves over time. It is influenced by operational policies, structures, operational culture and relationships within the team. A clear team identity can help consolidate the position of the team within overall services and can increase cohesion.

Team-building exercises that bring all team members into constructive activities can be valuable. These exercises are designed to assist the development of relationships through increasing member's understanding of their own professional and personal roles as well as those of colleagues (Woodcock, 1988; Dearling, 1991).

Delivering a specialist service

The primary purpose for the development of CLDTs was to enhance the delivery of a specialist and co-ordinated service to people with learning disabilities and their families. However, some doubt exists as to the degree of success teams have had in achieving this primary objective (Brown, 1992; Braye and Preston-Shoot, 1995).

No member of the current Health or Social Services can be in any doubt that their future depends on their ability not only to deliver a specialist service, but also to demonstrate clearly that they are delivering a high-quality, effective specialist service. This will not be an easy task for several reasons.

Difficulties exist in identifying conclusive measures of quality across professional groups that reflect the complexity of the work involved. Unfortunately, many of the current measures such as the number and duration of contacts, codes for the type of intervention and the often-limited space to record details, do not articulate the true nature of the work of team members. Clearer measures require development that provides accurate information on aspects such as changes in abilities and needs; the degree of competence achieved by people with learning disabilities and their families; the extent to which monitoring involvement averts crisis situations; and overall improvement in health status and quality of life. Further to this, additional information is required to demonstrate that the CLDT can achieve these targets more effectively than other service arrangements.

It is no longer practical or wise to believe that CLDTs will continue to exist without question. The very existence of CLDTs in some areas could be under threat from GP fundholding practices who may decide to purchase services for people with learning disabilities from outside the CLDT, or indeed have the practice nurse undertake this work. Increasing specialization within community nursing services has seen the growth of services such as the specialist health visitor for people with learning disabilities; community children's nurses; child and adolescence psychiatry teams; and disability teams who work with all people with disabilities, including people with learning disabilities. With time, some or all of these services may undertake some of the work that CLDTs currently carry out. It is essential that clear channels of communication for the exchange, networking and joint planning are developed between all community-based services. Strenuous efforts must be made to prevent the fragmentation of services to people with learning disabilities. All services should work together to provide a comprehensive resource to people with learning disabilities and their families. There is much more to be gained in working together than will ever be achieved by the blind defence of one's perceived professional territory.

Central to proving the value of the CLDTs are accurate records of intervention. There is an urgent need to reduce the duplication between computer-based record systems and written client notes. It is also necessary to reduce overlap between records held by team members. The use of a single central record would reduce this overlap and may increase the quality of communication among team members. It is important in all circumstances to work within the clear constraints of confidentiality. Records must show the specialist contribution of team members to the life of people with learning disabilities and their families. Short repetitive notes that contain little or no detail and do not clearly identify the objectives for intervention have no place in future services. All interventions should be based on agreed objectives that are evaluated at least every 3 months, including interventions to people with learning disabilities who are visited over a lengthy period of time. Without clear objectives the involvement of any team members may be easily challenged as vague and will be difficult to justify.

Records must be up-to-date and objective. All team members must recognize the legal and professional importance of accurate records. When team members delay recording in their notes by any more than a few days, the information recorded is often a record of what can be remembered rather than what actually happened. The use of dictaphones, either as a personal aid to memory, or for transcribing by a secretary should be investigated.

The services provided by the CLDT should be based on accurate information sought from a variety of sources including local Health and Social Services Departments; people with learning disabilities and their families; independent services; and national and local demographic information. Team members need to remain up-to-date in their knowledge and skills in relation to the changes in legislation, local and national policies, and clinical skills from their respective professions. New approaches to intervention should be investigated and evaluated as a strategy to remain innovative and creative. Valid and reliable research into the achievements of the CLDT is urgently required at local and national level. The findings of this research must be disseminated through professional publications, conferences, word-of-mouth and other forms of media to make them accessible to as many interested people as possible.

Research findings that are found to be reliable and valid after a careful critique can be a valuable source of support for the actions of team members. They can also provide a strong position from which to question any policy or operational decisions imposed on the team members. It is ironic that many of the decisions made about how services should be developed are not based on, or supported by, the research evidence available.

It is only by a continuous commitment to listening, reflecting, planning, responding and evaluating provision that CLDTs will retain their central contribution in services for people with learning disabilities. Some recent evidence exists to show the value of this process and how it may be further developed (Aylott and Todcaram, 1996; Simon and Roy, 1996). Above all, team members must be open to question and challenge by colleagues, people with learning disabilities, carers, and purchasers of services.

Indicators for Effective Teamwork

Stephen Brown, in the first edition of this text, identified a series of simple but robust indicators for evaluating the effectiveness of interprofessional teamwork amongst staff working with people with learning disabilities. Although the indicators do not genuinely measure the final outcomes of teamwork, they provide opportunity for professionals to consider the effectiveness of intermediate outcomes of team intervention; whether team members have managed to organize themselves in such a way as to collaborate effectively with the aim of enhancing the quality of life for people with learning disabilities and their families.

The primary aim of effective teamwork will be to co-ordinate the individual inputs from a range of learning disability support staff and to maximize their effectiveness in the planning, delivery and evaluation of care to people with learning disabilities. The work of CLDTs may be divided into two specific categories: activities concerned with the delivery of support or care to people with learning disabilities and their families; and the development of new service responses designed to meet the specific needs of clients in local communities. Together, these two specific functions form the baseline of activity for CLDTs in their aim to ensure that service users and their families have a quality of access to Health and Social Services provided for the citizens in society, and to supplement mainstream services through the provision of specialist responses directly to clients and families.

The indicators expressed in this section are presented as questions – questions that refer to the kind of procedures and processes which teams use to regulate their work and the responsibilities of their members. Some of the questions ask about relatively formal procedures: for example what kind of case referral system is in place, or what evidence exists to confirm that interprofessional client planning processes are in place? Others ask about the *culture* that the team has developed: for example how the leadership of the team operates while conflicts are resolved. Our belief is that these latter questions deserve more attention in order to assure maximum co-ordination amongst team members. Prevailing ideologies tend to concentrate on the mechanics of care planning and provision. However, it should be remembered that systems of care are driven by people; these motivations, morale and relationships do not follow idealized notions in professional or organizational behaviour. Rather, they are an accumulation of past history, professional and territorial values and personal aspirations.

Consequently, in asking questions about effective teamworking, it is important that we identify how best CLDTs manage to make effective use of the limited resources at their disposal. With very few exceptions, teams have only the time and the skills of their staff in their control, and rarely have the opportunity to manage the financial resources that underpin their allocation. In these circumstances, the ways in which team members relate to each other professionally (and interpersonally) may become the key indicators for effective teamwork.

Some of the key issues that influence teamworking have to do with the ways that teams construct an identity for themselves. In organizations terms, this reflects a relationship between CLDT members and their colleagues working in more traditional cultures in Social Service Departments and Health Service Trusts. In some cases other agendas operate to militate against effective teamwork, such as adherence to traditional values that were part of disestablished specialist long-stay hospitals.

Perhaps one of the most important indicators of effectiveness in teamwork relates to the extent to which individual team members work to enhance the individual autonomy and independence of service users and their families. Consequently, questions must be asked about advocacy, the promotion of autonomous decision-making and shared action planning (Brechin and Swain, 1987). Decision-making

procedures and accountability arrangements for service users and their professional supporters also require careful examination in this context.

However, in terms of the operational culture of the team, an examination of effectiveness must also relate to the way in which team members have or have not managed to create 'free space' for themselves – a 'free space' in which they are able to move beyond existing agency tensions (or outdated service policies and procedures) and to renegotiate roles and responsibilities with their colleagues across different agencies (including the independent voluntary and private sectors).

The purpose of the indicators presented in this chapter is to prompt enquiry about the relationships between team members and service users. They aim to ask whether staff who are involved in CLDTs fully understand the contribution that service users, families and carers and other team members are able to make, how they aim to promote and manage individual care responses, and how they view their work with clients and the responsibilities they carry from their employing agencies.

The indicators also ask about the dynamics within teams, including questions about leadership, roles and conflict resolution. It is these that we consider to be most difficult for team members to address and to resolve, but to be crucial in enhancing the quality of effective teamwork. In particular, consideration must be given to the implementation of effective (negotiated) risk-taking policies and procedures.

Precisely because multidisciplinary teamwork challenges deeply held beliefs about the scope of professional authority and activity (and the relative status of professional groups), it poses problems for staff who are involved in teamworking. Furthermore, it is not always apparent that team members and, importantly, team managers have established methods that promote co-operation. A measurement of effectiveness in teamwork must therefore include questions directly related to issues such as: How does the referral process work? How are cases allocated and reviewed? How are conflicts resolved? Multidisciplinary teamwork demands that these elements of the care process are examined critically, to see whether common and cohesive approaches are adopted across agency boundaries.

Bringing together staff from diverse professional backgrounds and with different agency loyalties is not sufficient to produce joint working. According to Brown and Wistow (1990) many CLDTs failed to promote innovative approaches to inter-agency teamwork, preferring to depend on traditional and separate approaches to professional practice that previously existed between Health and Social Service staff. In some teams, members continue to work together with only the most rudimentary co-operation. Other difficulties appear to exist outwith traditional Health and Social Service team structures. For example, many CLDTs do not include representatives from Education Departments or from local housing associations or from local council environmental groups. In contemporary society, community development and action approaches will also require co-operation between the statutory services and the voluntary and private sector, with the aim of developing flourishing and responsible alternatives to traditional care services. The extent to which these are facilitated may therefore be regarded as important indicators of team effectiveness.

Not all teams operate cohesively with the result that some degree of separation between team members may occur, characterized as follows:

- different referral routes for clients between different agencies;
- little opportunity for interprofessional case review;
- rigid demarcation criteria and guidelines for the allocation of clients between professionals;
- failure to maintain integrated interprofessional records;
- the absence of negotiated risk-taking procedures;
- fragmentation of service response between the generic primary healthcare teams (including GP fundholders) and specialist CLDTs and paediatric teams.

Whatever advantages there may be in organizing staff to work together within the context of a CLDT that operates like this, they are not ones which generate a common approach to professional practice. However, although such teams do not display a commitment to joint work in an operational sense, they may nevertheless develop as a kind of operational policy forum. That is to say, team members (and managers) may use the existence of team structures to clarify broad issues about agency responsibilities and priorities.

Clearly, effective teamwork depends on the clarification of individual team responses, and the transparency of effective interprofessional operational practices which indicate that joint working is taking place. It is instructive to consider in detail how teams adopt collaborative risk as methods of work and what kinds of influences prevent them from doing so.

Working Across the Boundaries

In order to achieve maximum effectiveness, CLDTs and their members will need to operate in close liaison with a range of other service providers. Perhaps the most important of these will be the primary healthcare team, co-ordinated by the local GP or GP fundholder. Today's Health Service is becoming increasingly focused on a primary healthcare service model, and places considerable reliance on the development of service responses that derive from the local community and neighbourhood setting. Conversely, reliance on the acute and specialist hospital sector is now reducing in accordance with Government policy. Indicators of effective teamwork in community learning disability must, therefore, refer to the following:

- The extent to which the CLDT explores opportunities to promote the health and social well-being of clients, and thus reduces the impact of disability and impairment.
- The effectiveness of negotiated arrangements for interprofessional networking between a specialist community learning disability service and the primary health care team (general practice team).
- The extent to which intraprofessional liaison is effective between fieldwork, residential and day care social work staff, and between various groups of nursing staff including district nurses, health visitors, community learning disability nurses and residential care specialists, etc.
- The extent to which opportunities have been developed to promote a positive working relationship among service users, their representatives and advocates.

Effective teamwork across service/agency boundaries demands the development of a seamless service striving towards the achievement of a common goal that maximizes opportunities for service users to integrate and participate in the day-to-day life of their local community. In so doing, networks and alliances between day care workers, residential care staff, fieldwork staff, respite care providers and the many gate keepers to generic community health and social services should be visible.

Some teams have employed project workers or development officers to assist in the discovery and implementation of more appropriate service responses. This has become particularly evident following the implementation of care management programmes and the identification of the actual needs of service users. As a result many traditional service responses are now being challenged as team members become more aware of the actual needs and preferences of users and their carers. The extent to which traditional services are challenged, and new innovative service responses developed, must therefore be accepted as a key indicator of effectiveness in contemporary learning disability teamwork.

Before leaving this section, it is also important to note that effective teamwork will demand that service managers from various agencies engage in collaborative negotiation and interaction. Inter-agency planning teams should be evident in each locality and these should be charged with responsibilty for designing, implementing and evaluating the effectiveness of inter-agency community care plans for people with learning disabilities and their families. They should also be responsible for ensuring that the teams' resources are effectively audited and utilized in accordance with the needs and wishes of users and their representatives. Inter-agency planning teams should include representatives from the voluntary and private sectors and from other community groups, and should measure the extent to which services meet their stated aims and objectives. In addition, by engaging in systematic dialogue with service users and voluntary groups, inter-agency teams can also act as a catalyst for data collection and information sharing between service users and providers, thus providing projective feedback on the effectiveness of interprofessional team activity.

Teamwork and Crisis Intervention

Each team should identify in its operational policy a formal statement declaring its approach to providing immediate responses to service users and their families in times of crisis or declared sudden need. In accordance with the *Patients' Charter* (Department of Health, 1992), teams should publish their standards and response times, thus providing users with an indication of expected response times. In many cases care management teams have assumed responsibility for needs identification and will often publish standards for the provision of responses to emergency situations within 24 hours of acceptance of the referral. The majority of crisis intervention services are co-ordinated by Social Services Departments in accordance with the statutory requirement to respond to persons in need. Some CLDTs discharge this responsibility on behalf of the Social Service Department and Health Service Trust, and operate a 24-hour crisis intervention/emergency service. Modern technology provides opportunities for immediate access and information to be conveyed to designated teamworkers through the provision of telecommunications equipment (e.g. mobile phones). Where such schemes are in operation, they have been positively regarded by service users, their representatives and other professionals with the result that admission into residential care has often been prevented.

In order to reduce the responsibilities associated with crisis work, teams should be organized in such a way as to provide on-call rotas. The provision of such schemes aims to reduce pressure on any one individual case worker, thus providing them with the opportunity to monitor and advise clients and their families during the course of their everyday work.

Other benefits associated with the provision of crisis intervention by CLDTs have been acknowledged by non-specialist service agencies such as the police. In some areas, court diversion schemes are now in operation for people with learning disability who commit minor offences. Such schemes are dependent on having immediate access to professional case workers, such as community learning disability nurses (and specialist social workers) who are able to negotiate and advocate on behalf of clients who may be called in for questioning following an alleged offence. Other examples of crisis intervention work may be associated with clinical emergencies, such as the alleviation of status epilepticus through the administration of anti-convulsive medication. Other examples include the intervention of CLDTs following the occurrence of disturbed behaviour in the home, or in the case of self-injurious behaviour.

Measuring the Effectiveness of Professional Work

This chapter has attempted to identify some of the factors that shape teamworking. These have centred around one of the key issues affecting professional practice: clarity about professional roles. As the care professions are drawn ever more firmly into interprofessional frameworks, definitions of responsibility and of the professional 'core task' become more necessary. The ability of professionals to co-operate with colleagues from other disciplines depends in large measure on shared or mutual understandings about what each other does and how. Professional boundary disputes are often aroused because of misunderstandings or vagueness about professional roles.

In this chapter we have attempted to bring some light to the matter by measuring how staff undertake their work in CLDTs. This has been an exercise in clarifying the operational rules and tasks which team members perform. In so doing, it is important to remember that team members and their managers, after all, are crucially concerned with clarifying how and why teamwork is shaped.

This exercise forms part of the quality appraisal of service provision. However, we enter a cautionary note. The scrutiny of professional practice may be challenging to professionals if their field of practice is too loosely defined. It questions assumptions and prejudices about professional goals or methods. It may be taken as an erosion of professional autonomy. For understandable reasons, such critical questioning may provoke anxiety amongst team members. Nevertheless, the emphasis placed on multidisciplinary teamwork amongst the care professions gives an urgency to the examination of roles and tasks. The appraisal of the professional role in the context of multidisciplinary work threatens to expose uncertainties about the limits of professional intervention. In these circumstances, professional self-confidence may be damaged, and in its place the emergence of true interprofessional teamwork based on mutual respect and positive regard for people with learning disabilities may emerge.

In order to prompt further discussion about the operational roles and tasks of professionals in teams, we offer some examples of instruments to measure professional work. These identify with some precision the ways in which staff manage cases and have been used in our studies to highlight similarities and differences in the patterns of work that different professions adopt.

Brown (1987) suggests some obvious differences in the ways that team members go about their work. Community learning disability nurses, for example, are much more inclined than are social workers to select younger clients. Their clients seem to be more disabled than those of their social work colleagues and they appear to work with individuals, whereas social workers have a more family-orientated style of work (Brown, 1987). Differences like these no doubt reflect the different professional traditions and training of team members. However, these illustrations suggest that the decision-making processes that govern case management in teams are neither explicit nor systematic.

Indeed, this analysis may point to three propositions about professional orientations to tasks within multidisciplinary teams:

- First, without clear specifications as to the roles of team members, members would drift towards the common ground between them.
- Second, where team members have no actual or perceived authority to co-ordinate services, they will create their own service niche to fill.
- Third, where a team has little direct control over service resources, its own role will be limited to using its personnel as resources.

Factors such as these point to an arena of decisions which importantly affect the patterning of services for people with learning disabilities. In reality, therefore, if operational policies or role expectations are unclear, and if teams are given little authority in resource control, it is reasonable to expect team members to adopt a modest and low-key way of providing services. This is not to decry the ways in which CLDTs develop roles for themselves or contribute to the overall pattern of services. In showing that clients and families are kept routinely in contact with services and keeping a routine eye out for problems (tasks which CLDTs commonly undertake) continuity of casework is necessary, and may be an important way of filling gaps identifying in service provision. But, this often does not utilize the concentrations of specialist skills that teams are intended to represent.

Challenges for the Future

Studies of CLDTs identify that the work undertaken by team members is diverse and directly related to local circumstances and organizational structures. Many teams have now assumed responsibility for care management functions, and for ensuring that care is systematically planned, implemented and evaluated. Many staff work intensively with clients and families deploying the distinctive professional skills for which their training has prepared them: social workers undertaking sustained case work and community learning disability nurses implementing behavioural change programmes, etc.

However, each method of teamwork will naturally vary in accordance with the local needs of the community and the operational context of the professional agencies that support clients and families. Whatever their method of operation, there appears to be agreement that the CLDT has now been established as the cornerstone of specialist service provision for clients, providing a reservoir of skills for deployment whenever the need arises.

It might be appropriate therefore to regard the CLDT team as a strategy for preserving a specialist resource for people with learning disabilities and their families. The strategy has relied on persuasive arguments about the need for interprofessional co-operation and about the development of more responsive community services as part of care management provision. CLDTs, we believe, focus attention on these policy goals. That they have been so successful in becoming established across the country is a sign that these arguments have maintained a prominence on the broad policy agenda of Health and Social Service Authorities/Trusts.

We have also called for further action in respect of clarifying the roles of various professional team members and mutual understanding about the contribution that staff from different disciplines may make to the care process; the importance of operational cultures in shaping the formal procedures adopted by teams; and the need for a careful scrutiny of patterns of work and for the re-alignment of professional boundaries.

There are signs that CLDTs are now embarking on this new phase of development and are contributing to the development of evidence-based practice to validate the effectiveness of both individual and team contributions to enhancing health and social gain for people with learning disabilities and their families. If there is a widespread commitment to refining the roles and operational tasks of teams, they will continue to lead the way forward in interprofessional approaches to service provision for Health and Social Service users and their carers.

However, a number of key issues have been raised in this chapter that suggest that operational policies and models of effective teamwork continue to require attention and modification in response to major policy changes and heightened awareness and demand for more responsive, local services. If the CLDTs are to continue to fulfil their role of integrating different professional skills into an operationally specific resource, then teams must evolve to demonstrate their further integration with primary health care activity and GP fundholders.

Discussion Questions

- What are the main advantages of effective teamwork for both people with learning disabilities and their carers?
- What are the main barriers to the promotion and maintenance of effective teamwork?
- Outline and compare the three main levels of collaboration as described by Pritchard and Pritchard (1994).
- Outline your interpretation of the indicators for the measurement of successful teamworking and confirm how you would apply them in practice.
- What is your vision for the future of interprofessional teamwork with regard to the delivery of integrated care for people with learning disabilities and their families?

References

Aylott, J. and Todcaram, J. (1996). Community Learning Disability Teams. *British Journal of Nursing*, **5**(8), 488–91.

Audit Commission (1986). *Making a Reality of Community Care*. HMSO, London.

Belbin, R.M. (1993). *Team Roles at Work*. Butterworth-Heinemann, Oxford.

Braye, S. and Preston-Shoot, M. (1995). *Empowering Practice in Social Care*. Open University Press, Buckingham.

Brechin, A. and Swain, J. (1987). *Changing Relationships. Shared Action Planning for People with a Mental Handicap*. Harper & Row, London.

Brown, S. (1987). *Case Management Practice: An Examination of Casework in CMHTs*. Available from CRSP, London.

Brown, S. (1990). *Variations on a Theme*. Available from CRSP, London.

Brown, S. (1992). Profession in teams. In *Standards and Mental Handicap, Keys to Competence* (eds T. Thompson and P. Mathais), pp. 371–85. Baillière Tindall, London.

Brown, S. and Wistow, G. (1990). *The Roles and Tasks of CMHTs*. Gower, London.

Carrier, J. and Kendall, I. (1995). Professionalism and interprofessionalism in health and community care: some theoretical issues. In *Interprofessional Issues in Community and Primary Health Care* (eds P. Owens, J. Carrier and J. Horder), pp. 9–36. Macmillan, London.

Dearling, M. (1991). *Effective Use of Team Building*. Longman, London.

Department of Health (1992). *The Patients' Charter*. HMSO, London.

Hattersley, J. (1995). The survival of collaboration and co-operation. In *Services for People with Learning Disabilities* (ed. N. Malin), pp. 260–73. Routledge, London.

Hayes, N. (1997). *Successful Team Management*. Thomson Business Press, London.

Hennemann, E.A., Lee, J.L. and Cohen, J.L. (1995). Collaboration: a concept analysis. *Journal of Advanced Nursing*, **21**(1), 103–9.

Hudson, B. (1995). A seamless service? Developing better relationships between the National Health Service and Social Services Departments. In *Values and Visions. Changing Ideas in Services for People with Learning Difficulties* (eds T. Philpot and L. Ward), pp. 106–22. Butterworth-Heinemann, Oxford.

Janis, I.L. (1983). *Groupthink*, 2nd edn. Houghton Mifflin, Boston.

Jenkins, J. and Johnson, B. (1991). Community nursing learning disabilities survey. In *The Community Mental Handicap Nurse: Specialist Practitioner in the 1990s*. Mental Handicap Nurses Association.

Leathard, A. (1994). *Going Interprofessional. Working Together for Health and Welfare*. Routledge, London.

McGrath, M. (1991). *Multidisciplinary Teamwork*. Avebury Studies of Care in the Community, Aldershot.

McGrath, M. and Humphreys, S. (1988). *The All Wales CMHT Survey*. University College of North Wales, Bangor.

Moorhead, G., Ference, R. and Neck, C.P. (1991). Group decision fiascoes continue. Space shuttle Challenger and a revised groupthink framework. *Human Relations*, **44**(6), 539–50.

Mullins, L. (1996). *Management and Organisational Behaviour*, 4th edn. Pitman Publishing, London.

Øvretveit, J. (1993). *Co-ordinating Community Care. Multidisciplinary Teams and Care Management*. Open University Press, Buckingham.

Owens, P., Carrier, J. and Horder, J. (eds) (1995). *Interprofessional Issues in Community and Primary Health Care*. Macmillan, London.

Pritchard, P. (1995). Learning to work effectively in teams. In *Interprofessional Issues in Community and Primary Health Care* (eds P. Owens, J. Carrier and J. Horder), pp. 205–232. Macmillan, London.

Pritchard, P. and Pritchard, J. (1994). *Teamwork for Primary and Shared Care. A Practical Workbook*, 2nd edn. Oxford Medical Publications, Oxford.

Rawson, D. (1994). Models of interprofessional work: likely theories and possibilities. In *Going Interprofessional. Working Together for Health and Welfare* (ed. A. Leathard), pp. 38–63. Routledge, London.

Simon, F. and Roy, M. (1996). Consumer audit of Community Learning Disability Teams. *British Journal of Learning Disabilities*, **24**(4), 145–9.

Woodcock, M. (1988). *50 Activities for Teambuilding*. Gower, London.

CHAPTER 22

The Social Educator in Western Europe

Haydn Davies Jones

Key Issues

- Social pedagogy
- Comparative systems
- Provision of primary care
- Shared living
- Group work
- Creative activities

Social Pedagogy

Workers in the social, medical and educational fields will be surprised to find in most Western European countries an important profession functioning in their domain for whom in the UK there is no counterpart. This is the *Socialpedagogue* of Northern Europe and the *éducateur spécialisé* of French-speaking countries with a host of other variants available in the different European languages (Kalcher, 1986; see also Table of Titles, etc. in Davies Jones, 1994a). The German term is derived from *pedagogus*

the slave who in classical times took the children of a Roman household to school, theatre and often for outings, standing in the place of their parents and occasionally undertaking a little instruction.

Social emphasizes that this professional is the agent of society (representing Central and Local Government or the voluntary bodies who undertake similar responsibilities), working not only with individual clients but widely with groups, communities and social organizations and part of a team of helping professionals offering a collective action. Nowadays the title 'social pedagogue' hardly fits the person concerned with wider problems than those of children. As a result, in some circles it is being replaced by the term *sozialagoge* which conveys the enlarged role described later in these pages (Greek *Agoge* – Leader).

The French form of *éducateur* is a reminder of the earlier English usage which conveyed a wider meaning to 'educator' and education than that linked with teachers and classrooms. The educator in 1618 was defined as 'the person responsible for bringing up his/her charge from childhood so as to form habits, manners, mental and physical attributes'. This would certainly include parents, friends, the clergy and many youth workers. From its Latin root (*educe*) the emphasis is on bringing out, educating and developing – processes at the heart of the European conception of the *éducateur*.

For the purposes of this chapter we will conveniently bring the German and French forms together, using the term 'social educator' to describe the group. An understanding of this profession's role and functions is vital if we are to make sense both of the daily work of the helping professions in Western Europe and also of the development of wider policies and goals in this area.

Despite problems of nomenclature and national variations due to different history, ideology and culture it is not difficult to identify this group of professional workers who distinctively help clients by sharing substantially in their living. 'Living with others as a profession' was in fact the somewhat ambiguous subtitle used by a small band of European scholars when presenting their published survey of this group in 1986 (Courtioux *et al.* 1986). The emergence of these 'life-space workers', to use Redl's (1966) striking phrase, in the last four decades has not been confined to Western European countries: there are beginnings in the USA, an established system in French-speaking Canada, interesting variations in Israel and some achievements also in Eastern Europe, especially in Hungary, Czechoslovakia and Poland. The core growth, however, has been in Western Europe and particularly within EU countries such as Denmark, Holland, Belgium, Luxembourg, France and Germany (Courtioux *et al.*, 1986).

Surprisingly little notice has been taken of this phenomenon in Britain and the USA. The impressive professional literature already existing in French, German and the Scandinavian languages contrasts starkly with the few articles and monographs in English. Even important policy statements concerning the future of training in the social–educational field give little recognition of the existence of this profession. The reasons for the English silence are probably complex. The difficulties of understanding the group's complicated historical background and of finding an appropriate English nomenclature to describe its work are certainly factors. With the EU impetus to secure some harmonization of professional training between member states, this is likely to change.

The profession historically grew out of the coalescing of a number of interests with a nucleus lying for most countries in the field of residential child care. Long before World War II, care workers in many countries could be seen groping towards an identity and even preparing their own training schedules. It was, however, the aftermath of that struggle in Europe with its appalling legacy of orphaned children and family dislocation that provided the impetus for a new profession. Many of its precursors were among the workers who staffed the children's homes, the residential schools, nurseries and hostels, the camps and the children's villages of post-war Europe.

At the same time another stimulus came from the social climate of that period with its accent on securing radical change. In the decade following the war, reports, official and unofficial, were published in most Western European countries critical of much traditional institutional care, recommending instead novel approaches. An example in the UK was the report of the Curtis Committee (1946). These reports set in motion the strong movements for 'de-institutionalization' and 'normalization' which were features of later development. From the outset many of the emerging social educators, themselves residential workers, identified vigorously with those forces which were later to lead to alternative systems of care and a diminished residential sector. In Maier's shrewd analysis 'the workers followed the clients' (Maier, 1981).

Today, although social educators work in settings often far removed from the initial child care base, the earlier component of their intervention still remains important, although practised on a smaller scale. The task of providing an alternative nurturing experience for children unable to be reared in their natural homes or substitute family settings remains firmly their responsibility. In this category, which includes some of the deeply disturbed, seriously maladjusted, chronically delinquent, psychotic and autistic clients, will be children whose behavioural and relationship problems are not amenable to treatment within the community. The very existence of this group has placed great pressure on the social educators to develop the requisite therapeutic skills and methods.

At the same time residential care remains also in some European countries a provision for more normal young people as is seen in hostel and comparable accommodation for adolescents. The Danish system provides many examples (Rasmussen, 1970). Another illustration is the survival of homes for children coming from the families of 'shippers' on the Rhine which allows them to attend local schools. Social educators will have responsibilities for these residential centres which exist in Belgium, Switzerland, Germany, France and Holland (Davies Jones, 1986a).

The history of the profession shows how this work has been extended to include an increasing range of clients in need of the distinctive caring, shared living, educational and therapeutic approaches of the social educators. Their early childhood intervention will now be in nurseries, kindergartens, pre-school groups as well as care centres. Their child care, nurturer and

therapist roles will be in children's homes and villages, professional foster homes, residential schools and treatment homes. As diagnosticians they will serve in the observation and assessment centres and linked clinics. Working with families and communities they will be based in family centres, independence units, leisure-time centres, youth clubs, community centres, street theatres, hostels and kindred organizations. Sometimes they will be found in adult training centres, hospitals, prisons, after-care hostels, homes and centres for the elderly and occasionally as detached workers in the community, unsupported by traditional and formal organizational structures. How has this profession broken free from the confines of its earlier restricted environment? What rationale makes this expansion both understandable and credible? In seeking to answer these questions it is not assumed that the expansion noted here has been even and consistent in all the countries concerned. In some the process is highly developed and the profession large and influential as a result, in others the social educators are working substantially as they did two or three decades ago.

To make sense of these changes it is necessary to examine the nature of the social educators' work as life-space workers/child nurturers in the residential child care centres. As a starting point this will help us to identify the methods and skills which were later adapted and developed for use with other client groups in quite different settings. In this sense child care practice was a fertile source of theories and interventions.

The shared life of workers with children provided many opportunities for caring, education and therapy. This can be described in a number of ways:

- the provision of primary care;
- the clinical exploitation of day-to-day events in shared living;

- group-work in the setting of ordinary life;
- the use of creative activities.

It should be emphasized that these opportunities, although present in a striking way in residential child care, are available in some form wherever the worker participates substantially in the life of clients, whether they are young or old, living in a restricted residential setting or in the wider community. It is, as we shall see, the principle of shared living with its therapeutic and educational implications, that provides the thread linking together the social educator's activities in so many different fields.

The Provision of Primary Care

Both Maier (1963) and Bedell (1962) have described the significance of primary, caring relationships to children deprived of contact with their natural parents or surrogates. Sharing the intimate moments of daily life with the child will enable the educators to help in many ways. Using Maier's language they will be able to support the dependency, independency and expressive needs of the child. These of course continue long after infancy and extend into adult life becoming critically important again in the case of the elderly. A range of dependency needs may show themselves at almost any point in the child's daily life. Rising times may be critical for some who wish to withdraw from the pressing demands of the day ahead by developing disordered defences. Bedtime too for others will see the onset of infantile fears and disturbing recollections. In round-the-clock care at literally any time and with any type of activity the child may need the adult's supportive help.

The same is true of the opportunities that occur to establish the child's independence. Educators are alert to find new areas where children can make decisions for themselves

and reach towards a greater freedom. The process is rarely simple and straightforward; for most children their hesitant, groping steps forward call for genuinely sensitive adult support.

Children too need adults with whom they can safely confide their thoughts and feelings, especially when these are worrying and threatening. Feelings of personal inadequacy, fears for the future, despair, and difficulties in coping with some authority figures are examples of problems which should be discussed with caring grown-ups whom children trust.

Finally, good primary experience means that children should not only receive support but should be enabled in daily life to give support to others, to peers and indeed to adults. This reciprocal factor is what transforms care, ultimately making it into the great dynamic, liberating influence of human experience.

The Clinical Exploitation of Day-to-Day Events in Shared Living

The writings of Fritz Redl, translated into the main European languages, have been influential in the development of this aspect of the social educator's work (Redl and Wineman, 1965). His concept of the 'life space interview' has helped to clarify many of the therapeutic elements of the task. This is the term he uses to characterize some of the interactions between the child and a significant adult figure who is part of the natural habitat. In a colourful but artificial vocabulary, he shows how for the seriously disturbed child a 'strategically wise use' and 'technically correct handling' of that interview is of critical clinical importance. The issues are built around the child's direct life experience and the total therapy will depend substantially on how the worker copes with them. This view of the therapist with clear roles and influence in the child's daily life contrasts sharply with the conventional image of the clinician.

Despite Redl's language – the 'reality rub in', 'symptom estrangement' and the 'massaging of numb value areas' – his work shows how the clinical exploitation of everyday issues makes possible the use of passing life experiences to promote therapeutic objectives. It indicates too how 'educational first aid' is possible at times of crisis to relieve guilt, pain, anger, fury and to help the child regain afterwards a sense of proportion. To sustain work of this intensity places acute strains on relationships and communications. A number of strategies, techniques and supports have been shaped to help.

Group Work in the Setting of Ordinary Life

In residential life the social educators work not only with individual children but with the 'living group'. As group workers they have the opportunity to do much more than supervise routines and programmes. Group life provides countless conflicts and situations which can be used positively to help its members. The careful restructuring of small groups often enables children who are constricted in their role performance to develop versatility and expansiveness. It may contribute also to a 'social climate' amenable to treatment and growth. The seemingly endless conflicts of the peer group may be used constructively to improve awareness, develop fresh learning and to teach coping skills. The peer learning processes may be facilitated by social educators who know of their value. Group living

and conflict as the venue and arena for therapy have been the subjects of important texts in English as well as in the main Western European languages, Konopka's (1949) account of work in a children's home has been influential.

The Use of Creative Activities

Because they share much of the life of clients, social educators become involved in a wide range of activities. These are not ends in themselves but constitute the means by which workers and clients develop the shared interests and understanding that make growth possible. Sometimes as in play, art and music there will be additionally a specific therapeutic intent.

The importance attached to creative activities can be judged by the time devoted to this subject in the professional curriculum of the social educator, most colleges giving about a quarter of the course to the study. This includes the main areas of art, drama, music, formal and informal play as well as outdoor education. It does not, however, take into account the range of extracurriculum pursuits followed by social education students in addition. National culture plays an important part in the choice of these subjects. In 1976 at a main Austrian school for social training, students were expected to learn to play the guitar and one other musical instrument (piano accordian or recorder) as well as to become competent in skiing and skating. In the same year at a Swiss residential centre for disturbed children in the *Valais*, social educators needed an understanding of viniculture to work with children in tending their vineyard – *therapie par le vin*, you might say.

The range of creative subjects pursued by the social educators is extensive, although of course they are not expected to reach a proficiency in each. Linton (1971), after his study tour in 1969, listed the following: painting, graphic arts, design, collage, wood and metal work, sculpturing, print-making, weaving, ceramics, activities with puppets and marionettes, dramatics, dance, choral work and music. In the last decade the importance of informal play has been further recognized and also the value of making films and audiovisual pro-grammes. Apart from the direct help afforded to children by the expressive media, in the release of tension, the expression of feeling, the furthering of exploration and the growth of self-confidence, the creative skills are used to develop the residential living environment.

Outdoor education sees much time given to mountaineering, rock climbing, camping, canoeing, skiing, skating, fishing and field excursions as well as to physical education and the conventional sports. Often conducted in small groups these activities have real potential in educational development. In skilled hands they are sometimes used therapeutically, as in helping maladjusted children with substantial unresolved authority problems to learn some accommodation to the 'discipline of circumstance' imposed by weather conditions in a mountaineering expedition.

Vocational studies are widely used and in some countries there is a strong tradition of 'handyman' training. The earlier trade instructors working in residential child care in Great Britain, the *maîtres professionelles* of Switzerland and the *éducateurs techniques* of France are a reminder that this approach was thought sufficiently important at one time to produce its own specialists. Vocational training ensures for the group an important contact in ordinary life, with the common skills, values and attitudes of people outside the immediate environment. Normally too, people are highly motivated to take part and this helps in the creation of a purposive way of life in

settings where apathy and despair can easily prevail.

Finally, what Linton referred to two decades ago as the development by social educators of 'personal reinforcement techniques', plays a much greater part today than he could have envisaged. The acquisition of types of personal behaviour which are likely to be effective as 'motivational or accelerating devices' in work with clients has become especially important with the growth of behaviour modification approaches in residential settings (Linton, 1971).

The social educator then, whilst sharing substantially in the life of others, has opportunities to offer clients primary caring, a clinical exploitation of life events, a distinctive group work approach and a widely ranging activity contact.

With this background it is now possible to understand how the social educators were able to move away from their initial residential child care field to other settings. For a more detailed account of this process see Davies Jones (1986b). Some examples will be given. In Denmark the residential child care workers and the staff who worked in the pre-school field (in nursery, kindergarten and pre-school) have been able in recent years to find a professional identity. At one time the Ministry of Social Welfare was responsible for the colleges training child care pedagogues and the Ministry of Education for those educating pre-school staff. The professional preparation was different leading to separate qualifications and careers. Today the colleges work with both types of student following a common basic curriculum but with opportunities for specialization. There is one qualification and a sense of commitment among students to a single profession. It is not difficult to see how the training programmes of both groups, each with its emphasis on individual caring, group work and the use of the creative arts could be brought together. Above all, the pre-school pedagogue, like the residential worker, shares in much of the children's life. Small children sleep for a few hours in the kindergarten; as part of the educational scheme they go shopping with the pedagogue, help in the preparation of food, eat together with the staff, all vital ingredients in the process of shared living.

Denmark also had a group of leisure time pedagogues (*Fritidshiem Pedagoger*) working with children after school hours, at weekends and in the holidays. From their social and recreational centres they have played an important preventive role in Danish society. They too trained originally in separate colleges awarding specialist qualifications. Today they too are securely part of the integrated pedagogue profession established by legislation in 1991.

The social educator's involvement in community work is another illustration of the same process. In some countries like Norway and Denmark, a number will be found working in youth service and club settings. As in Great Britain, many youth workers enter into the lives of their groups in ways which resemble the intervention of the social educator. The *milieu ouvert* of the French and Swiss *éducateur* is a parallel development. Here the workers will use the natural environment of delinquent adolescents (usually for periods of 6 months) with a freedom to forge suitable living and working links with their clients. They operate more like detached youth workers than conventional social therapists.

Work with families also follows some interesting lines. The social educator in the residential child care setting always needed close contact with the families of children. This alone would ensure that the alternative nurturing arrangements of the children's home were consistent with the child's earlier upbringing and future. Some residential workers went further actively seeking to bring about improved attitudes and practice in family life.

The social educators' role in relation to the family of the children they nurture is not normally the same as that of the family case worker. In caring for the child they enter to some extent the matrix of family relationships and share in its secrets and legends. In a sense they become part of the set-up and because of this special relationship have been able to operate in a distinctive way. In some countries entire families are sometimes brought into residential care allowing the social educator to work with the whole group, parents and children. Stein Lasson's pioneering therapy in his Danish residential centre is a good example (Lasson, 1978).

Sweden provided an example of another important innovation. Not without opposition, the workers of the Children's Village of Ska began to act directly with families in the community itself. They entered family units for short intensive periods offering help as 'quasi members'. These peripatetic family care workers had their critics. Some saw the approach as an unacceptable intrusion into the private life of individuals, stressing the risks that occurred when educators forgot the social context in which they worked. Others stressed the dangers of teaching families 'to over-adapt to their environment and lose the beneficent results of protest' (Lindby, 1977). Yet the work continued and early results were said to be encouraging.

Although most of the social educators' early work was with the general population of children in care and delinquents, the strong trend in many countries has been to involve them increasingly in the areas of mental and physical handicap and with other special categories. They will be found therefore in hospitals, special schools and in a variety of training centres.

Poised between education on the one hand and social work on the other, it is instructive to examine the relationship of social educators to neighbouring professions. For a more detailed analysis see Davies Jones (1986c). Currently they enjoy in most Western European countries an independent professional status. The European standpoint is that social educators represent a separate profession bringing together many important helping groups who might otherwise remain isolated and relatively unprotected. In some countries the division from social work is complete. In Denmark, France and Austria, for example, the professional schools are separate, the training schemes and qualifications quite different. The same applies to career structures and membership of professional associations. In other countries such as Germany there is a common basic training scheme for social workers and educators but for 2 years only of a 4-year course. One suspects that the *Sozialpedagog* and the *Sozialarbeiter* might eventually merge into an integrated profession but probably not for some years. Another group of countries such as Switzerland and Norway often bring social workers and educators together to train in the same college but with restricted sharing of courses.

Links with the teaching profession tend to be more distant save in the case of nursery and pre-school workers who also stand uneasily poised between being regarded either as teachers of the young or as social educators. In many residential schools, teachers have traditionally been responsible for pastoral and nurturing work. Some interprofessional rivalry has been inevitable in these settings. But modern systems of teacher education often give greater prominence to social and child-rearing questions. A sociological study of the infant classroom in Great Britain during the late 1970s describes an underlying ideology which would be close to that of many child care workers (King, 1978) In a period of teacher unemployment many young teachers have found jobs and fulfilment in the child care sector working as social educators.

The profession has been supported in many countries by the growth of vigorous trade unions and professional associations. The Danish, French and Swiss unions are good examples. Their main concerns lie with developing a known and credible image, using pressure groups for professional purposes, providing in-service training and study and publishing lively and informative journals. Most European social educators spend a considerable part of their income on union membership fees. Ideological issues are often keenly felt by social educators; in countries like Denmark they tend to have a radical image. But everywhere one meets a concern to examine the social, economic and political structures supporting contemporary life. This arises partly because the pathologies which interest the social educator are not only located in individuals; their roots lie in the social system of the day. Many urgent and pressing problems – of delinquency, alienation, social deprivation – are in fact symptoms of a wider social pathology which some educators wish to tackle at a more fundamental level. To grapple with these problems inevitably means a preparedness to wait for solutions in the middle and long term.

Meanwhile, clients need immediate help and workers have a responsibility to answer 'the knock at the door'. The dilemma for the social educator is often one of reconciling their commitment to helping individuals with that of a wider social intervention.

The emphasis on their responsibility to seek an improvement in the damaging areas of the client's social system leads to the view that they are the natural advocates of handicapped groups and change agents in society. In the contemporary children's rights movement they often take a promi-nent part.

For some radical educators the prospect of working with the very young child may have ideological attractions. So much of the helping process with the older child and adult is thought of as a 'patching' operation, or at best a palliative. With the very young, however, the social educators have oppor-tunities to work in a more fundamental way. They may still be able to shape atti-tudes and contribute to more tenacious value systems. In seeking to provide a caring, sharing (non-competitive) society among their young charges are they pursu-ing professional or political objectives?

In this context, the professional prepara-tion and socialization of the social educator becomes a key issue. For a more detailed analysis see Davies Jones (1986d, 1994b). Although practice is not standardized most countries offer training over a 3- or 4-year period in specialized schools of social pedagogics and/or social work. Here and there, as in Germany, training has also begun in the universities and asso-ciated higher institutions of learning. The tradition is for the school or college to be a relatively small unit (300–500 students) with its own staff and premises. Most schools enjoy a considerable measure of autonomy; some have become major cen-tres of influence and excellence. They are the repositories (and custodians) of profes-sional learning and skills. A study group of Directors of Training for Schools of Social Educators identified the following strengths of the system:

- A staffing ratio to students which allows for credible, professional training with its focus on individual growth and on the value of the small group process. Schools guard against their courses becoming occasions for developing academic knowledge only.

- A system which works closely to practice, drawing a high proportion of its teachers from the ranks of experienced workers and placing a special emphasis on prac-tice training and associated learning through supervision.

- An organization which is single-minded in pursuing professional goals and which becomes an important factor in the life and development of the profession in the local area. This is partly achieved by the schools offering, in addition to basic training, supplementary and further courses, part-time, occasional and full-time. Professional teachers too have a central reference (to practice both inside and outside the school) and do not dis-sipate their energies in too many other directions.

- Buildings, premises, equipment and other resources which are developed to fit the needs of specialized training. Adaptation and makeshift plans tend to be less used.

On the other hand, the small schools run the risk of becoming isolated in a world of large complex organizations. Their research output to date has been small. In many countries research is considered a preserve of the university and certain accredited institutes.

A comparative study of the schools' cur-ricula show that the following studies are normally included in most courses although the categories and subject names may differ according to a country's own traditions of scholarship.

- individual and social development including relevant studies in psychology, sociology, the associated behavioural and human sciences, education, social work theory and health;
- group dynamics;
- organizational theory;
- social administration and legal studies;

- social politics, philosophy and ethics (related to the professional task);
- creative work in music, art, drama, play, etc.

The substantive studies listed above are closely linked with the development of professional practice and skills. Approximately one-quarter of the course is devoted to the creative work area. One-third of the training consists of supervised professional practice which is evaluated.

In some countries, part-time in-service training courses leading to professional qualification exist. Recruitment tends to allow for a number of entry points to the profession recognizing the importance of admitting people from other fields who often bring experience of an exceptional order.

The chequered development of training, in some countries, at different levels has caused difficulty and resentment. To find an adequate rationale for the allocation of roles and functions to differently qualified workers has sometimes been impossible. The problem is made more acute by the differing status levels, conditions of salary and service, and career prospects determined by the qualification itself.

In the field under review the directions taken by Western Europe and Britain are different. In Europe the residential and 'life space workers' are moving towards an enlarged separate profession standing side-by-side with social work. In Britain some residential workers have been absorbed into the social work profession, others stand uneasily on the periphery. A number of related para-professional groups remain in an isolated and vulnerable situation. A sharing of experiences, some early comparative study and a preparedness to re-examine contemporary policies would be opportune during the next decade (Vanderven and Davies Jones, 1990).

DISCUSSION QUESTIONS

- What are the key features of Social Pedagogy?
- Do you think that there is any use or application for this approach in UK?
- What skills and knowledge are required of the social educator/ pedagogue?
- Do you have them? How could they be acquired?

References

Bedell, C. (1962). *Residential Life with Children.* Routledge & Kegan Paul, London.

Courtioux, M. *et al.* (eds) (1986). *The Socialpedagogue in Europe.* Fice, Zurich.

Curtis Committee (1946). *Report of the Care of Children Committee.* HMSO, London.

Davies Jones, H. (1986a). The profession at work in contemporary society. In *The Socialpedagogue in Europe* (eds M. Courtioux *et al.*), pp. 74–108. Fice, Zurich.

Davies Jones, H. (1986b). In *The Socialpedagogue in Europe* (eds M. Courtioux *et al.*), pp. 92–105. Fice, Zurich.

Davies Jones, H. (1986c). Conclusions. In *The Social-pedagogue in Europe* (eds M. Courtioux *et al.*), pp. 188–94. Fice, Zurich.

Davies Jones, H. (1986d). Professional training. In *The Socialpedagogue in Europe* (eds M. Courtioux *et al.*), pp. 128–64. Fice, Zurich.

Davies Jones, H. (1994a). The social pedagogues in Western Europe – some implications for European interprofessional care. *Journal of Interprofessional Care,* 8(1), 19–29.

Davies Jones, H. (1994b). *Social Workers or Social Educators? The International Context for Developing Social Care.* National Institute for Social Work, London.

Kalcher, J. (1986). Professional nomenclature. In *The Socialpedagogue in Europe* (eds M. Courtioux *et al.*), pp. 40–73. Fice, Zurich.

King, R. (1978). *All Things Bright and Beautiful*. Wiley, Chichester.

Konopka, G. (1949). *Therapeutic Groupwork with Children*. University of Minnesota Press, MN.

Lasson, S. (1978) *Anxious Children – A Family Matter*. Unpublished MSS. Aby, Denmark.

Lindby, K. (1977). Problems and trends in the field of juvenile delinquency. *International Child Welfare Review*, (*Geneva*), **December**.

Linton, T.E. (1971) The educator model: a theoretical approach. *Journal of Special Education* (*New York*), 3(4), 319–27.

Maier, H.W. (1963). Child care as a method of social work. In *Training for Child Care Staff*. Child Welfare League of America, New York.

Maier, H.W. (1981). Essential components in care and treatment environments for children. In *Group Care for Children* (eds F. Ainsworth and L. Fulcher), pp. 19–70. Tavestock, London.

Rasmussen, H. Chr. (1970). *Doginstitutioner*. Gyldendals Paedagogiske Bibliotek, Copenhagen.

Redl, F. (1966). *When We Deal with Children*. Collier & Macmillan, London.

Redl, F. and Wineman, D. (1965). *Controls from Within*. Free Press, New York.

Vanderven, K. and Davies Jones, H. (1990). Education and training for child and youth care practice: The view from both sides of the Atlantic. *Child and Youth Care Quarterly*, **19**(2).

Chapter 23

The Changing Practitioner Support Systems

Tony Thompson and Peter Mathias

Key Issues

- The changing world of work
- European influences on vocational education and training
- International influences on health and social care
- The Health for All Targets (WHO)
- The European Generalist Nurse Initiative

Introduction

Those involved in providing services for people with learning difficulties practice in an uncertain and changing world of work. The fundamental function remains the ability to assist people who have reduced ability to understand new or complex information due to impaired intellectual function to:

- learn new skills
- cope independently.

Overall impairment is likely to have commenced prior to adult maturation and will have an enduring effect upon the development of the person. Learning disability practitioners in the UK have a lot in common with their peers within other professions in Europe in that they are working in a state of rapid transition, which includes changes aligned to the community economy; the value systems of their community; fast information networks; and high technology changes which have their roots in:

- increased expectations of improved social conditions;
- expectations that work skills will be rewarded;
- greater egalitarian approaches to community presence;
- an expectation to be able to work outside geographic boundaries in order to meet the demands of competition for employment provision.

For example, since the revision of the learning disabilities nurse training syllabus in 1982, together with the expectations of a curriculum which expects to prepare nurses for working in the next millennium, nurses have had particular pressure to balance the risks and opportunities that can arise from meeting the demands of change. Therefore, in order for practitioners of the various professions to develop, it is imperative that they have a firm grasp of the features of the type of changes they are to face, which are likely to be quite complex. In this chapter we illustrate these general points by:

- considering the issues associated with the European curriculum development for the concept of a 'generalist nurse';
- describing the broad influences emerging from the European Union which impact upon the future of the learning disability nurse and other practitioners;
- describing the European vocational policies which impact upon the changing practice development;
- recognizing aspects of policy formation in the World Health Organization (WHO) and identifying the implications of *Health for All*.

General Trends

Most of the traditional professions have felt the effects in the last decade of the removal of barriers to competition which are concerned with the delivery of trade and industry. It has been the intention to remove such barriers in order to improve workforce and labour opportunities. However, this can simultaneously threaten specific aspects of employment and most importantly alongside this alter the arrangements for welfare protection, health and safety protection, together with safeguarding specific occupational interests. The technologies and methodologies which have emerged to assist in the production of new services are often associated with a search for different and varied methods of working. This in itself creates new risks and challenges which can have social implications which are not discovered until after the change process has commenced.

One result of the above phenomena on the professions and occupational groups is that pressures for change build up and the pace of competition within a specific service is accelerated. It is at this time that professions, organizations and occupational interests which have held a monopoly on services can find that they have to face great demands in order for them to add value to their services if they are to flourish. Another result of this phenomena is that the challenges that have arisen because of these conflicting demands, such as increasing job insecurity in the more developed world and the levels of stress-induced problems, together with an unstable future for professional groups, bring about a differing expectation from society as to the way those professionals will have to work if they are to continue to provide a relevant service.

The socio-political culture now emerging within the UK is one in which there seems to be general recognition that the growing emphasis on community may lead professions to re-assess the level of their own resources and whether they can now survive alone as single groups. One result of this is a greater and accelerated move towards interprofessional development and this probably marks a more informed understanding of needs in relation to associated occupational groups. There are many reasons why the professions have to become less insular and more open about their own limitations. As this phenomena unfolds, it is likely that the sharing of experiences and values which will be necessary for effective working may result in far more appropriate ways to facilitate service provision, together with increased problem-solving abilities as practitioners.

It is becoming more accepted that effective levels of co-operation and collaboration alongside strategic working practices will be required if the global problems associated with health and social care provision are to be tackled with any degree of optimism.

Reforming the Professions

The reformation of health and social care systems appears on most of the political agendas of the developed European countries. Amongst these are the following:

- operational, organizational and structural changes within the delivery of service;
- the introduction of the market philosophy into public sector organizations;
- the introduction of value for money methods for containing costs whilst at the same time seeking to make services user focused.

These changes are amongst those which have been responsible for pushing the developments in the health and social care fields towards delivery taking place at a primary level and which have subsequently led to the reconfiguration or reconstruction of the acute care services. They have brought in their wake a drive for more cost-effective training solutions which has led to the provision of individualized, distance, modular, computer-based and open learning.

This sort of approach supports professional work patterns since it allows a degree of flexibility within access to programmes and the time spent on achieving the outcomes of the programmes. These rapid flows of information are increasing the opportunities for multimedia applications and, in turn, training and education providers are tending to introduce these methodologies into their programmes. One result of this is the increasing range of opportunities for self-development and the acquisition of transferable skills. One of the major features of the transition of professionals during the late 1990s has been the notion of such transferable skills. The professionals concerned with learning disabilities have much in common with their colleagues within the wider commercial and industrial worlds in that they are now attempting to develop new skills in order to make the most of the challenges and opportunities offered by the diverse demands of the purchasers of their services.

The events that have affected the services pertaining to the public sector of the late 1980s have been quite revolutionary and there is little doubt that the traditional perception of professional status has become eroded and this has been quite traumatic to many of the professions. There is an increasing realization that the members of the care professions are required to address the issues associated with the growing importance of developing a range of skills which include wide networking, marketing, negotiation, value added client care, project management skills, team and cross-functional working practices. One consequence of this phenomena is that the strategic and policy direction which emerges for health and social care within Europe is demanding the translation of the growing awareness into displays of competent performance for the future.

There is a raging debate amongst strategists who now tend to agree that it is important to balance market forces and social responsibility, and this is reflected in the arguments of the advocates of social responsibility and the controlled developments or otherwise of the interactions of the free market.

In the UK the debate about introduction of measures such as the European Union's

Social Chapter is an indication of the elements of such arguments. The professional carers have to extend the depth and breadth of their existing knowledge and the range of their skills or face the prospects of seeing the results of failing to adapt and watching others exploit the reserves of skill transfer (Thompson and Mathias, 1997).

Those practitioners who are at the leading edge of the learning disability care sector know that they are having to work in an ever-changing and stressful professional environment. They are being required to develop new abilities, including those which are associated with living with uncertainty, and at the same time they have to project positive views to the benefit of the service user. They are expected to increase their continuing professional development and ensure that their skills are updated on a frequent basis. Another important factor for them is that they may have to increasingly respond to demands from a service which calls upon skills that are beyond the immediate competence in the professional employment base.

These major changes and expectations mean that professionals require trans-disciplinary approaches to their education and training, and this in turn means that those people who are in support posts are increasingly having to adapt to the occasional lack of clarity regarding specialist or shared roles. This demands skills of the professionals which are not narrow cognitive and subject-specific but are in future much broader ones. Primarily, future education and training associated with responding to health and care targets must offer the developing professional skills to adapt to change and concentrate on the fundamental principles that are likely to underpin the development of specialist expertise.

International Influences on Practice

A lot of the demands being placed upon health workers and the associated public policy factors that affect them are rooted in the work of the European Union. The Union is a unique grouping of member states which are committed to economic, social and political integration. These form the largest trading entity and cover a population of over 350 million people which makes them instrumental in being a growing force for an increase in democracy and international co-operation. The aims of the European Union are set out in its founding treaties, which are essentially economic. These revolve around activities which form unitary economic regions in which goods, services, people and capital can move across boundaries.

The various treaties developed by the member states have given institutions the ability to act and to legislate at a European level in specified economic, social and associated areas. The unique nature of the European Union is reflected in its four governing institutions: the Council of Ministers, the European Parliament, the Commission and the Court of Justice. The Council of Ministers is the major decision-making body. The Council consists of one minister for each of the member states with the participating ministers varying according to the topic under discussion.

The community works in partnership with international organizations such as the World Health Organization, the United Nations and the Red Cross, together with the many voluntary aid organizations within its own member states. Amongst the implications for the forthcoming initiatives are the need for co-operation amongst the professions and include the fact that those initial efforts which heralded the way for change within Europe have in some respects brought about other reforms. These reforms have often fractured previous professional organizational structures, and in turn have demanded a change in the way in which professions function and also a change in the values that they may have previously held. Evidence of a reform of professional attitude and values can be seen by looking at the outcomes of some of the initiatives lodged within the European Union. It is increasingly the case that programme planners working within the domain of vocational training and education consider the following as important in the predicted outcomes of the European initiatives:

- learning from the experience of others who are engaged in meeting the challenge of similar health and social problems;
- the impact that economic policies have on the quality of life standards of ordinary citizens;
- the resultant worker mobility within Europe is likely to identify problems which can only be overcome with assistance from their home country;
- an increasing number of professionals who wish to exercise their rights to practise their trade, occupation or profession in other countries;
- comparative visits and human resource exchange between practitioners, teachers and students will become increasingly common;
- the European legal effects, the conventions and policies will have a growing impact on the service users and professionals in the contributing countries.

As indicated in previous chapters, a number of these factors have clear implications for the development of the professions associated with learning disabilities, for

example the removal of technical barriers including the mutual recognition of qualifications. This means that within specific criteria the qualifications thought to be necessary to pursue a particular profession will be recognized in the member states. The professions need to collaborate effectively with the objective of reducing the gap between the advantaged and those from weaker areas of the community.

Aspects of European Vocational Training

In Article 118 of the Treaty of Rome it states that the Commission has the responsibility to promote co-operation between member states in the area of basic and advanced vocational training. Later in this Treaty, Article 128 states that the community can lay down general principles for implementing a common vocational training policy. It is interesting to note that the legal framework of the European Union in the field of vocational training is interpreted in such a way that it includes the whole of higher education. Effective collaboration and co-operation between the professions will enable the development of the field of education and training as it applies to the European perspectives to be achieved by effective joint working rather than trying to harmonize or standardize the systems of vocational preparation or professional practice.

The vocational training initiatives that have been spawned in the European Union are likely to continue to grow in the future. One example of this is the memorandum which the Commission issued in 1990 which referred to the rationalization of Community Vocational Training programmes (CMO, 1990). This memorandum is important as it aims to establish an overall framework for all community initiatives in the area of vocational training. A specific objective of the rationalization is to design general objectives for the whole sector, thereby bringing a greater coherence to the management of programmes within each state. As we move towards the effects of a single European Act it will be possible for the professions to see the physical and technical barriers, which have hitherto acted to impede progress, be eliminated in order to create an arena without internal frontiers, in which free movement of persons, services and capital is assured.

This politically intense activity may appear somewhat remote to those who work within direct service provision. In fact it is not; the contributing nations face many of the same contemporary social problems such as immunosuppressive diseases, an ageing population, child abuse, racism and chronic unemployment. We have a lot to learn from each other in the member states and to share with each other the effects that these negative influences may have within the development of learning disability services.

The World Health Organization – *Health for All* Targets

The World Health Organization is a specialized agency of the United Nations with a primary responsibility for international health matters and public health. Through this organization, created in 1948, the health professions of some 165 countries exchanged their knowledge and experience with the aim of attaining a level of health for all citizens of the world, by the year 2000, which will permit them to lead a socially and economically productive life.

The region of Europe covers some 850 million people in an area which reaches from Greenland in the north, the Mediterranean in the south to the Pacific shores of Russia. It is unique in that a large proportion of its countries are industrialized with advanced medical services. The European programme of the World Health Organization differs from that of other regions as it concentrates on the problems associated with industrial society. A lot of the policy that is created on a national basis in contributing states has its roots in the strategy of the World Health Organization of *Health for All by the Year 2000* (see, for example, WHO, 1978). Yet again the professions are being pushed forward towards effective collaboration in order that these targets are attained. It is likely that the demands on the professions will become even greater as the three main areas of activities associated with *Health for All* are pursued. These are:

- the promotion of lifestyles conducive to health;
- the reduction of preventable conditions;
- provision of care that is adequate, accessible and acceptable to all.

The overall perspective of the *Health for All* Policy for Europe (WHO, 1991), which consists of 38 targets, means that it is of particular importance that the contributing professionals work together in achieving the aims. It is clear that no singular profession has the monopoly on the raising of the health status of any particular nation. It is not possible to consider health issues in isolation from the social, educational and economic activities which are associated with the broader concepts of health. To summarize, the health policy for Europe targets three main areas:

- the improvements in health status which are expected over the 20-year period 1980 to 2000;

- the changes in lifestyles, improvements in the environment and the developments in the prevention, treatments, care and rehabilitation which will make it possible to attain the targets;
- policy formulation and sustained implementation on the basis of political, managerial and institutional support and co-ordination.

The outcomes of the *Health for All* movement in the European region aims to achieve progress on four dimensions:

- ensuring equity in health by reducing disparities in health status between countries and between groups within countries;
- adding life to years by helping people to achieve and use their full physical, mental and social potential;
- adding health to life by reducing disease and disability;
- adding years to life by increasing life expectancy.

Of all these strategies, it is likely to be the provision of high-quality services for prevention, treatment, care and rehabilitation that is likely to be most effective.

Health for all, which is the official European health policy, remains an important social goal for the new millennium. A renewal of this policy and its related targets will take place and will continue to reflect the fundamental principles of the World Health Organization. Any new policies that emerge will take full account of recent developments and challenges that have occurred in Europe. They will retain the essential features of the current policies with a greater emphasis being placed upon equity, decentralization and intersectoral co-operation, as well as further accountability for health. It will be recognized that there are a number of important developments in ecology, technology, geopolitics, economy, demography, political structures and social relations that have important consequences for health. At the

time of writing, the World Health Organization European member states were commenting upon the update of the draft global policy.

WHO Targets – An Example of Influence

Target 27 Rationale and preferential distribution of resources according to need

By 1990 in all member states the infrastructures of the delivery systems should be organized so that resources are distributed according to need and so that services ensure physical and economic accessibility and cultural acceptability to the population.

In 1990 a report on the WHO consultation document curriculum development for the 'generalist nurse' was distributed by the regional office for Europe. This document had been selected for review because it highlights how more global initiatives are affecting the concerns of professions who have direct responsibilities in the areas of specialized care such as learning disabilities; professions sometimes experience confusion and controversy because of not understanding some of the roots of the policy changes.

We know that many changes have taken place in health care and in health care systems in the last decade. An increasingly ageing population, ever-advancing technology, and more discerning and demanding public expectations have caused almost all Governments across the European Union to look critically at their current health care systems. This means that they also look at new ways of delivering health care within a climate of a reduced gross domestic product. It is because of this that getting the best value for the invested finance and containing costs is high on the agenda. Clinical effectiveness is increasingly an expectation from Government agencies and this means that professionals have to scrutinize their own practice and leave their practice open for scrutiny by others.

The search for evidence-based practice means that there is a requirement for the professions to demonstrate that they are making a difference in terms of meeting peoples' needs, and influencing the health gain process. Multiprofessional and inter-professional working has been perceived as the key to progress with every effort being made to give control back to the con-sumer of services and their family for their own health. A new focus is being placed on the determinants of health with profes-sionals being encouraged to adopt a multi-disciplinary approach to their work.

It was in October 1989 that Government chief nursing officers first met and adopted a 6-year plan for the development of the 'generalist nurse' project which would include the development of a basic nursing curriculum.

The overall purpose of the project therefore was to provide advice to the Eur-opean nursing unit relevant to the develop-ment of an educational programme which would provide assistance at country level on basic nursing curriculum development. These moves have had a great impact upon the way in which learning disability nurses are being prepared and are likely to be pre-pared in the future. Not least of all was the launch of a project in the UK called Project 2000 which resulted in a 146-week training programme based upon a common founda-tion preparation with a period of time being devoted to what became known as the branch programme for learning disabilities.

The consultative group in relation to the 'generalist nurse' project was expected to consider and agree any amendments to the proposed role, functions and competencies of the 'generalist nurse' as set out in the first draft profile. These were:

- identification of education models exist-ing in member states which may be adopted or adapted to develop the 'gen-eralist nurse' programme within member states;
- advising on appropriate curricula struc-ture and content for consideration by countries;
- suggesting strategies which may be deployed:
  1. to prepare nurse teachers and man-agers to develop the 'generalist nurse' programme in their own settings;
  2. to ensure support from:
     (a) other health care workers
     (b) consumers
     (c) local influential persons;
  3. to ensure enactment of any needed legislation changes;
- identifying schools and departments of nursing which may be approached to participate as pilot sites for the imple-mentation and evaluation of experimen-tal programmes.
- proposing a realistic time schedule for this component of the nursing pro-gramme.

Having first worked out definitions of such areas as primary health care, health personnel, levels of care, community-orientated education, community-based education, community-based learning activ-ities, and community-based educational programmes, the first draft of the profile of the 'generalist nurse' was sent out from the nursing unit to all 32 member states of the World Health Organization's European Region for debate at national level. At the end of this period, members set about defining the various components of the 'generalist nurse's' role. These tended to reflect the following:

- *The role of the 'generalist nurse'.* The group agreed that the role of the 'generalist nurse' should be developed in the context of a health care system of each country. Nursing education programmes must fit into the country's long-term plans for health and workforce development. It was recognized that change would be subject to a variety of social, demographic, economic and political factors.

- *The direct care provider.* The direct provision of care has always been an important feature of nursing. Accordingly, the 'generalist nurse' needs to have a variety of clinical skills and be able to carry out all stages of the nursing process. As a direct provider, he or she must participate fully in all the essential components of primary health care, hence their additional roles as an educator and as a facilitator and a manager of health care.

- *The teacher and educator.* The 'generalist nurse's' central concerns should be the promotion of health and rehabilitation, the prevention of disease and disability, as well as the provision of supportive and curative care. They should educate individuals and families on healthy lifestyles and the community on the primary prevention of ill health and on protective and supportive health measures. Their role as a teacher also involves training health care personnel, including professional colleagues and auxiliary staff.

- *The supervisor and manager.* The 'generalist nurse' must exercise leadership. Their duties include supervising other personnel in providing care, planning health services for the community in conjunction with other members of the health team, and organizing and administering community health services. In these functions the 'generalist nurse' assesses the health needs of the community, listens to the communities' views on these needs and communicates with the community, acting as its advocate. As a community organizer, they involve people in their own care and enlist the co-operation of other sectors of society concerned with health (e.g. the housing, sanitation, agriculture, industry and in education sectors). From being a direct provider of care to individuals, the 'generalist nurse' thus becomes a manager of care on a wider scale.

- *The researcher and evaluator.* Health needs and services are not static. The 'generalist nurse' should monitor, observe, analyse and study health conditions and services in their area. As a primary contact for people when they are sick, they are in a position to determine health needs and to understand the problems involved in meeting these needs.

- *The generalist nurse in relation to auxiliaries.* As well as teaching auxiliaries, it was agreed that nurses should also supervise and manage them. This was considered to be extremely important in the context of nursing team mixes. Therefore, all in-service training, as well as initial preparation, should be slanted toward preparing auxiliaries as generalists also able to work in both hospitals and communities.

It was on the basis of discussions of these aspects of the nurses' profile that the European group in 1990 agreed several amendments, drawing up a new structure. The changes revolved around the need for the education of the 'generalist nurse', particularly in considering the orientation of basic education of nurses to the primary health care approach. They drew attention to the fact that the nursing curriculum needed to be revised to prepare nurses with the clinical and other skills necessary for them to provide primary health orientated care wherever people were living. This meant that they needed to have epidemiological knowledge to detect and prevent disease, dysfunctions and disabilities as far as possible. They also included an understanding of behavioural responses required in order to promote healthy lifestyles, and the organizational ability to plan, manage and evaluate community health as well as curative programmes.

Those nurses working within the learning disability services may take exception to the notion of a 'generalist nurse' but they must realize that it is these large political influences that govern their present situation. Across Europe the members of the consultative group discussed the experiences of their own countries in trying to re-orientate curricula to emphasize primary health care and the problems that they encountered during the process. These were primarily:

- lack of a clear definition of the role of nursing in primary health care;
- lack of a nucleus of nursing education planners imbued with the will to develop nursing personnel equipped for primary health care;
- lack of retraining for teachers, who need practical experience of working with the community as part of their re-orientation to primary health care;
- the extreme isolation of nurse education planners, who rarely consult persons from other branches of health care or other sectors about educational programmes;
- lack of material resources to support the re-orientation of curricula;
- lack of involvement of community groups who represent the public interests in curriculum planning.

This aspect of policy is being chosen because it stresses that the re-orientation of nursing education systems and curriculum reflects primary health care approaches and

is relevant to a planned and deliberate restructuring process.

The Deployment of the Strategy

A three-pronged approach was suggested by the planning group for the dissemination of the 'generalist nurse' concept. This was to take place at three levels: national, regional and local. At the regional level it was believed that the World Health Organization should communicate with and seek support from all relevant international agencies such as the International Labour Organization, and the Commission of European Communities, together with the International Council of Nurses.

The participants recognized the value of intercountry workshops for nurse teachers and managers which could serve the basis for securing the required changes at a national level. They believe that intercountry networking would also be helpful. In relation to the need for changes in regulatory mechanisms and national legislation, the group suggested that the World Health Organization should develop a pool of legal experts who could be called upon by any other member states as required and that the organization should make better known its existing literature on the subject of the 'generalist nurse'.

At the national level the first stage would include the production of surveys in order to:

- analyse the present situation and identify the changes needed as well as the procedures to be employed to achieve these changes;
- identify the deficits in the practice and education of nurse managers and teachers;

- analyse the existing legal framework and political scenarios;
- identify the changes needed in national legislation and regulatory mechanisms.

It was felt that organizational actions should also be taken at local and national levels to disseminate information on the 'generalist nurse' to professional associations, educational authorities and other professional bodies or agencies.

It can be clearly seen that the initiative proposed with regard to the 'generalist nurse' can overlap and in some respects contradict some of the more pressing concerns in terms of the models of multidisciplinary teamwork occurring in the area of specialist learning disability practice. These are legitimate areas of concern for the learning disability nurse and those in the other professions associated with the client group. Our response to them has to reflect the nature of the client's interests and to some extent of who the client actually is in terms of who has a legitimate claim upon the traditional and emerging skill base.

The values associated with learning disability nursing would appear to be based upon individualism and those of the 'generalist nurse' appear to be concerned with collective, structural and political dimensions. It is sometimes the case that diversity of values even within single professions can be an asset for clients, but it is important for us to understand some of the consequences that are emerging as a result of the European push for these generalist dimensions. The reality for those people who are concerned with delivering publicly accountable care and those that are in supporting conditions include the following:

- the delivery of services has moved at a pace, but sometimes the contemporary training has trailed behind;
- there are problems in shifting the training dimensions at the interface of care;

- there is a lack of clarity about specialist and shared roles within professions, disciplines and agencies in health and social care;
- there is a deficit in relation to a core curriculum;
- there are ongoing questions about the generic versus the specialist balance of both training and care practice;
- in the UK we have a uniprofessional training but strive towards multidisciplinary working;
- the focus for training is on traditional rather than primary health care based structures;
- the user or carer perspective is quite under-developed;
- there are difficulties in balancing the care and the health and social service control functions.

Whilst there are revised guidelines for training both in health and social care sectors, these are often unclear in relation to their translation at the interface of care delivery and there are questions to be asked regarding the skills of academic and vocational staff which relate to the delivery of contemporary care practices.

It can be identified in other relevant chapters of this book that in order to progress these issues the development of explicit occupational standards becomes increasingly important. We may have to rethink the nature of learning disability nursing and the nature of specialism in other professions. We may have to search for a common core of training in health and social care which underpins specialist roles. There will have to be a mechanism established for benchmarking post-qualifying multidisciplinary training.

These factors then beg the question – who will safeguard these standards of both care and training? It may be that new agencies will emerge in the future which have a greater collective responsibility for meeting and addressing some of the common problems and challenges for professional systems which are designed to have a greater degree of influence first in the European Union and then more globally in health and social care policy.

Discussion Questions

- What are the key influences/ pressures on your work, practices or occupational group:
  a) from within the UK
  b) from European Initiatives
  c) from international movements or   agreements?
- What opportunities do they make available to you; what support do you need to make best use of them?

- Who should safeguard standards?
- Review the plan at Chapter I in the light of the above.

References

CMO (1990). *Commission Memorandum on the Rationalisation and Co-ordination of Vocational Programmes at Community Level (34 Final, 21 August 1990).* European Communities, Brussels.

Thompson, T. and Mathias, P. (1997). The World Health Organization and European Union: occupational vocational and health initiatives and their implications for co-operation amongst the professions. In *Interprofessional Working for Health and Social Care* (eds J. Øvretveit, P. Mathias and T. Thompson), pp. 201–225. Basingstoke, Macmillan.

WHO (1978). *Primary Health Care. The Declaration at Alma Ata: Health for All, Series 1.* Geneva, WHO.

WHO (1991). *The Health Policy for Europe – Summary of the Updated Edition.* Copenhagen, WHO Regional Office for Europe.

Index